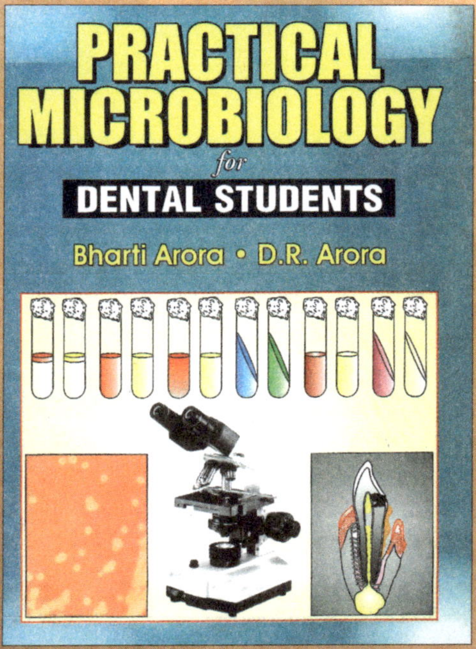
PRACTICAL MICROBIOLOGY
for
DENTAL STUDENTS
Bharti Arora • D.R. Arora

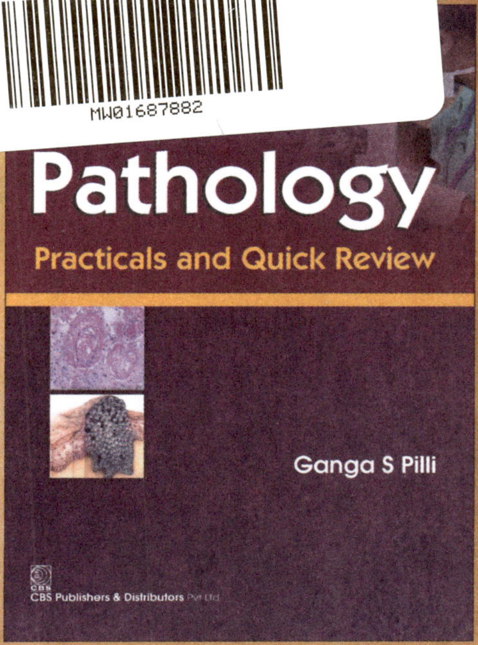
Pathology
Practicals and Quick Review
Ganga S Pilli
CBS Publishers & Distributors Pvt Ltd

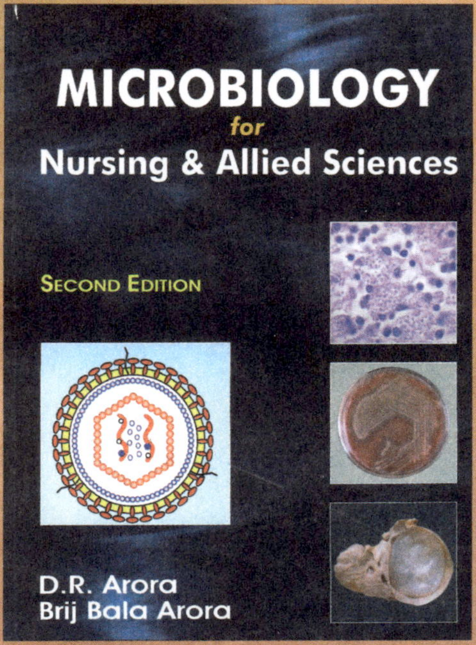
MICROBIOLOGY
for
Nursing & Allied Sciences
SECOND EDITION
D.R. Arora
Brij Bala Arora

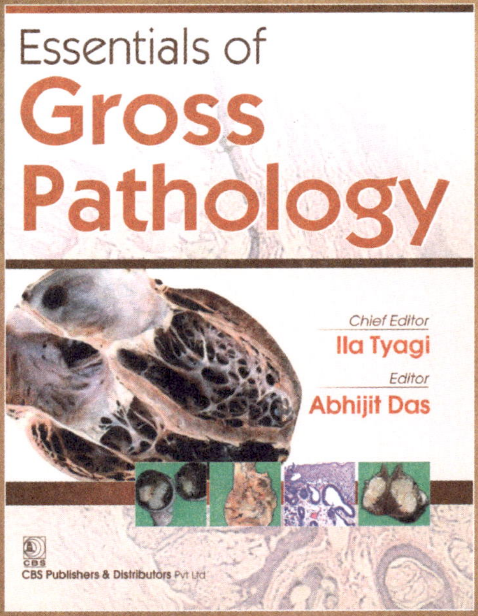
Essentials of
Gross
Pathology
Chief Editor
Ila Tyagi
Editor
Abhijit Das
CBS Publishers & Distributors Pvt Ltd

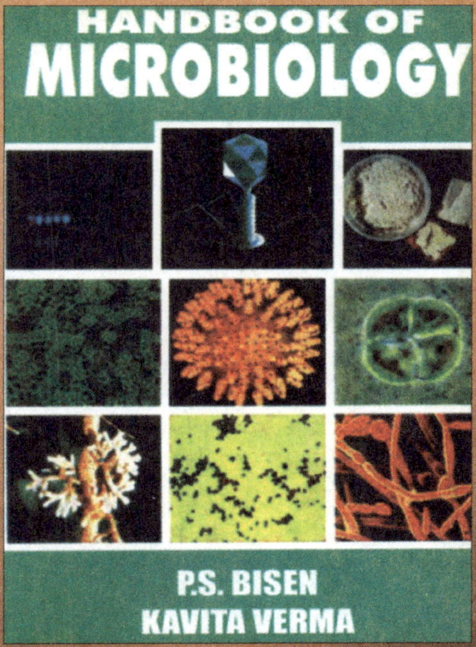
HANDBOOK OF
MICROBIOLOGY
P.S. BISEN
KAVITA VERMA

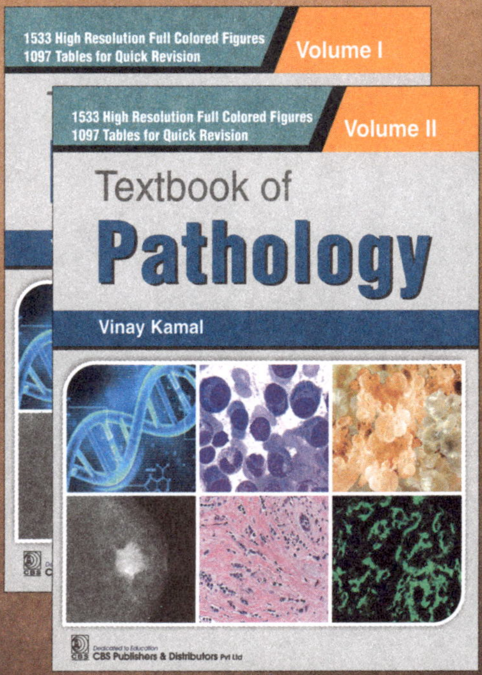
1533 High Resolution Full Colored Figures
1097 Tables for Quick Revision
Volume I
1533 High Resolution Full Colored Figures
1097 Tables for Quick Revision
Volume II
Textbook of
Pathology
Vinay Kamal
CBS Publishers & Distributors Pvt Ltd

MEDICAL PARASITOLOGY

Fifth Edition

Other Books by Dr. D.R. Arora

- Textbook of Microbiology, 5th ed.
- Textbook of Microbiology for Dental Students, 4th ed.
- Medical Mycology, 2nd ed.
- Essentials of Microbiology for B. Sc. Nursing Students
- Exam–Oriented Microbiology (Questions & Answers)
- MCQs in Microbiology and Parasitology (with Explanations)
- Practical Microbiology
- Practical Microbiology for Dental Students
- Microbiology for Nursing & Allied Sciences, 2nd ed.

MEDICAL PARASITOLOGY

Fifth Edition

Dr. D.R. Arora M.D., Ph.D., M.N.A.M.S.

Ex-Professor & Head, Department of Microbiology,
Postgraduate Institute of Medical Sciences, Rohtak, Haryana (India), and
Maharaja Agarsen Medical College, Agroha, Haryana (India)

Ex-Professor & Head, Department of Microbiology,
Medical Superintendent, and Dean Faculty of Allied Health Sciences,
SGT University, Gurgaon, Haryana (India)

Ex-W.H.O. Fellow; and Visiting Professor, University of Mauritius

Lead Assessor and Member, Accreditation Committee,
National Accreditation Board for Testing and Calibration Laboratories (NABL), Gurgaon, Haryana (India)

Principal Assessor, National Accreditation Board for Hospitals &
Healthcare Providers (NABH), New Delhi (India)

Assessor, National Accreditation Board for
Education and Training (NABET), New Delhi (India)

Dr. Brij Bala Arora M.D.

Ex-Senior Professor & Head, Department of Pathology,
Postgraduate Institute of Medical Sciences, Rohtak, Haryana (India)

Ex-Director-Principal and Senior Professor & Head,
Department of Pathology, SGT Medical College, Hospital & Research Institute,
Gurgaon, Haryana (India)

CBS

CBS Publishers & Distributors Pvt Ltd

New Delhi • Bengaluru • Chennai • Kochi • Kolkata • Mumbai
Hyderabad • Jharkhand • Nagpur • Patna • Pune • Uttarakhand

Disclaimer

Science and technology are constantly changing fields. New research and experience broaden the scope of information and knowledge. The authors have tried their best in giving information available to them while preparing the material for this book. Although, all efforts have been made to ensure optimum accuracy of the material, yet it is quite possible some errors might have been left uncorrected. The publisher, the printer and the authors will not be held responsible for any inadvertent errors, omissions or inaccuracies.

ISBN: 978-93-86827-55-5

Fifth Edition : 2018

First Edition : 2001

Reprint : 2002, 2003

Second Edition : 2005

Reprint : 2005, 2007, 2008 (twice), 2009

Third Edition : 2010

Reprint : 2010, 2011, 2012, 2013

Fourth Edition : 2014

Reprint : 2015, 2016

Published by Satish Kumar Jain and produced by Varun Jain for

CBS Publishers & Distributors Pvt Ltd

4819/XI Prahlad Street, 24 Ansari Road, Daryaganj, New Delhi 110 002, India.

Ph: 23289259, 23266861, 23266867 Website: www.cbspd.com

Fax: 011-23243014 e-mail: delhi@cbspd.com; cbspubs@airtelmail.in.

Corporate Office: 204 FIE, Industrial Area, Patparganj, Delhi 110 092

Ph: 4934 4934 Fax: 4934 4935 e-mail: publishing@cbspd.com; publicity@cbspd.com

Branches

- **Bengaluru:** Seema House 2975, 17th Cross, K.R. Road, Banasankari 2nd Stage, Bengaluru 560 070, Karnataka
  Ph: +91-80-26771678/79 Fax: +91-80-26771680 e-mail: bangalore@cbspd.com
- **Chennai:** 7, Subbaraya Street, Shenoy Nagar, Chennai 600 030, Tamil Nadu
  Ph: +91-44-26680620, 26681266 Fax: +91-44-42032115 e-mail: chennai@cbspd.com
- **Kochi:** Ashana House, No. 39/1904, AM Thomas Road, Valanjambalam, Ernakulam 682 016, Kochi, Kerala
  Ph: +91-484-4059061-65 Fax: +91-484-4059065 e-mail: kochi@cbspd.com
- **Kolkata:** 6/B, Ground Floor, Rameswar Shaw Road, Kolkata-700 014, West Bengal
  Ph: +91-33-22891126, 22891127, 22891128 e-mail: kolkata@cbspd.com
- **Mumbai:** 83-C, Dr E Moses Road, Worli, Mumbai-400018, Maharashtra
  Ph: +91-22-24902340/41 Fax: +91-22-24902342 e-mail: mumbai@cbspd.com

Representatives

- **Hyderabad** 0-9885175004
- **Jharkhand** 0-9811541605
- **Nagpur** 0-9021734563
- **Patna** 0-9334159340
- **Pune** 0-9623451994
- **Uttarakhand** 0-9716462459

Printed at International Print-O-Pac Limited, Noida, UP, India

Dedicated to the Sweet Memories of
Our Loving Daughter,
Dr. Hina Arora

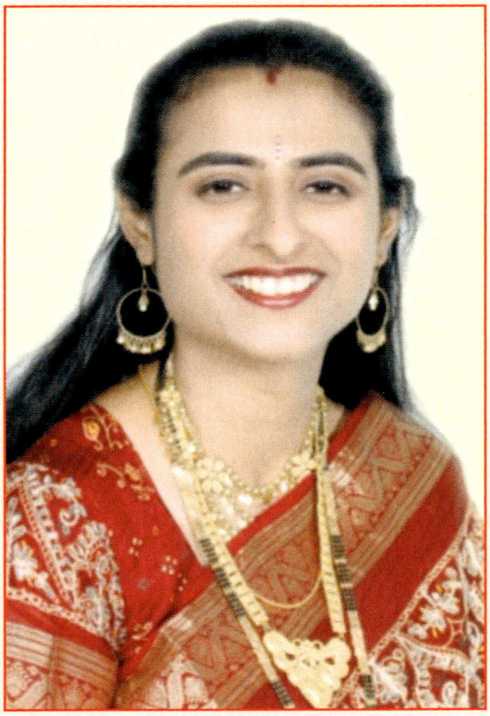

Dr. Hina Arora
BDS, IDES 2001
09-04-1976 to 02-11-2009

Foreword

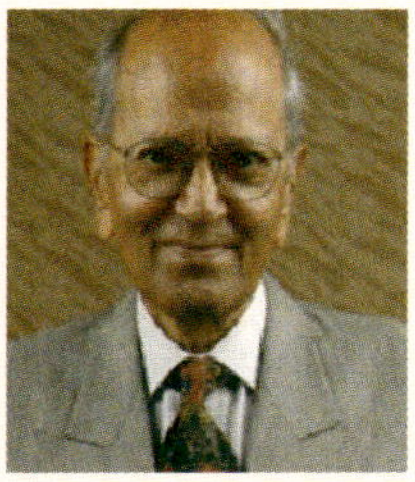

Infectious diseases have been with us for centuries and cause high mortality and morbidity all over the world, more so in the developing world. The emergence of new infectious diseases and re-emergence of some old diseases in endemic and epidemic forms have been a matter of great concern for medical community.

Parasitic infections afflict more than half the world's population with a major health burden particularly in developing world where they are most common. These are closely related to travel to areas of high endemicity and certain occupations. We need to have a knowledge of geographic distribution and life cycles of parasites to understand the diseases caused by them and their diagnosis.

The present book deals with intestinal, and blood and tissue parasites in relation to human diseases.

The well-illustrated life cycles and pathologic lesions caused by them make the understanding easy for the medical students, microbiologists, pathologists and clinicians. The reach of various parasitic diseases, in spite of global efforts, has been increasing because of increasing number of immunocompromised hosts, lack of any effective vaccines and global travels.

The authors have done full justice to the subject of parasitology and made the understanding of the subject easy and interesting. I hope the students, research scholars, microbiologists, pathologists and clinicians alike will find it useful and will be benefited.

T.D. Chugh
National Emeritus Professor
National Academy of Medical Sciences
(India)

Book Review

Arora D.R., Arora Brij Bala Medical Parasitology, 2nd ed. CBS Publishers & Distributors, Darya Ganj, New Delhi, 2004. Rs. 275.00

Rapidly increasing information in medical science requires that textbooks be revised and updated to keep pace. The authors, Dr. D.R. Arora and Dr. Brij Bala Arora, have revised their textbook in keeping with the times. Improvement from the first edition is worth noting. The authors have revised almost all chapters and yet have not made the book unwieldy or bulky with additional information. The hardbound book comes with an attractive jacket. The first chapter on General Parasitology has an interesting table comparing a parasite with a human embryo. Subsequent chapters have retained the general pattern of the previous edition but improved with colour highlights of salient features and important information. The black & white and coloured diagrams are uncomplicated and clear, as also the pictures of gross and histopathological sections. Diagrams of life cycles have been improved with simple line sketches. Number of references at the end of each chapter have, however, been reduced, perhaps to bring down the bulk of the book. The language remains lucid and easy to understand. Rapid diagnostic tests have been included in many chapters, one example being antigen detection and quantitative buffy coat examination in malaria, illustrated with diagrams for easy comprehension. Nosocomial parasitic infections is an additional feature of the chapter on parasitic opportunistic infections. This is a relevant addition in view of the growing importance of hospital-acquired infections. Diagrammatic representation of relative sizes and morphology of protozoa and helminthic eggs, added at the end of the book, has good visual impact and will help in understanding the importance of micrometry in diagnostic parasitology.

Applied and analytical approach to solving clinical problems could have been introduced along with multiple choice and essay questions, by including problem-based questions. An attempt has been made with a few questions but it needs to be improved. This edition may well replace the older one as a textbook for MBBS, and Laboratory Technology students and may be recommended for the same. It will also help postgraduate students of Medical Microbiology, as additional Indian data have been included in some of the chapters. Authors need to be congratulated on the second edition of their book on Medical Parasitology.

Reba Kanungo
Department of Clinical Microbiology
Pondicherry Institute of Medical Sciences
Pondicherry - 605 006, India
email: rebakanungo2001@hotmail.com

Preface to the Fifth Edition

Parasites are one of the five **P**'s constituting "Nature's Hangmen". Other four include **P**athogens, **P**arasitoids, **P**ests and **P**redators. Parasitic diseases continue to be a major public health problem all over the world with associated high degree of morbidity and mortality, and man-day loss.

International travel and shifting patterns of immigration have increased the importance of awareness of major clinical syndromes associated with infections due to parasites. Parasites cause over two billion infections every year worldwide.

Parasitic infections continue to present a major challenge to the health and well-being of millions of people across the world, particularly those living in the poorest regions, mainly the tropics and subtropics. Global unrest, floods and famine, the migration of huge populations, and spread of HIV infection have added to the already serious problems not only in terms of increased parasite burdens but also in terms of interactions between parasites and other infectious agents. Out of 60 million deaths in the world, more than 25% are accounted to parasites.

There is currently no vaccine against any parasitic infection in humans. Parasites also have capacity to develop resistance to the few effective drugs available, resistance to antimalarials being the most spectacular. Furthermore, attempts to control parasites by attacking their vectors have been hampered by the development of insecticide resistance. Parasitic infections, therefore, present enormous challenges.

Although, enteroparasitic infections constitute a serious public health problem in developing countries with inadequate sanitary conditions, they are not exclusive to them. Many types of helminths and protozoal intestinal parasites affect man, provoking a wide range of symptoms that are generally associated with the gastrointestinal tract.

Patients with some type of immunocompromised condition and those on immunosuppressive therapy have an increased probability of acquiring parasitic infections, generally with a higher degree of severity. Parasitic infections that cause self-limited diarrhoea in immunocompetent individuals may cause profuse diarrhoea in immunocompromised individuals, generally accompanied by loss of weight, anorexia, malabsorption syndrome and in some cases fever and abdominal pain. In such patients, parasites such as *Cryptosporidium parvum*, *Enterocytozoon bieneusi*, *Encephalitozoon intestinalis* and *Strongyloides stercoralis* may disseminate to other organs such as the bronchi and liver ducts producing symptomatology specific to the organ affected.

Rapidly increasing information in medical science requires that textbooks be revised and updated to keep pace. Earlier editions of Medical Parasitology received an overwhelming response from undergraduate and postgraduate students, and the teachers. This has played a vital role in bringing out fifth edition of the book. Almost all chapters of the book have been revised and yet have not made the book unwieldy or bulky with additional information. Classification of parasites and treatment of parasitic infections have been updated. Opportunistic parasitic infections in AIDS cases and nosocomial parasitic infections have been described in one of the chapters. New multiple choice questions have been added. Diagrams are coloured, uncomplicated and clear, as also the pictures of gross and histopathological sections. Diagrams of life cycles are computer-drawn with simple line sketches. New parasitic figures have been added. Diagrammatic representation of relative sizes and morphology of protozoa and helminthic eggs at the end of the book has good visual impact and will help in understanding the importance of micrometry in diagnostic parasitology. Indian data have been given in most of the chapters. The book has been divided into four sections.These are General Parasitology, Protozoology,

Helminthology, and Applied Parasitology, Diagnostic Procedures and Overview. The language is lucid and easy to understand. This book shall be highly useful to undergraduate and postgraduate students, clinicians, and medical laboratory technology students.

I express my sincere thanks to Dr. Paramjeet Singh Gill, Professor, Department of Microbiology, Postgraduate Institute of Medical Sciences, Rohtak, for meticulously drawing all the figures, adding new figures, and for contributing chapter on Trematodes.

I am grateful to Mr. B.M. Singh for meticulous proof-reading and valuable professional help and support. I am also grateful to Mr. Anurag Trivedi for designing the book. I honestly acknowledge the most sincere and dedicated support and advice of Mr. Dharmvir.

The readers are requested to send suggestions for the improvement of the book which will be incorporated in subsequent editions. Shortcomings, if any, may please be communicated at draroradr@rediffmail.com

D.R. Arora

Preface to the First Edition

Parasites affect over half the world's population and are a major cause of mortality in the developing world. In the developed world, they represent a threat to those undergoing immunosuppressive therapy or suffering from HIV infection. In recent years parasitology has undergone revolutionary changes. It has drawn heavily from different areas of basic sciences for its enrichment and embellishment. The advances made have led to enhancement of diagnostic skills, better exploration of transmission dynamics, clearer understanding of pathophysiology, and formulation of effective strategy against parasitic diseases.

In 1976, WHO drew attention to the magnitude of the problem that parasitic diseases cause and listed five parasitic infections – malaria, trypanosomiasis, leishmaniasis, schistosomiasis and filariasis presenting the greatest challenges in the developing world. A number of parasites are now worldwide in their distribution and many infections once thought to be harmless are now known to be life-threatening in immunocompromised individuals and those suffering from acquired immunodeficiency syndrome (AIDS). These include *Toxoplasma gondii*, *Cryptosporidium parvum*, *Isospora belli* and microsporidia.

The laboratory diagnosis of parasitic infections mainly rests upon the direct demonstration of the parasites, detection of specific antibodies in serum and body fluids and/or detection of parasitic antigen/DNA in various samples. Currently no vaccine against any parasitic infection, in humans, is available. Parasites also have capacity to develop drug resistance and vectors transmitting certain parasitic infections have developed insecticide resistance. Therefore, parasitic infections present enormous challenges. No up-to-date book on medical parasitology is currently available that conforms to the requirements of undergraduate and postgraduate students.

This book gives all essential details of general parasitology (Section I), description of various protozoa (Section II) and helminths (Section III) i.e. geographical distribution, habitat, morphology, life cycle, pathogenicity, immunity, epidemiology, laboratory diagnosis, treatment and prevention. Section IV deals with opportunistic infections in AIDS cases, diagnostic methods and overview of medical parasitology.

There is a well-known saying, prevention is better than cure, therefore, methods of prevention of each parasite have been described. However, if the disease has established then an early and accurate diagnosis is essential. The same has been described in proper details giving all latest methods of diagnosis. All the chapters in this book are followed by important essay type questions, multiple choice questions and references for further reading.

This book will be highly useful to undergraduate and postgraduate students. It is also hoped that it will serve as a useful resource for teachers of parasitology. The readers are requested to write any shortcomings and give us suggestions for the improvement of the book in the subsequent editions.

D.R. Arora
Brij Bala Arora

Contents

SECTION 3
Helminthology

SECTION 1

General Parasitology

1

General Parasitology

- *Parasite*
- *Why a human embryo or foetus is not a parasite?*
- *Host*
- *Host-parasite relationships*
- *Sources of infection*
- *Portal of entry into the body*
- *Life cycle of human parasites*
- *Pathogenicity*
- *Immunity in parasitic infections*
- *Laboratory diagnosis*
- *Classification of parasites*

Parasitology is the study of invertebrate animals capable of causing disease in humans and other animals.

It is concerned with 200 or so species of helminth worms and about 80 species of protozoa that infect humans. Many of these are rare and accidental parasites, but about 100 species of protozoa and helminths are commonly found in humans. They range in size from tiny protozoa as small as 1–2 μm in diameter to tapeworms that may measure up to 10 metres in length.

PARASITE

A parasite is an organism that is entirely dependent on another organism, referred to as its host, for all or part of its life cycle and metabolic requirements. Strictly speaking, the term parasite can be applied to any infectious agent but, by convention, it is generally restricted to infections caused by protozoa and helminths and excludes the viruses, bacteria and fungi.

On the basis of their location, parasites may also be divided into two types:

- Ectoparasites
- Endoparasites

Ectoparasites

Organisms which live on the surface of the body, e.g., the human louse, *Pediculus humanus*, are known as ectoparasites. The infection by these parasites is known as *infestation*. They are important as vectors transmitting pathogenic microorganisms.

Endoparasites

Organisms that live within the body of the host (in the blood, tissues, body cavities, digestive tract and other organs) are known as endoparasites. All protozoan and helminthic parasites of man are endoparasites. The invasion by endoparasites is known as *infection*. These can be further subdivided into following types:

- ***Obligate parasites:*** Organisms that cannot exist without a host (e.g., *Toxoplasma gondii*).
- ***Facultative parasites:*** Organisms that under favourable circumstances may live either a parasitic or free-living existence (e.g., *Naegleria fowleri, Acanthamoeba* spp. and *Balamuthia mandrillaris*).
- ***Accidental parasites:*** Organisms that attack an unusual host (e.g., *Echinococcus granulosus* in man).
- ***Aberrant parasites:*** Organisms that attack a host where they cannot live or develop further (e.g., *Toxocara canis* in man).
- ***Free-living:*** The term free-living describes the non-parasitic stages of existence which are lived independently of a host, e.g., hookworms have active free-living stages in the soil.

WHY A HUMAN EMBRYO OR FOETUS IS NOT A PARASITE?

Human embryo or foetus develops inside the uterus of the mother for more than nine months deriving its nourishment from the mother. In spite of this it is not treated as a parasite (Table 1.1).

HOST

It is defined as an organism which harbours the parasite and provides the nourishment and shelter to the latter. It is of following types:

Definitive host

The host which harbours the adult parasite, the most highly developed form of a parasite or where the parasite replicates sexually. When the most highly developed form is not obvious, the definitive host is the mammalian host.

Intermediate host

This is the host which alternates with the definitive host and harbours the larval or asexual stages of a parasite. Some parasites require two intermediate hosts for completion of their life cycle. These are referred to as first and second intermediate hosts respectively.

Paratenic host

It is a host in which larval stage of a parasite survives but does not develop further. It is often not a necessary part of the life cycle.

Table 1.1. Comparison between parasite and human embryo or foetus

	Parasite	Human embryo or foetus
1.	A parasite is an organism of one species living in or on an organism of other species (a hetero-specific relationship) and deriving its nourishment from the host.	A human embryo or foetus is an organism of one species (*Homo sapiens*) living in the uterine cavity of an organism of the same species and deriving its nourishment from the mother. This is a dependent relationship, but not a parasitic relationship.
2.	A parasite is an invading organism coming to parasitize the host from an outside source.	A human embryo or foetus is formed from a fertilized egg coming from an inside source, being formed in the ovary of the mother from where it moves into the oviduct where it may be fertilized to form the zygote, the first cell of the new human being.
3.	A parasite is generally harmful to some degree to the host.	A human embryo or foetus developing in the uterine cavity does not usually cause harm to the mother, provided proper nutrition and care is maintained by the mother.
4.	A parasite makes direct contact with the host's tissues, often holding on by mouth parts, hooks or suckers to the tissues involved (intestinal lining, lungs, connective tissue, etc.).	A human embryo or foetus makes direct contact with the uterine lining of the mother for only a short period of time. It soon becomes isolated inside its own amniotic sac and makes indirect contact with the mother only by way of the umbilical cord and placenta.
5.	When a parasite invades host tissue, the host tissue sometimes responds by forming a capsule of connective tissue to surround the parasite and cuts it off from other surrounding tissues.	When the human embryo or foetus attaches and invades the lining tissue of the mother's uterus, the lining tissue responds by surrounding the human embryo but does not cut it off from the mother. Rather it establishes a means of close contact (the placenta) between the mother and the new human being.
6.	When a parasite invades a host, the host usually responds by forming antibodies in response to the somatic antigens (molecules comprising the body of the parasite) or metabolic antigens (molecules secreted or excreted by the parasite). Parasitism usually involves an immunological response on the part of the host.	Mother does react to the presence of the embryo by producing humoral antibodies, but the trophoblast (the jacket of cells surrounding the embryo) blocks the action of these antibodies and, therefore, the embryo or the foetus is not rejected. This reaction is unique to the embryo–mother relationship.

Reservoir host

It is a host that harbours the parasite and serves as an important source of infection to other susceptible hosts.

Compromised host

A compromised host is one in whom normal defence mechanisms are impaired (e.g., AIDS), absent (e.g., congenital deficiencies), or bypassed (e.g., penetration of skin barrier). Such hosts are extremely susceptible to a variety of common as well as opportunistic pathogens.

Zoonosis

This term is used to describe an animal infection that is naturally transmissible to humans either directly or indirectly via a vector. Examples of parasitic diseases that are zoonoses include leishmaniasis, South American trypanosomiasis, rhodesiense trypanosomiasis, japonicum schistosomiasis, trichinosis, fascioliasis, hydatid disease, and cryptosporidiosis.

Vector

A vector is an agent, usually an insect, that transmits an infection from one human host to another. It is of two types:

1. *Mechanical vector:* The term mechanical vector is used to describe a vector which assists in the transfer of pathogens between hosts but is not essential in the life cycle of the parasite, e.g., a housefly that carries parasite cysts and eggs, bacteria or viruses from infected faeces to food that is eaten by humans. Vector-borne parasitic human infections are given in Table 14.3.
2. *Biological vector:* A vector in which the pathogens multiply or undergo developmental changes with or without multiplication. Biological vectors are of three types:
   - *Propagative vector:* When a pathogen undergoes no cyclic change but multiplies in the body of the vector, transmission is said to be propagative, e.g., plague bacilli in rat fleas.
   - *Cyclo-propagative vector:* The pathogen undergoes a cyclic change and multiplies in the body of the arthropod, e.g., malaria parasites in female *Anopheles* mosquito.
   - *Cyclo-developmental vector:* When pathogen undergoes cyclic changes but does not multiply in the body of the vector, e.g., filarial parasite in *Culex* mosquito and guinea worm larvae in cyclops.

HOST-PARASITE RELATIONSHIPS

Host-parasite relationships are of following types:

Symbiosis

An association in which both host and parasite are so dependent upon each other that one cannot live without the help of the other. Neither of the partners suffers from any harm from this association.

Commensalism

An association in which only parasite derives benefit without causing any injury to the host. A commensal lives on food residues or waste products of the body and is capable of leading an independent life.

Parasitism

Parasitism is a relationship in which a parasite benefits and the host provides the benefit. The host gets nothing in return and always suffers from some injury. The degree of dependence of a parasite on its host varies.

SOURCES OF INFECTION

Although many infectious diseases are caused by **endogenous** organisms that are part of the normal flora of the human host, this is not the case with most diseases caused by protozoan and helminthic parasites. These organisms are virtually always acquired from an **exogenous** source and as such have evolved numerous ways to enter the body of the human host:

1. ***Contaminated soil and water:*** Soil polluted with human excreta acts as a source of infection with *Ascaris lumbricoides, Trichuris trichiura, Ancylostoma duodenale, Necator americanus* and *Strongyloides stercoralis*. Before acquiring infectivity for man, eggs of these parasites undergo certain development in the soil. These are known as **soil-transmitted helminths**.

   Water polluted with human excreta may contain viable cysts of *Entamoeba histolytica, Giardia lamblia, Balantidium coli*, eggs of *Taenia solium, Hymenolepis nana*, and the infective cercarial stage of *Schistosoma haematobium, S. mansoni* and *S. japonicum.*
2. ***Freshwater fishes*** constitute the source of *Diphyllobothrium latum* and *Clonorchis sinensis.*
3. ***Crab and crayfishes*** are the sources of *Paragonimus westermani.*
4. ***Raw or undercooked pork*** is the source of *Trichinella spiralis, Taenia solium, T. asiatica* and *Sarcocystis suihominis.*

5. ***Raw or undercooked beef*** is the source of *T. saginata*, *Toxoplasma gondii* and *Sarcocystis hominis*.
6. ***Watercress*** is the source of *Fasciola hepatica*.
7. ***Blood-sucking insects*** transmit *Plasmodium* spp., *Wuchereria bancrofti*, *Brugia malayi*, *Onchocerca volvulus*, *Trypanosoma brucei gambiense*, *T. b. rhodesiense*, *T. cruzi*, *Leishmania* spp. and *Babesia* spp.
8. ***Housefly*** (mechanical carrier) is the source of *E. histolytica*.
9. ***Dog*** is the source of *Echinococcus granulosus* (hydatid cyst), and *Toxocara canis* (visceral larva migrans).
10. ***Cat*** is the source of *T. gondii*.
11. ***Man*** is the source of *E. histolytica*, *Giardia lamblia*, *Enterobius vermicularis* and *H. nana*.
12. ***Autoinfection*** may occur with *Enterobius vermicularis* and *S. stercoralis* leading to **hyper-infection**.

PORTAL OF ENTRY INTO THE BODY

Mouth

The commonest portal of entry of parasites is oral, through contaminated food, water, soiled fingers or fomites. Many intestinal parasites, e.g., *E. histolytica, G. lamblia, Balantidium coli, E. vermicularis, T. trichiura, A. lumbricoides, T. spiralis, T. solium, T. saginata, T. asiatica, D. latum, Fasciola hepatica, Fasciolopsis buski, C. sinensis* and *P. westermani,* enter the body in this manner.

Skin

Entry through skin is another important portal of entry of parasites. Infection with *A. duodenale, N. americanus* and *S. stercoralis* is acquired when filariform larvae of these nematodes penetrate the unbroken skin of an individual walking over faecally contaminated soil. Schistosomiasis caused by *S. haematobium, S. mansoni* and *S. japonicum* is acquired when the cercarial larvae, in water, penetrate the skin. A large number of parasites, e.g., *Plasmodium* spp., *W. bancrofti*, *B. malayi*, *O. volvulus, T. brucei gambiense, T. b. rhodesiense*, *T. cruzi*, *Leishmania* spp. and *Babesia* spp. are introduced percutaneously when blood-sucking arthropods puncture the skin to feed.

Sexual contact

Trichomonas vaginalis is transmitted by sexual contact. *E. histolytica* and *G. lamblia* may also be transmitted by anal-oral sexual practices among male homosexuals.

Kissing

E. gingivalis is transmitted from person-to-person by kissing or from contaminated drinking utensils.

Congenital

Infection with *T. gondii* and *Plasmodium* spp. may be transmitted from mother to foetus transplacentally.

Inhalation

Airborne eggs of *E. vermicularis* may be inhaled into posterior pharynx leading to infection.

Iatrogenic infection

Malaria parasites may be transmitted by transfusion of blood from the donor with malaria containing asexual forms of erythrocytic schizogony. This is known as **trophozoite-induced malaria** or **transfusion malaria**. Malaria parasites may also be transmitted by the use of contaminated syringes and needles. This may occur in drug addicts.

LIFE CYCLE OF HUMAN PARASITES

On the basis of their life cycles human parasites can be divided into three major groups (Table 1.2).

PATHOGENICITY

A parasite may live in or on the tissues of its host without causing evident harm. However, in majority of cases the parasite has the capacity to produce damage. With the advent of AIDS there is an increase in the incidence of newer parasitic infections caused by *Cryptosporidium parvum, Isospora belli, Cyclospora cayetanensis* and other hitherto unheard of parasites. These parasites also cause infections in patients who are immunocompromised, e.g., patients receiving cytotoxic drugs or organ transplant. Following are the ways in which the damage may be produced by the parasites:

Traumatic damage

Relatively slight physical damage is produced by entry of filariform larvae of *S. stercoralis, A. duodenale* and *N. americanus*, and cercarial larvae of *S. haematobium, S. mansoni* and *S. japonicum* into the skin. Migration of several helminthic larvae through the lung produces traumatic damage of pulmonary capillaries leading to

Table 1.2. Life cycle of human parasites

NO INTERMEDIATE HOST	
Protozoa	**Helminths**
• *Entamoeba histolytica*	• *Enterobius vermicularis*
• *Giardia lamblia*	• *Trichuris trichiura*
• *Chilomastix mesnili*	• *Ascaris lumbricoides**
• *Trichomonas vaginalis*	• *Ancylostoma duodenale**
• *Balantidium coli*	• *Necator americanus**
	• *Hymenolepis nana*
ONE INTERMEDIATE HOST	
Intermediate host	**Parasite**
Pig	• *Taenia solium*
	• *T. asiatica*
	• *Trichinella spiralis*
Cow	• *Taenia saginata*
Man	• *Echinococcus granulosus*
	• *Plasmodium* spp.
Flea	• *Dipylidium caninum*
	• *Hymenolepis diminuta*
Triatomine bug	• *Trypanosoma cruzi*
Mosquito	• *Wuchereria bancrofti*
	• *Brugia malayi*
Snail	• *Schistosoma* spp.
Copepod	• *Dracunculus medinensis*
Fly	
Sandfly	• *Leishmania* spp.
Tsetse fly	• *Trypanosoma* spp.
Chrysops	• *Loa loa*
Simulium	• *Onchocerca volvulus*
TWO INTERMEDIATE HOSTS	
Intermediate hosts	**Parasite**
Snail, crustacean	• *Paragonimus westermani*
Cyclops, fish	• *Diphyllobothrium latum*
Snail, fish	• *Clonorchis sinensis*
Snail, plant	• *Fasciola* spp.

* Require a period of maturation in the soil after passage before they are infective.

extravasation of blood into the lung. Similar damage in cerebral, retinal or renal capillaries may lead to serious injury.

Eggs of *S. haematobium* and *S. mansoni* cause extensive damage with haemorrhage as they escape from vesical and mesenteric venules, respectively, into the lumen of the urinary bladder and the intestinal canal.

Attachment of hookworms (*A. duodenale* and *N. americanus*) to the intestinal wall results in traumatic damage of the villi. They ingest blood and, moreover, move from site to site in the gut mucosa, leaving small bleeding lesions. These two facts are responsible for the chief pathological manifestation of heavy infection with hookworms – iron-deficiency anaemia.

Mechanical blockage

Many of the pathogenic consequences of helminthic infections are related to the size, movement, and longevity of the parasites. The host is exposed to long-term damage and immune stimulation, as well as the sheer physical consequences of being inhabited by large foreign bodies. The most obvious forms of direct damage from helminthic parasites are those resulting from mechanical blockage of internal organs or from the effects of pressure exerted by growing parasites. Large adult *Ascaris* organisms can physically block the intestine and the bile ducts.

Likewise, blockage of lymph flow, leading to elephantiasis, is associated with the presence of adult *Wuchereria* parasites in the lymphatic system. Some neurologic manifestations of cysticercosis are due to the pressure exerted by the slowly expanding larval cysts of *Taenia solium* in the central nervous system (CNS) and eyes. Migration of helminths (usually larval forms) through body tissues such as skin, lungs, liver, intestines, eyes, and CNS can damage the tissues directly and initiate hypersensitivity reactions.

Lytic necrosis

E. histolytica secretes lytic enzyme which lyses tissues for its nutritional needs and helps it to penetrate into the tissues of the colon and extraintestinal viscera. Obligate intracellular parasites, e.g., *Plasmodium* spp., *Leishmania* spp., *Trypanosoma cruzi* and *Toxoplasma gondii* cause necrosis of parasitized host cells during their growth and multiplication.

Physiological effects

Large numbers of *Giardia lamblia* covering the walls of the small intestine can lead to malabsorption, especially of fats.

Competition for specific nutrients

Diphyllobothrium latum competes with the host for vitamin B_{12} leading to **parasite-induced pernicious anaemia**. Other forms of anaemia result from blood loss, especially in hookworm infection, and from red blood cell destruction in malaria.

Inflammatory reaction

Most of the parasites provoke cellular proliferation and infiltration at the site of their location. In many instances, the host reaction walls off the parasite by fibrous encapsulation. In metazoan and in some protozoan parasitoses, there is a moderate-to-notable eosinophilia. *E. histolytica* may produce inflammation of the large intestine leading to the formation of amoebic granuloma or **amoeboma**. Parasitization of fixed macrophages in the spleen, bone marrow, and lymph nodes by *L. donovani* causes proliferation of reticuloendothelial cells.

Allergic manifestations

In certain helminthic infections, the normal secretions and excretions of the growing larvae and the products liberated from dead parasites may give rise to various allergic manifestations, e.g.:

- Schistosomes cause cercarial dermatitis and eosinophilia
- *D. medinensis* and *T. spiralis* infections cause urticaria and eosinophilia, and
- Rupture of hydatid cyst may precipitate anaphylaxis.

Neoplasia

The parasitic infection may contribute to the development of neoplastic growth, e.g., *C. sinensis* and *Opisthorchis viverrini* have been associated with **cholangiocarcinoma** and *S. haematobium* with **vesical carcinoma**.

Secondary infection

In some helminthic infections (e.g., strongyloidiasis, trichinosis and ascariasis), the migrating larvae may carry bacteria and viruses from the intestine to the blood and tissues leading to secondary infection.

IMMUNITY IN PARASITIC INFECTIONS

There are two main types of immunity – innate and acquired:

Innate immunity

Innate immunity is not dependent on prior contact with the parasites or their products. It is due to genetic and constitutional make up of an individual. Examples of genetic innate immunity of man to human parasitic infections are as under:

- West Africans are more resistant than white Americans to hookworm infection.
- Presence of **abnormal haemoglobin** like thalassemia haemoglobin and foetal haemoglobin confers resistance against all *Plasmodium* spp., while sickle cell anaemia trait and haemoglobin E protect against *P. falciparum* and *P. vivax* respectively.
- A genetic deficiency known as **glucose-6-phosphate dehydrogenase (G6PD) trait** confers some protection against *P. falciparum* infection. This enzyme is essential for respiratory process of the parasite.
- The presence of **Duffy factor** on red blood cells increases the susceptibility to malaria. It is believed that Duffy factor present on red blood cells acts as receptor for attachment of malaria parasite.

Acquired immunity

Because of their biochemical and structural complexity, protozoa and helminths present a large number of antigens to their hosts. Protozoa are small and multiply within their vertebrate host, often inside cells, thus posing an immediate threat unless contained by an appropriate immune response. Helminths are large and do not multiply within their vertebrate host. Thus they do not present an immediate threat after initial infection. However, the host must protect itself from large infections and reinvasion by infective stages by eliciting an appropriate immune response. Therefore, immune responses to protozoa and helminths are different from one another.

Like other infectious agents, parasites also elicit both humoral as well as cellular responses. But immunological protection against parasitic infections is much less efficient than it is against bacterial and viral infections. This is due to following factors:

- As compared to bacteria and viruses, parasites are large and more complex structurally and antigenically so that immune system may not be able to mount immune response against the protective antigens.
- Many protozoan parasites (e.g., *Leishmania* spp., *T. cruzi* and *T. gondii*) are **intracellular**. This protects them from immunological attack.
- Many parasites, both protozoa and helminths, live inside the intestines. This location limits the efficiency of immunological attack and also facilitates dispersal of the infective forms of the parasites.
- *T. brucei gambiense* and *T. b. rhodesiense* exhibit **antigenic variations** within the host. When antibody response to one antigenic type reaches peak, antigenic variation of the parasite occurs by mutation. The new antigenic type is unaffected by the antibodies against the parent strain. This enables the prolonged persistence of the parasite in the host.

- *Plasmodium* spp., the cause of malaria, also change their surface antigens and are poorly antigenic. Malaria may continue for several months in a person before the immune response is sufficiently strong to reduce the number of the parasites.
- Blood flukes of humans, *Schistosoma* spp., adsorb host-produced molecules onto their surface so that the host fails to recognize the worms as nonself. The blood flukes can remain alive in the blood vessels of the human host for 20–30 years at least in part by utilizing this mechanism.
- Many nematodes have a cuticle which is antigenically inert and evokes little immune response.
- *L. donovani* causes extensive damage to the reticulo-endothelial system thus leading to immunological tolerance.
- *E. vermicularis* does not breach the integrity of gut wall, thus immune system is not stimulated.
- In most of the parasitic infections, immunity lasts only till original infection remains active. This is known as **concomitant immunity** (previously called **premunition** or **infection-immunity**). A possible exception is cutaneous leishmaniasis in which the ulcer heals leaving behind good protection against reinfection.

All the above mechanisms have made the production of vaccine against eukaryotic parasites extremely difficult.

The protective immune response to parasitic infections has four arms:

1. Cytotoxic T (Tc) cells.
2. Natural killer (NK) cells.
3. Activated macrophages.
4. Antibodies (produced by B-cells).

The first three constituting 'cell-mediated immunity' and the last constituting 'humoral immunity'. The main classes of antibodies (immunoglobulins) produced are IgM, IgG and IgE. The first to appear is IgM which marks the presence of acute infection. IgG antibodies are usually the most abundant type in parasitic infections. Helminths and ectoparasites also provoke high titres of IgE antibodies.

LABORATORY DIAGNOSIS

Laboratory diagnosis of parasitic infections can be carried out by:

- Demonstration of parasite.
- Immunodiagnosis.
- Molecular biological methods.

Demonstration of parasite

The diagnosis of parasitic infections may be very difficult, particularly in non-endemic setting. The clinical manifestations of parasitic diseases are seldom specific enough to raise the possibility of these processes in the mind of the clinician, and routine laboratory tests are seldom helpful. Although **peripheral eosinophilia** is widely recognized as a useful indicator of parasitic disease, this phenomenon is characteristic only of helminthic infection and even in these cases it is frequently absent. Proper diagnosis requires that:

(a) the physician considers the possibility of parasitic infection,
(b) appropriate specimens be obtained and transferred to the laboratory in a timely fashion, and
(c) the laboratory competently performs the appropriate procedures for the recovery and identification of the etiological agent.

For most parasitic diseases, appropriate test selection and interpretation is based on an understanding of the life cycle of the parasite, as well as the pathogenesis of the disease process in humans. Although the mainstay of diagnostic clinical microbiology is the isolation of the causative pathogen in culture, the diagnosis of parasitic diseases is accomplished almost entirely by morphologic (usually microscopic) demonstration of parasites in clinical material.

Blood

In those parasitic infections, where the parasite itself, or in any stage of its development, circulates in the blood stream, the examination of blood film forms the main procedure for specific diagnosis, e.g., demonstration of *Plasmodium* spp. and *Babesia* spp. inside the erythrocytes, *L. donovani* inside monocytes, trypomastigotes of *T. b. gambiense, T. b. rhodesiense* and *T. cruzi*, and microfilariae of *W. bancrofti* and *B. malayi* in the blood.

Stool

Examination of stool is important for the diagnosis of intestinal parasitic infections and helminthic infections of the biliary tract in which eggs are discharged in the intestine. In protozoal infections, the trophozoites (during active phase) and cysts (during chronic phase) of *E. histolytica, G. lamblia* and *B. coli* can be demonstrated by wet mount of stool in normal saline and Lugol's iodine. In helminthic infections eggs, larvae and adult worms may be demonstrated (Table 1.3).

Table 1.3. Parasites found in stool

CYSTS / TROPHOZOITES	
Protozoa	
• *Entamoeba histolytica*	• *Giardia lamblia*
• *Dientamoeba fragilis*	• *Balantidium coli*
• *Sarcocystis hominis*	• *S. suihominis*
• *Isospora belli*	• *Cyclospora cayetanensis*
• *Cryptosporidium parvum*	• *Encephalitozoon intestinalis*
• *Enterocytozoon bieneusi*	
EGGS	
Cestodes	
• *Diphyllobothrium latum*	• *Taenia solium*
• *T. saginata*	• *T. asiatica*
• *Hymenolepis nana*	• *H. diminuta*
• *Dipylidium caninum*	
Trematodes	
• *Schistosoma mansoni*	• *S. japonicum*
• *Fasciolopsis buski*	• *Fasciola hepatica*
• *F. gigantica*	• *Clonorchis sinensis*
• *Gastrodiscoides hominis*	• *Watsonius watsoni*
• *Heterophyes heterophyes*	• *Metagonimus yokogawai*
• *Opisthorchis* spp.	
Nematodes	
• *Trichuris trichiura*	• *Ancylostoma duodenale*
• *Necator americanus*	• *Enterobius vermicularis*
• *Capillaria philippinensis*	• *Trichostrongylus orientalis*
LARVAE	
• *Strongyloides stercoralis*	• *Trichinella spiralis* (rarely)
ADULT WORMS	
Cestodes	
• *Taenia solium*	• *T. saginata*
• *T. asiatica*	• *Diphyllobothrium latum*
Nematodes	
• *Ascaris lumbricoides*	• *Ancylostoma duodenale*
• *Necator americanus*	• *Enterobius vermicularis*
• *Trichinella spiralis*	

When direct stool smears are repeatedly negative for ova and cysts then the concentration methods such as salt floatation or formalin-ether sedimentation may be used. *Cryptosporidium parvum*, *Isospora belli* and other coccidia in stool specimens may be detected by **modified Ziehl-Neelsen staining** of the fixed smear (see Chapter 13). *Demonstration of parasites in the stool confirms the diagnosis and is the gold standard in the diagnosis of intestinal parasitic infections.*

Perianal and perineal skin scrapings may show the eggs or adult worms of *E. vermicularis*.

Urine

When the parasite localises in the urinary tract, the examination of urine is useful in establishing the parasitological diagnosis, e.g., eggs of *S. haematobium* and trophozoites of *T. vaginalis* may be demonstrated in the urine. In case of chyluria caused by *W. bancrofti*, microfilariae are often demonstrated in chylous urine.

Genital specimens

Trophozoites of *T. vaginalis* may be demonstrated in the vaginal and urethral discharge and in the prostatic secretions.

Cerebrospinal fluid (CSF)

Trypomastigotes of *T. brucei gambiense* and *T. b. rhodesiense*, and trophozoites of *Naegleria fowleri*, *Acanthamoeba* spp. and *Balamuthia mandrillaris* may be demonstrated in the CSF.

Sputum

In cases where the habitat of the parasite is in the respiratory tract, as in paragonimiasis, the eggs of *Paragonimus westermani* may be demonstrated in the sputum specimen. Rarely, migrating larvae of *A. lumbricoides*, *S. stercoralis*, *A. duodenale*, and *N. americanus* may be found in the sputum. In amoebic abscess of lung or in the case of amoebic liver abscess bursting into the lungs, the trophozoites of *E. histolytica* can be detected in the sputum.

Tissue biopsy and aspiration

1. Scolices and brood capsules may be demonstrated in the fluid aspirated from hydatid cyst.
2. Amastigote forms of *L. donovani* may be demonstrated inside the reticuloendothelial cells in the aspirates of spleen, bone marrow, liver and lymph nodes.
3. Larvae of *T. spiralis, T. solium* and *T. multiceps* may be demonstrated in the muscle biopsy.
4. Trophozoites of *G. lamblia* may be demonstrated in the bile aspirated from duodenum by intubation.
5. Trophozoites of *E. histolytica* may be demonstrated in pus aspirated from amoebic liver abscess and in the necrotic tissue obtained from the base of the ulcers in the large intestine.

Culture

Some parasites like *Entamoeba histolytica*, *Naegleria fowleri*, *Acanthamoeba* spp., *Balamuthia mandrillaris*, *Leishmania* spp., *Trypanosoma* spp., *Trichomonas vaginalis*, *Giardia lamblia* and *Balantidium coli* can be cultured in the laboratory. Cultures of parasites grown in association with an unknown microbiota are referred to as **xenic cultures**. A good example of this type of culture is stool specimens cultured for *E. histolytica*. If the parasites are grown with a single known bacterium, the culture is referred to as **monoxenic**. An example of this type of culture is clinical specimen cultured with *Escherichia coli* as a means of recovering species of *Acanthamoeba* and *Naegleria*. If parasites are grown as pure culture without any bacterial associate, the culture is referred to as **axenic**. An example of this type of culture is the use of media for isolation of *Leishmania* spp. or *Trypanosoma cruzi*.

Animal inoculation

Animal inoculation is a sensitive means of detecting infection caused by blood and tissue parasites such as *Toxoplasma gondii*, *Trypanosoma brucei gambiense*, *T. b. rhodesiense*, *T. cruzi*, and *Leishmania* spp.

Xenodiagnosis

The technique of xenodiagnosis employs the use of laboratory-raised arthropod vectors to detect low levels of parasites in infected individuals. Classically this approach was used to diagnose Chagas' disease by allowing an uninfected reduviid bug to feed on an individual suspected of having the disease. Subsequently the bug was dissected and examined microscopically for the evidence of developmental stages of *T. cruzi*. This technique may be used in endemic areas.

Immunodiagnosis

Immunological tests are of two types:

1. Skin tests.
2. Serological tests.

Skin tests

These tests are performed by intradermal injection of parasitic antigens and are read as under:

1. ***Immediate hypersensitivity reaction:*** It reveals wheal and flare response within 30 minutes of injection. This reaction is seen in cases of hydatid disease, filariasis, schistosomiasis, ascariasis and strongyloidiasis.
2. ***Delayed hypersensitivity reaction:*** It reveals erythema and induration after 48 hours of injection. This reaction is seen in cases of leishmaniasis, trypanosomiasis, toxoplasmosis and amoebiasis.

Serological tests

These tests detect antibodies or antigens in the patient serum and other clinical specimens (Table 1.4).

Table 1.4. Important serological tests used for the diagnosis of parasitic infections

Test	Applications
Enzyme-linked immunosorbent assay and radioimmunoassay	Toxoplasmosis, toxocariasis, leishmaniasis, Chagas' disease, malaria and schistosomiasis
Indirect haemagglutination test	Amoebiasis, hydatid disease, filariasis, cysticercosis and strongyloidiasis
Indirect fluorescent antibody test	Amoebiasis, malaria, toxoplasmosis and schistosomiasis
Complement fixation test	Paragonimiasis, Chagas' disease and leishmaniasis
Agglutination tests	
• Direct agglutination	Visceral leishmaniasis
• Bentonite flocculation	Trichinellosis and hydatid disease

Molecular biological methods

These include DNA probes and polymerase chain reaction (PCR).

DNA probes

DNA probe is a radiolabelled or chromogenically labelled piece of single-stranded DNA complementary to a segment of parasitic genome and unique to a particular parasitic strain, species and genus. Specific probe is added to the clinical specimen. If the specimen contains the parasitic DNA, probe will hybridize with it which can be detected. DNA probes are available for the detection of the infection with *P. falciparum, W. bancrofti, T. b. gambiense, T. b. rhodesiense, T. cruzi* and *Onchocerca* spp.

Polymerase chain reaction (PCR)

PCR is a DNA amplification system that allows molecular biologist to produce microgram quantities of DNA from picogram amounts of starting material. It has been employed for the diagnosis of infections caused by *Giardia lamblia*, *Entamoeba histolytica*, *Plasmodium falciparum*, *Leishmania donovani*, *Toxoplasma gondii*, *Trichomonas vaginalis*, *Cryptosporidium parvum*, etc.

CLASSIFICATION OF PARASITES

Human parasites are classified within four eukaryotic kingdoms – Protozoa, Stramenopila, Fungi and Animalia (Tables 1.5 and 1.6). Kingdom is the highest taxonomic category. It is subdivided as follows:

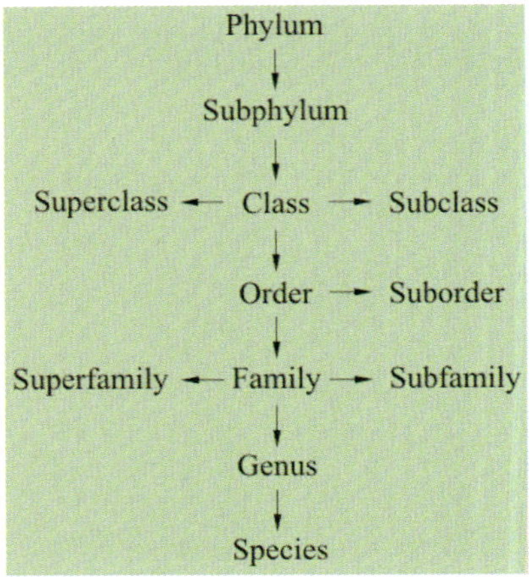

NOMENCLATURE OF PARASITES

It refers to the naming of parasites. Each parasite possesses a generic and a specific name. The genus name is capitalized followed by species name which is not capitalized. Both the genus and species are italicized. Often the genus name is abbreviated by using the first letter of the genus followed by a period and the full species name, which is never abbreviated, such as *A. lumbricoides*, *E. histolytica*.

Traditionally, parasite classification has taken into account the morphology of intracytoplasmic structures, such as the nucleus, the type of locomotive organelles, and the mode of reproduction. The Protozoa and

Table 1.5. Classification of medically important unicellular parasites

Kingdom	Phylum	Class	Order	Parasites
Protozoa	Metamonada	Trepomonadea (intestinal flagellates)	Diplomonadida	*Giardia lamblia*
			Enteromonadida	*Enteromonas hominis*
		Retortamonadea	Retortamonadida	*Chilomastix mesnili*, *Retortamonas intestinalis*
	Parabasala (flagellates)	Trichomanadea (intestinal and related flagellates)	Trichomonadida	*Dientamoeba fragilis*, *Trichomonas vaginalis*, *T. hominis*, *T. tenax*
	Percolozoa (flagellates)	Heterolobosea	Schizopyrenida	*Naegleria fowleri*
	Euglenozoa (flagellates)	Kinetoplastidea (Kinetoplastid flagellates)	Trypanosomatida	*Lesishmania donovani*, *L. infantum*, *L. major*, *L. tropica*, *L. braziliensis*, *L. mexicana*, *L. aethiopica*, *L. peruviana*, *L. chagasi*, *Trypanosoma brucei gambiense*, *T. b. rhodesiense*, *T. cruzi*, *T. rangeli*
	Amoebozoa (amoebae)	Amoebaea (amoebae)	Acanthopodida	*Acanthamoeba castellanii*, *A. culbertsonii*, *A. polyphaga*, *Balamnthia mandrillaris*
		Entamoebidea (intestinal amoebae)	Euamoebida	*Entamoeba histolytica*, *E. coli*, *E. dispar*, *E. hartmanni*, *E. gingivalis*, *E. polecki*, *Endolimax nana*, *Iodamoeba bütschlii*
	Sporozoa (sporozoans)	Coccidea	Eimeriida	*Cryptosporidium parvum*, *C. hominis*, *C. felis*, *C. meleagridis*, *C. canis*, *C. muris*, *Toxoplasma gondii*, *Cyclospora cayetanensis*, *Isospora belli*, *Sarcocystis hominis*, *S. lindemanni*, *S. suihominis*
			Piroplasmida	*Babesia microti*, *B. divergens*, *B. bovis*
			Haemosporida	*Plasmodium vivax*, *P. falciparum*, *P. malariae*, *P. ovale*, *P. knowlesi*
	Ciliophora (ciliates)	Litosmomatea	Vestibuliferida	*Balantidium coli*
Stramenopila	Bigyra	Blastocystea		*Blastocystis hominis*
Fungi	Microspora (microsporidians)	Microsporea		*Encephalitozoon cuniculi*, *E. hellem*, *E. intestinalis*, *Enterocytozoon bieneusi*, *Microsporidium ceylonensis*, *Nosema ocularum*, *Pleistophora ronneafiei*, *Trachipleistophora hominis*, *T. anthrophthera*, *Vittaforma corneae*, *Anncaliia* (formerly *Brachiola*) *algerae*, *A. connori*, *A. vesicularum*

Table 1.6. Classification of medically important parasites of kingdom Animalia

Phylum	Class	Superfamily	Family	Parasites
Nemathelminthes (roundworms)	Adenophorea	Trichnelloidea	Trichinellidae	*Trichinella spiralis*
			Trichuridae	*Trichuris trichiura, Capillaria philippinensis, C. aerophila, C. hepatica*
	Secernentea (Phasmidea)	Ancylostomatoidea	Ancylostomatidae	*Ancylostoma duodenale, A. braziliense, A. caninum, A. ceylanicum, Necator americanus*
		Ascaridodiea	Ascaridodiae	*Ascaris lumbricoides, A. suum, Toxocara canis, T. catis*
			Anisakidae	*Anisakis simplex*
		Dracunculoidea	Dracunculidae	*Dracunculus medinensis*
		Filariodea	Onchocercidae	*Wuchereria bancrofti, Brugia malayi, B. timori, Loa loa, Onchocerca volvulus, Dirofilaria immitis, D. repens, D. tenuis, D. ursi, Mansonella ozzardi, M. perstans, M. streptocerca*
		Gnathostomatoidea	Gnathostomatidae	*Gnathostoma spinigerum*
		Oxyuroidea	Oxyuridae	*Enterobius vermicularis, E. gregorii*
		Rhabditoidea	Strongyloididae	*Strongyloides stercoralis*
		Strongyloidea	Chabertiidae	*Oesophagostomum bifurcum, O. aculeatum, Ternidens derminutus*
		Thelazioidea	Thelaziidae	*Thelazia callipaeda*
		Trichostrongyloidea	Trichostrongylidae	*Trichostrongyloides colubriformis, T. orientalis*
			Dioctophymatidae	*Dioctophyma renale*
Platyhelminthes	Digenea (Trematoda, flukes)		Schistosomatidae	*Schistosoma haematobium, S. japonicum, S. mansoni, S. mekongi, S. intercalatum*
			Fasciolidae	*Fasciola hepatica, F. gigantica, Fasciolopsis buski*
			Gastrodiscidae	*Gastrodiscoides hominis, Watsonius watsoni*
			Heterophyidae	*Heterophyes heterophyes, Metagonimus yokogawai*
			Opisthorchidae	*Clonorchis sinensis, Opisthorchis felineus, O. viverrini*
			Paragonimidae	*Paragonimus westermani*
	Cestoidea (Cestoda, tapeworms)		Diphyllobothriidae	*Diphyllobothrium latum*
			Dipylidiidae	*Dipylidium caninum*
			Hymenolepididae	*Hymenolepsis nana, H. diminuta*
			Taeniidae	*Taenia solium, T. saginata, T. asiatica, T. multiceps, Echinococcus granulosum, E. multilocularis, E .vogeli, Multiceps multiceps*

Stramenopila are animals whose life functions occur in a single cell. The microsporidians are also single-celled organisms and were previously classified among the protozoans; however, they are now thought to be more closely related to fungi than to Protozoa and have been reclassified with the Fungi (Table 1.5). The members of the kingdom Animalia (Table 1.6), also known as metazoans, are multicellular animals in which the life functions occur in cellular structures organized as tissue and organ systems.

Further Reading

1. Ash, L.R. and Orihel, T.C. 1980. *Atlas of human Parasitology.* Chicago, American Society of Clinical Pathologists.
2. Ash, L.R. and Orihel, T.C. 1987. *Parasites: A guide to laboratory procedures and identification,* ASCP Press, Chicago.
3. Ashford, R.W. and Crewe, W. 2003. *The parasites of Homo sapiens*, 2nd ed. London: Taylor and Francis.
4. Farmer, J.N. 1985. *The Protozoa: Introduction to Protozoology.* St. Louis, CV Mosby Co, 1985.
5. Fleck, S.L. and Moody, A.H. 1988. *Diagnostic Techniques in Medical Parasitology.* Wright, London.
6. Garcia, L.S. 2001. *Diagnostic Medical Parasitology*, 4th ed. Washington DC: American Society for Microbiology Press.
7. Sher, A. and Coffman, R.L. 1992. Regulation of immunity to parasites by T cells and T cell-derived cytokines. *Ann. Rev. Immunol.*, **10**: 385–409.
8. Warren, K.S., ed., 1993. *Immunology and Molecular Biology of Parasitic Infections*, Blackwell Scientific Publications, Oxford.
9. World Health Organization. 1991. *Basic Laboratory Methods in Medical Parasitology*. WHO, Geneva.

Important Questions

Write short notes on:

(a) Parasite
(b) Host
(c) Host–parasite relationships
(d) Sources of infection of parasites
(e) Portal of entry of parasites
(f) Pathogenicity of parasitic infections
(g) Immunity in parasitic infections
(h) Laboratory diagnosis of parasitic infections
(i) Classification of parasites

Multiple Choice Questions

1. Which type of vector of malaria parasite is female *Anopheles* mosquito?
   (a) Mechanical.
   (b) Propagative.
   (c) Cyclo-developmental.
   (d) Cyclo-propagative.
2. Blood-sucking insects may transmit:
   (a) *Ancylostoma duodenale.*
   (b) *Ascaris lumbricoides.*
   (c) *Wuchereria bancrofti.*
   (d) *Strongyloides stercoralis.*
3. Crab may transmit:
   (a) *Diphyllobothrium latum.*
   (b) *Clonorchis sinensis.*
   (c) *Paragonimus westermani.*
   (d) *Enterobius vermicularis.*
4. Undercooked pork may act as a source of:
   (a) *Taenia solium.*
   (b) *Taenia saginata.*
   (c) *Diphyllobothrium latum.*
   (d) *Ancylostoma duodenale.*
5. Which of the following parasites is transmitted by cat?
   (a) *Balantidium coli.*
   (b) *Toxoplasma gondii.*
   (c) *Echinococcus granulosus.*
   (d) *Toxocara canis.*
6. Which of the following parasites is transmitted by dog?
   (a) *Echinococcus granulosus.*
   (b) *Hymenolepis nana.*
   (c) *Taenia solium.*
   (d) *Diphyllobothrium latum.*
7. Which of the following parasites is transmitted congenitally?
   (a) *Toxoplasma gondii.*
   (b) *Wuchereria bancrofti.*
   (c) *Entamoeba histolytica.*
   (d) *Giardia lamblia.*
8. Parasite which may be transmitted by sexual contact is:
   (a) *Trichomonas vaginalis.*
   (b) *Trypanosoma cruzi.*
   (c) *Leishmania donovani.*
   (d) *Enteromonas hominis.*
9. Parasite transmitted by percutaneous route is:
   (a) *Entamoeba histolytica.*
   (b) *Giardia lamblia.*
   (c) *Babesia* spp.
   (d) *Naegleria fowleri.*
10. Obligate intracellular parasite is:
    (a) *Naegleria fowleri.*
    (b) *Acanthamoeba culbertsoni.*
    (c) *Toxoplasma gondii.*
    (d) *Balamuthia mandrillaris.*

1. Pernicious anaemia is seen in:
   (a) diphyllobothriasis.
   (b) malaria.
   (c) hookworm disease.
   (d) filariasis.
2. Cholangiocarcinoma is associated with:
   (a) *Clonorchis sinensis*.
   (b) *Schistosoma haematobium*.
   (c) *Paragonimus westermani*.
   (d) *Fasciola hepatica*.
3. Which of the following parasites can be demonstrated in blood film?
   (a) *Naegleria fowleri*.
   (b) *Leishmania donovani*.
   (c) *Endolimax nana*.
   (d) *Entamoeba histolytica*.
4. Which of the following parasitic eggs is excreted in urine?
   (a) *Schistosoma haematobium*.
   (b) *Schistosoma japonicum*.
   (c) *Schistosoma mansoni*.
   (d) *Clonorchis sinensis*.
5. Trophozoites of *Naegleria fowleri* can be demonstrated in:
   (a) CSF.
   (b) blood.
   (c) stool.
   (d) urine.
6. Larvae of which of the following parasites can be demonstrated in muscle biopsy?
   (a) *Trichinella spiralis*.
   (b) *Dracunculus medinensis*.
   (c) *Wuchereria bancrofti*.
   (d) *Brugia malayi*.
17. Animal inoculation is **not** useful for detection of:
   (a) *Toxoplasma gondii*.
   (b) *Babesia* spp.
   (c) *Leishmania donovani*.
   (d) *Trichomonas vaginalis*.
18. A parasite that must spend at least part of its life cycle on or in a host is called:
   (a) facultative parasite.
   (b) hyperparasite.
   (c) obligate parasite.
   (d) pathogenic parasite.
19. Parasites may damage their host's body by:
   (a) taking nutrients from the host.
   (b) triggering inflammatory response.
   (c) causing internal haemorrhages.
   (d) All of these.
20. Large parasites, such as helminths, are most likely attacked by:
   (a) neutrophils.
   (b) eosinophils.
   (c) basophils.
   (d) platelets.

ANSWERS TO MCQs

1 (d), 2 (c), 3 (c), 4 (a), 5 (b), 6 (a), 7 (a), 8 (a), 9 (c), 10 (c), 11 (a), 12 (a), 13 (b), 14 (a), 15 (a), 16 (a), 17 (d), 18 (c), 19 (d), 20 (b).

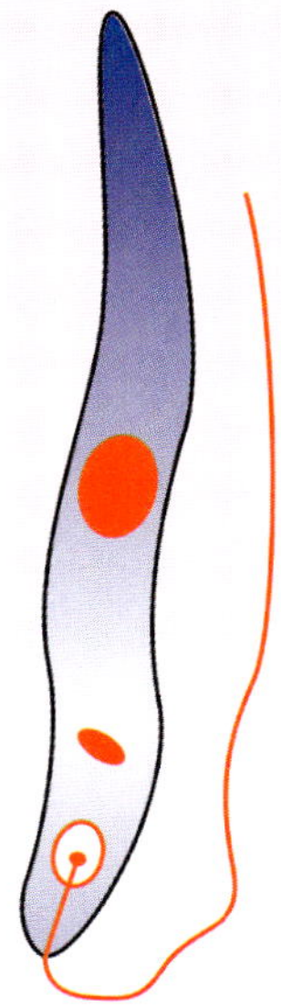

SECTION 2
Protozoology

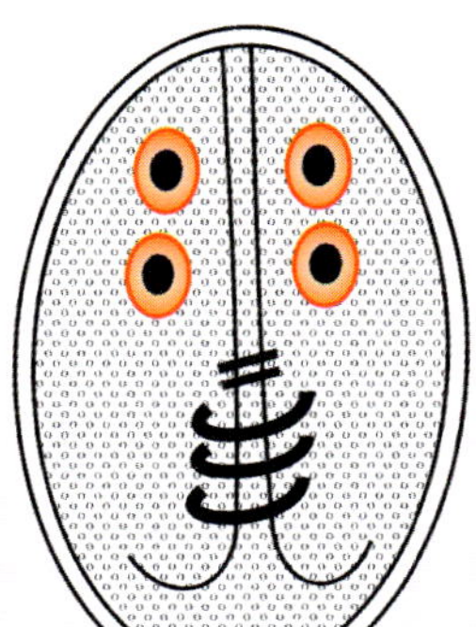

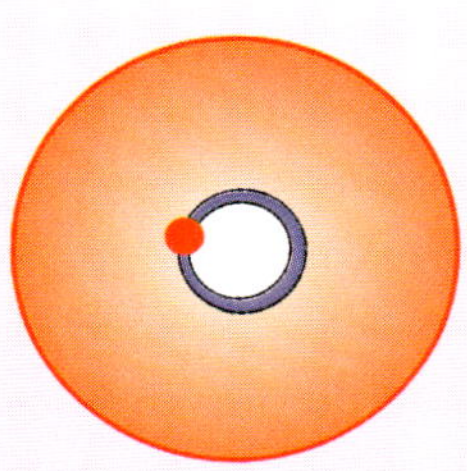

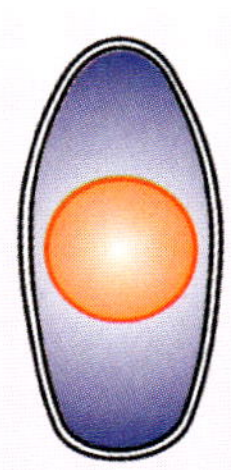

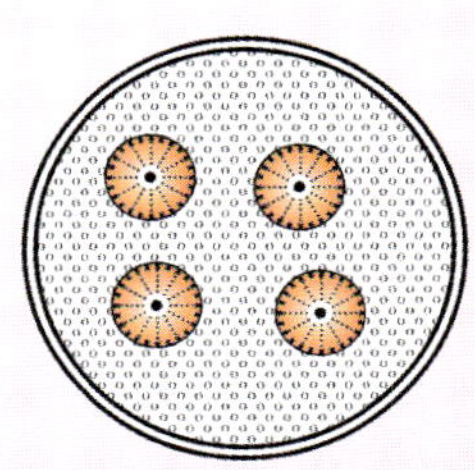

2

Unicellular Parasites

- *Kingdom Protozoa*
  - *Phyla Metamonada, Parabasala, Percolozoa and Euglenozoa*
  - *Phylum Amoebozoa*
  - *Phylum Sporozoa*
  - *Phylum Ciliophora*
- *Kingdom Stramenopila (formerly Chromista)*
  - *Phylum Bigyra*
- *Kingdom Fungi*
  - *Phylum Microspora (Microsporidians)*

Unicellular parasites are classified under three kingdoms – Protozoa, Stramenopila and Fungi (Table 1.5).

KINGDOM PROTOZOA

Protozoa are simple microorganisms that range in size from 2–100 μm. Their protoplasm is enclosed by a cell membrane and contains numerous organelles, including membrane-bound nucleus, endoplasmic reticulum, and food and contractile vacuoles. The nucleus contains clumped or dispersed chromatin and a karyosome. Organelles of locomotion vary from simple cytoplasmic extrusions or pseudopods to more complex structures, such as flagella or cilia. The kingdom Protozoa comprises 13 major subgroups, or phyla, 7 of which are the concern of medical parasitology (Table 1.5).

Phyla Metamonada, Parabasala, Percolozoa and Euglenozoa

These phyla were previously grouped under the former subphylum Mastigophora. The flagellates are now distributed under four phyla – Metamonada, Parabasala, Percolozoa and Euglenozoa. The organelles of locomotion of the flagellates are their **whiplike flagella**. The number and position of the flagella vary a great deal in different species. In addition, specialized structures associated with the flagella, e.g., **undulating membrane**, may produce a characteristic appearance that may be useful in species identification.

Phylum Amoebozoa

The phylum Amoebozoa contains amoebae. It is equivalent to the old subphylum Sarcodina. The organelles of locomotion of amoebae are the **pseudopodia** ("**false feet**"). Amoebae are phagocytic and contain mitochondria with tubular cristae.

Phylum Sporozoa

Phylum Sporozoa organisms are often referred to as

Apicomplexa or **Coccidia**. These organisms have a system of organelles at their apical end that produces substances to help the organism penetrate host cells and thus become intracellular parasite.

Phylum Ciliophora

Phylum Ciliophora consists of the ciliates. These include a variety of free-living and symbiotic species. Organelles of locomotion of ciliates are **hairlike structures**, or **cilia**. Cilia are structurally similar to flagella but are usually shorter and more numerous. *Balantidium coli* is the only ciliate parasite of man. It contains two nuclei – a large macronucleus and a small micronucleus.

KINGDOM STRAMENOPILA (formerly CHROMISTA)

Phylum Bigyra

The kingdom Stramenopila contains a number of plantlike organisms, mainly algae. Based on analysis of 18S rRNA and other molecular evidence, *Blastocystis hominis* is now placed in kingdom Stramenopila, phylum Bigyra, class Blastocystea.

KINGDOM FUNGI

Phylum Microspora (Microsporidians)

Microsporidia are now considered to be degenerate fungi. Further evidence for the fungal nature of microsporidia includes spores with walls of chitin and a mitotic mechanism that is indistinguishable from that of fungal ascomycetes. Microspora are small intracellular parasites. They possess a complex tubular extrusion mechanism (**polar tube**) used to inject the infective material (sporoplasm) into host cells.

Further Reading

1. Cavalier-Smith, T. 1993. Kingdom Protozoa and its 18 phyla. *Microbiol. Rev.,* **57**: 953–94.
2. Cox, F.E.G. 1991. Systematics of parasitic protozoa, *Parasitic Protozoa,* 2nd edn., Vol 1, eds. Kreier, J.P., Baker, J.R., Academic Press, San Diego, 55–80.
3. Cox, F.E.G. 1993. *Modern Parasitology,* 2nd edn., Blackwell Scientific Publications, Oxford, 1–2.

Important Questions

Discuss classification of unicellular parasites.

Multiple Choice Questions

1. Organelles of locomotion in *Balantidium coli* are:
   (a) flagella.
   (b) pseudopodia.
   (c) cilia.
   (d) fimbriae.
2. Which of the following protozoa belongs to phylum Amoebozoa?
   (a) *Cryptosporidium parvum.*
   (b) *Isospora belli.*
   (c) *Toxoplasma gondii.*
   (d) *Entamoeba coli.*
3. Intestinal flagellate is:
   (a) *Giardia lamblia.*
   (b) *Leishmania tropica.*
   (c) *Trypanosoma brucei.*
   (d) *Trypanosoma cruzi.*
4. Phylum Sporozoa contains:
   (a) malaria parasites.
   (b) ciliates.
   (c) flagellates.
   (d) amoebae.
5. Pseudopodium is the organelle of locomotion of:
   (a) *Entamoeba histolytica.*
   (b) *Giardia lamblia.*
   (c) *Leishmania donovani.*
   (d) *Balantidium coli.*
6. Which of the following parasites belongs to phylum Ciliophora?
   (a) *Balantidium coli.*
   (b) *Cryptosporidium parvum.*
   (c) *Plasmodium* spp.
   (d) *Entamoeba histolytica.*
7. Which of the following parasites belongs to the phylum Percolozoa?
   (a) *Cryptosporidium parvum.*
   (b) *Isospora belli.*
   (c) *Naegleria fowleri.*
   (d) *Cyclospora cayetanensis.*

ANSWERS TO MCQs

1 (c), 2 (d), 3 (a), 4 (a), 5 (a), 6 (a), 7 (c).

3

Amoebae and Naegleria fowleri

Entamoeba histolytica

Nonpathogenic amoebae

- *Entamoeba dispar*
- *Entamoeba hartmanni*
- *Entamoeba coli*
- *Entamoeba polecki*
- *Entamoeba gingivalis*
- *Endolimax nana*
- *Iodamoeba bütschlii*

Opportunistic protozoa

- *Naegleria fowleri*
- *Acanthamoeba* spp.
- *Balamuthia mandrillaris*

Amoebae belong to kingdom Protozoa, phylum Amoebozoa. Class Entamoebidea (intestinal amoebae) contains organisms of the genera *Entamoeba*, *Endolimax* and Iodamoeba. Class Amoebaea contains organisms of the genera *Acanthamoeba* and *Balamuthia*. *Naegleria fowleri* belongs to phylum Percolozoa (flagellates), class Heterolobosea (Table 1.5). During their trophic stage, amoebae characteristically form pseudopodia which constitute organelles of locomotion. Because of the extension and retraction of temporary pseudopodia they do not have constant shape.

Six species of amoebae are commonly found in the human gastrointestinal tract. Of these, four belong to the genus *Entamoeba* – *E. histolytica, E. hartmanni, E. coli* and the recently redescribed *E. dispar.* The rest represent separate genera – *Endolimax nana* and *Iodamoeba bütschlii*. Of these only *E. histolytica* is of medical importance. It causes amoebiasis. **However, other intestinal amoebae are of interest mainly because their trophozoites may be difficult to distinguish from those of *E. histolytica* by light microscopy.**

Dientamoeba fragilis, long considered another intestinal amoeba, has now been reclassified in kingdom Protozoa, phylum Parabasala.

ENTAMOEBA HISTOLYTICA

Entamoeba histolytica was first described by Losch in 1875 after being isolated in Russia from a patient with dysenteric stools. It derives its name from its ability to lyse virtually every tissue in the human body and in the bodies of experimental animals.

Geographical distribution

It is worldwide, with higher incidence of amoebiasis in tropical and subtropical regions that have poor sanitation and contaminated water. The average prevalence of infection in these areas is 10–15%, with as many as 50% of the population infected in some areas. Many of the infected individuals are asymptomatic carriers who represent a reservoir for the spread of *E. histolytica* to others. Risk groups include male homosexuals, travellers and recent immigrants, and institutionalized populations. **On a global scale, it ranks second after malaria as a cause of death among people with parasitic infections produced by protozoa.**

Habitat

Trophozoites of *E. histolytica* reside in mucosa and submucosa of large intestine of man.

Morphology

The parasite exists in three morphological forms (Fig. 3.1):

1. Trophozoite
2. Precyst
3. Cyst

Trophozoite

It measures 10–60 μm (average 20–30 μm) in diameter.

Cytoplasm

The cytoplasm of the trophozoite can be divided into **a clear outer ectoplasm and an inner finely granular endoplasm in which red blood cells, leucocytes and tissue debris are found within the food vacuoles.** The presence of ingested erythrocytes is the characteristic feature of *E. histolytica* but not of *E. dispar*. Trophozoites are motile with active, unidirectional and purposeful motility. Movement results from long finger-like pseudopodial extensions of ectoplasm into which endoplasm flows. Trophozoite is the only form present in the tissues. It usually appears only in diarrhoeic faeces in active cases and survives only for a few hours.

Nucleus

It is spherical in shape varying in size from 4–6 μm in diameter. In stained preparations it shows **a central dot-like karyosome** which is surrounded by a clear halo. The nuclear membrane is delicate and is lined by a single layer of **fine chromatin granules**. The space between the karyosome and the nuclear membrane is traversed by linin network (achromatic fibrils) having spoke-like radial arrangement.

Precyst

It is smaller in size, varying from 10–20 μm in dia-

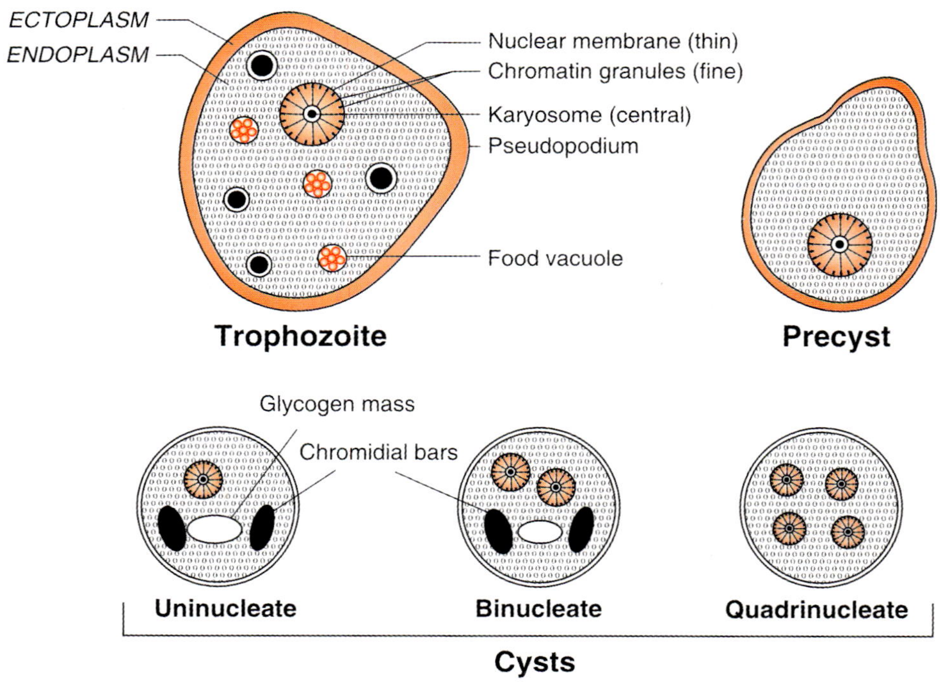

Fig. 3.1. Morphological forms of *Entamoeba histolytica*.

meter. It is oval with a blunt pseudopodium projecting from the periphery. Food vacuoles disappear. There is no change in the nucleus which shows characteristics of the trophozoite.

Cyst

It is spherical, 10–15 µm in diameter. It is surrounded by a **thick chitinous wall** which makes it highly resistant to the gastric acid, adverse environmental conditions and the chlorine concentration found in potable water. It starts as a uninucleate body, but later the nucleus divides to form two and then four nuclei. Uninucleate and binucleate cysts in addition also possess a **glycogen mass**, which stains brown with iodine, and 1–4 **chromidial or chromatoid bars**. These do not stain with iodine but appear as refractile oblong bars with rounded ends in normal saline preparations. With iron-haematoxylin stain they stain black in colour. **Cysts are present only in the lumen of the colon and in formed faeces.** Stools may contain cysts with 1–4 nuclei depending on their degree of maturation. ***E. histolytica* cysts are not produced in tissues.**

Cultivation

The first medium to be used for cultivation of *E. histolytica* was Boeck and Drbohlav's (1925) diphasic medium which consists of an egg slant base with an isotonic overlay. Other media used for cultivation of *E. histolytica* were described by Balamuth (1946) and Nelson (1947). In all these media, it is necessary to include certain associates such as enteric bacteria or the flagellate (*Trypanosoma cruzi*), as well as starch or rice flour for the amoebae to grow and multiply. These are known as **polyxenic media**.

In 1961, Diamond first reported the successful cultivation of *E. histolytica* in the absence of bacteria (**axenic cultivation**). In 1965, he described a clear liquid medium for maintenance and mass cultivation of the amoebae. This medium consists of trypticase, ox-liver digest, glucose, cysteine, ascorbic acid, and salts supplemented with horse serum and a vitamin mixture. This medium yields 100 million to 150 million *E. histolytica* from an inoculum of 10 million amoebae. Axenic cultivation of *E. histolytica* is essential for study of its:

- pathogenicity,
- immunological and biochemical properties,
- *in vitro* drug susceptibility testing, and
- preparation of axenic amoebic antigen for use in immunodiagnosis of amoebiasis.

Culture of stools yields higher positivity for *E. histolytica* as compared to direct examination. Therefore, it may also be employed for the diagnosis of amoebiasis. Fresh stools uncontaminated with urine are required. About 50 mg of formed stools containing cysts or about 0.5 ml of liquid stools containing trophozoites are inoculated into the medium and the culture is incubated at 37°C. Subcultures are usually made at 48 hour intervals. Examine a drop of culture under microscope for the motile trophozoites of the parasite. At times, original culture may be negative but the subculture is positive.

Life cycle

It passes its life cycle in **only one host** (Fig. 3.2). Cysts are passed in faeces. Man acquires the infection by ingestion of **mature quadrinucleate cysts** in faecally contaminated food or water. Trophozoites can also be passed in diarrhoeal stools, but are rapidly destroyed once outside the body, and if ingested would not survive exposure to the gastric environment. In contrast, **cysts may remain viable in a humid environment and stay infective for several days**. Infection may also be acquired by anal-oral sexual practices among male homosexuals. Flies and cockroaches can also serve as vectors for the transmission of *E. histolytica* cysts.

In the small intestine the cyst wall is lysed by trypsin and a single tetranucleate amoeba (**metacyst**) is liberated. Each nucleus divides by binary fission giving rise to eight nuclei. Almost immediately the cytoplasm becomes separated into as many parts as there are nuclei, thus from each mature cyst eight small amoebulae (**metacystic trophozoites**) are produced. This process is known as *excystation*. Metacystic trophozoites are carried in the faecal stream into the caecum. They invade the mucosa and ultimately lodge in the submucous tissue of large intestine. Here they grow and multiply by binary fission.

During growth, *E. histolytica* secretes a **proteolytic enzyme of the nature of histolysin** which brings about destruction and necrosis of tissue and produces flask-shaped ulcers (Fig. 3.3). The amoebae are mostly present at the periphery of the lesion. At this stage, a large number of trophozoites are excreted along with blood and mucus in the stool leading to amoebic dysentery. In a few cases, erosion of the large intestine may be so extensive that **trophozoites gain entrance into the radicles of portal vein** and are carried away to the liver where they multiply leading to amoebic hepatitis and amoebic liver abscess (Figs. 3.3–3.5).

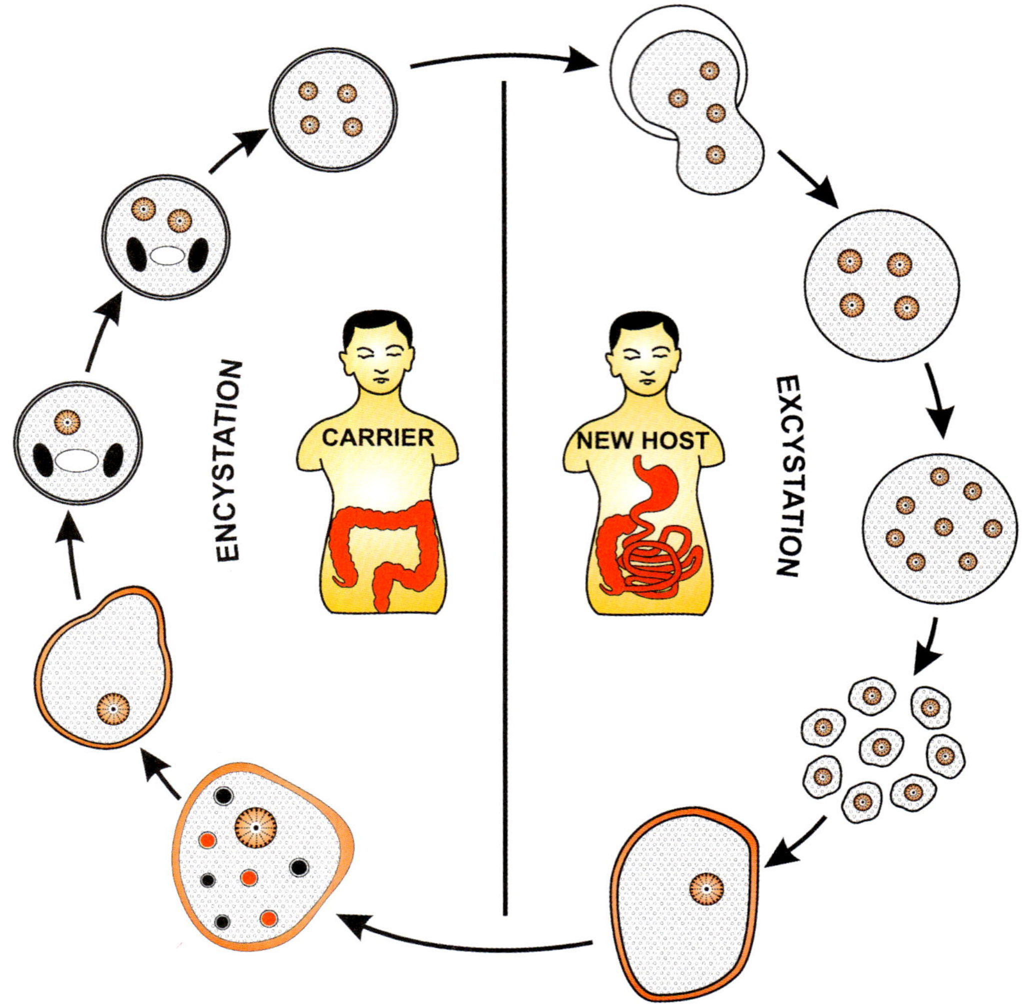

Fig. 3.2. Life cycle of *Entamoeba histolytica*.

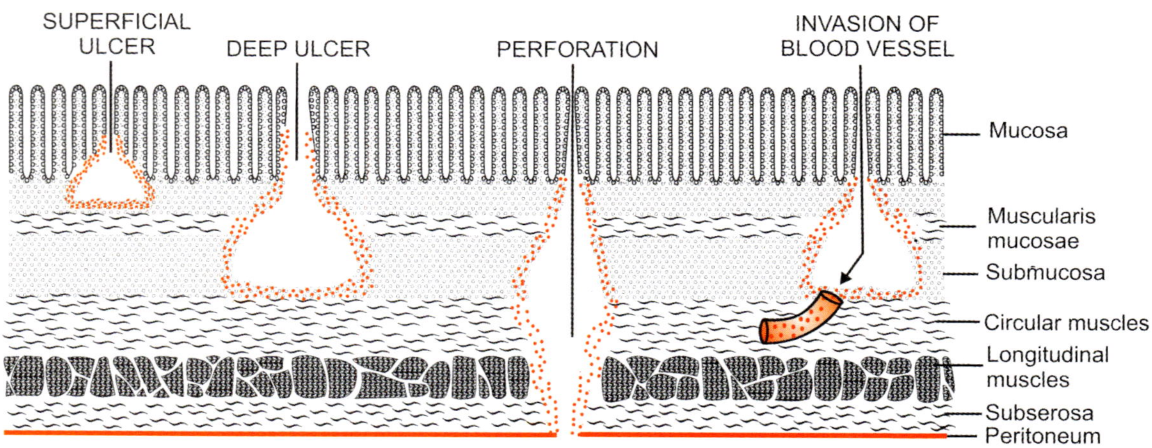

Fig. 3.3. Pathogenesis of intestinal amoebiasis.

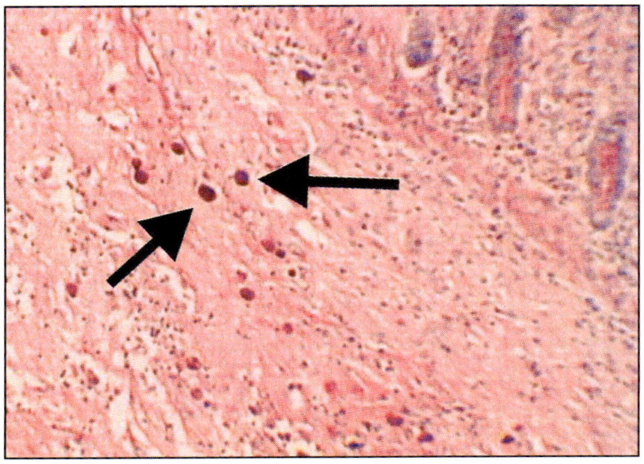

Fig. 3.4. Trophozoites of *Entamoeba histolytica* in submucosa of large intestine (PAS stain, × 100).

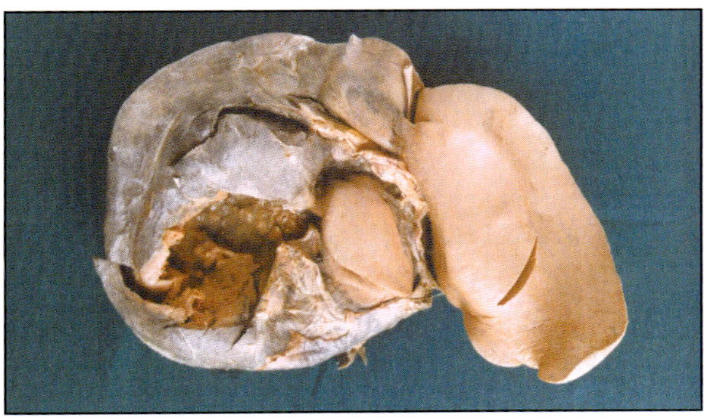

Fig. 3.5. Amoebic liver abscess.

After some time, when the effect of the parasite on the host is toned down and patient has developed resistance, the lesions start healing and patient starts passing normal (formed) stools. The trophozoites, in the lumen of the large intestine, discharge undigested food particles and transform into precysts and then into mature quadrinucleate cysts. These are the infective forms of the parasite. This process is known as *encystation*. **Cyst formation occurs only within the intestinal tract**; once the stool has left the body, cyst formation does not occur.

Pathogenicity

E. histolytica causes intestinal and extraintestinal amoebiasis. Epidemiologically, India can be divided into three regions depending on the prevalence of intestinal amoebiasis. These include the regions of high prevalence (> 30%), moderate prevalence (10–30%), and regions of low prevalence (< 10%). Maharashtra, Tamil Nadu and Chandigarh are in the region of high prevalence; Assam, Andhra Pradesh, Karnataka, Kerala, Punjab, Rajasthan, Uttar Pradesh, Bihar, Delhi and West Bengal are in the region of moderate prevalence; and Gujarat, Madhya Pradesh, Pondicherry, Himachal Pradesh, Haryana, Orissa and Sikkim remain the regions of low prevalence.

Pregnancy, malnutrition, underlying metabolic diseases, and corticosteroid therapy predispose to more serious disease.

Intestinal amoebiasis

Intestinal amoebiasis indicates that organisms are confined to gastrointestinal tract. After an **incubation period of 1–4 weeks**, the amoebae invade the colonic mucosa, producing characteristic ulcerative lesions and a profuse bloody diarrhoea (**amoebic dysentery**). The ulcers may be generalized involving the whole length of the large intestine or they may be localized in the ileo-caecal (caecum, ascending colon, ileo-caecal valve and appendix) or sigmoido-rectal (sigmoid colon and rectum) region. Ulcers are discrete with intervening normal mucosa. They vary in size from pin-head size to more than 2.5 cm in diameter (Fig. 3.6). They may be deep or superficial. Base of the deep ulcers is generally formed by muscular coat. However, superficial ulcers do not extend beyond muscularis mucosae (Fig. 3.3). When destruction is not limited to the submucosa but extends deeper into the muscular layer, the following complications may arise:

- Local peritonitis
- Perforation and generalized peritonitis
- Pericaecal or pericolic abscess
- Sloughing and gangrene of large gut.

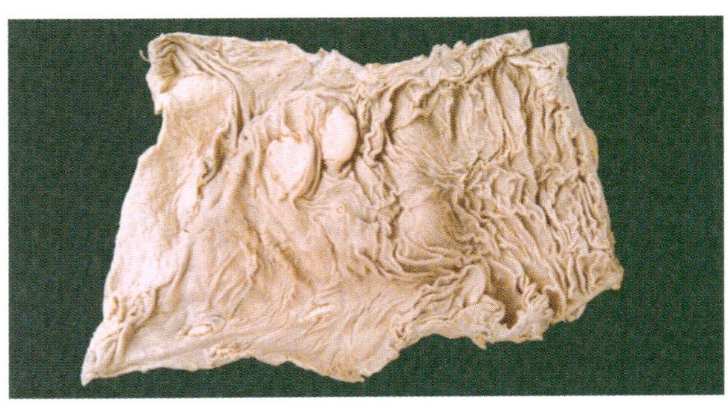

Fig. 3.6. Amoebic ulcers large intestine.

E. histolytica may also cause amoebic appendicitis and **amoebomas**. The latter are pseudotumoural lesions, whose formation is associated with necrosis, inflammation and oedema of the mucosa and submucosa of the colon. Amoebomas are generally single, but occasionally multiple masses usually found in the vertical segments of the large intestine – the caecum, the sigmoido-rectal region of the colon, the ascending colon, and the hepatic and splenic angles of the colon. The condition is usually acute with dysentery, abdominal pain and a palpable mass in the corresponding area of the abdomen.

Extraintestinal amoebiasis

About 5% individuals with intestinal amoebiasis, 1–3 months after the disappearance of the dysenteric attack, develop hepatic amoebiasis. Trophozoites of *E. histolytica* are carried as emboli by the radicles of the portal vein from the base of the amoebic ulcer in the large intestine (Fig. 3.3). The capillary system of the liver acts as an excellent filter and holds these parasites. They multiply in the liver and lead to cytolytic action (Fig. 3.7). The amoebae cause obstruction of the portal venules resulting in anaemic necrosis of hepatic cells. The destruction starts here and continues in concentric layers. Necrosis is followed by cytolysis. Small miliary abscesses coalesce to form big liver abscess (Fig. 3.5).

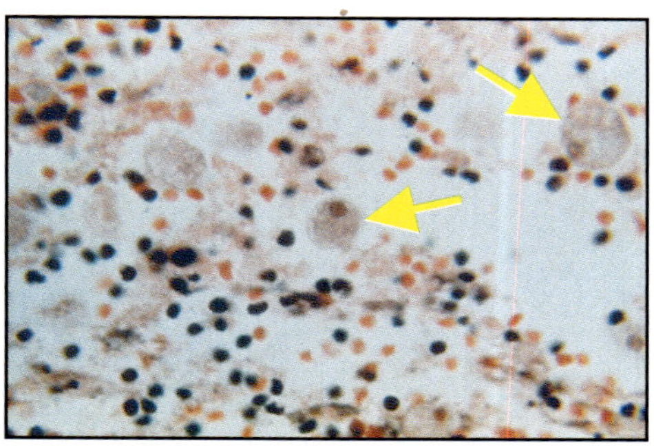

Fig. 3.7. Trophozoites of *Entamoeba histolytica* in liver aspirate showing cytolysis of liver cells (haematoxylin and eosin stain, × 400).

Amoebic liver abscess

It varies greatly in size. It has been reported in patients of all ages, but predominates in adults between 20–60 years. It has a marked preference for the right lobe of the liver and it is at least three times more frequent in males than in females. The wall of the abscess cavity is ragged with shreds of connective tissue running across the abscess cavity. A section through the margin of the liver abscess can be differentiated into three zones:

1. A necrotic centre filled with thick pus with no amoebae.
2. An intermediate zone consisting of degenerated liver cells, a few red blood cells, leucocytes and occasional trophozoites of *E. histolytica*.
3. An outer zone of nearly normal hepatic tissue just being invaded by amoebae.

Pus of liver abscess

The centre of an amoebic liver abscess contains a **viscous red-brown (anchovy sauce appearance)** or grey-yellow fluid consisting of cytolysed liver cells, red blood cells and leucocytes. It is referred to as 'pus' but contains very few pus cells. Since the amoebae actively multiply in the walls of the abscess, the last few drops of pus obtained from the lesion are most likely to yield recognizable trophozoites of the parasite.

The signs and symptoms of amoebic liver abscess vary but, in general, the onset is abrupt with pain in the right hypochondrium radiating towards the right shoulder and scapular area. The pain usually increases with deep breathing and coughing. Fever between 38° and 40°C is found in all patients with amoebic liver abscess. On palpation, the liver is soft and smooth in contrast to the rough hard irregular character of the liver in patients with cirrhosis and hepatocellular carcinoma. Jaundice is present in 8% of the patients. When jaundice is severe, multiple abscesses should be suspected.

Complications of amoebic liver abscess

With the continued lysis of liver tissue, the abscess may grow in various directions coming in contact with neighbouring organs through which its contents may be discharged (Fig. 3.8):

- **A right-sided liver abscess** may rupture externally. In such cases amoebae may cause infection of the skin leading to *granuloma cutis*. It may rupture into the lungs and the pus containing trophozoites of *E. histolytica* may be expectorated. It may also rupture into right pleural cavity leading to *empyema thoracis*, below the diaphragm causing *subphrenic abscess* and into the peritoneal cavity producing *generalized peritonitis*.
- **A left-sided liver abscess** may rupture externally through the anterior abdominal wall leading to *granuloma cutis*, into the stomach leading to *haematemesis*, and into pleural cavity and pericardial cavity leading to *empyema thoracis* and *pericarditis* respectively.
- **A liver abscess situated on the inferior surface** may rupture into bowel and peritoneal cavity, and the one situated on the posterior surface may rupture into inferior vena cava which is invariably fatal.

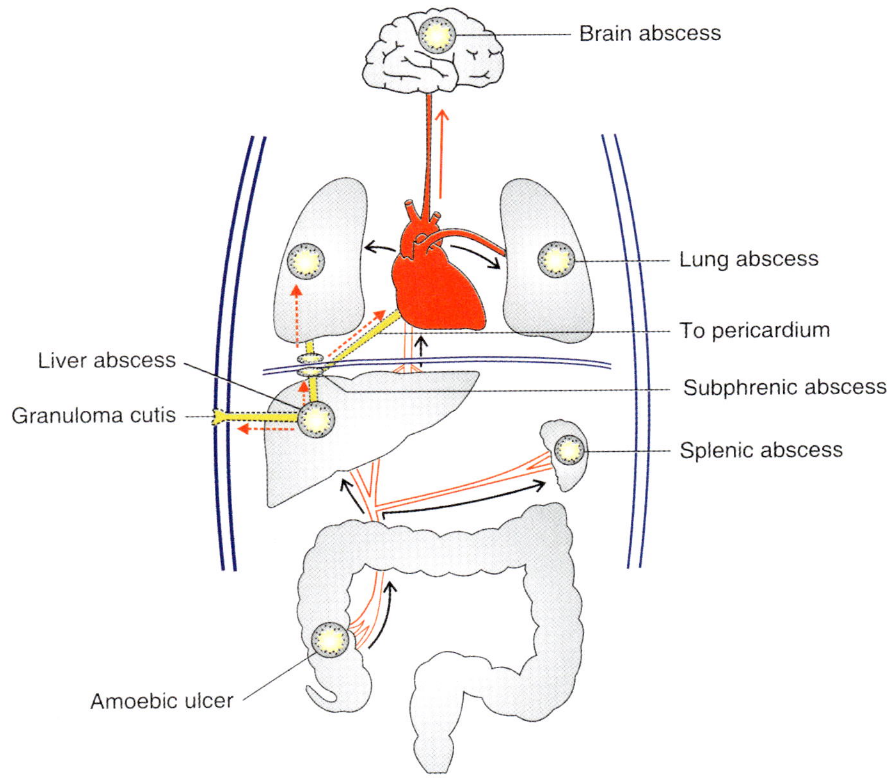

Fig. 3.8. Diagrammatic representation of routes of origin and locations of extraintestinal amoebiasis. Solid arrows indicate haematogenous spread and interrupted arrows indicate direct spread of amoebae.

From the liver, *E. histolytica* may enter into general circulation involving other organs of the body like lungs, brain, spleen, skin, etc. Both faecal and sigmoidoscopic examinations for the parasite are negative in approximately half of the patients in extra-intestinal disease.

Immune response

Both humoral and cellular immune responses are generated following infection with *E. histolytica*. Humoral immune response in patients with invasive intestinal amoebiasis is initiated by a short and transient local secretory response, followed by an increase in systemic antibodies. IgA anti-*E. histolytica* antibodies have also been found in human milk, colostrum and saliva. Circulating antibodies to *E. histolytica* can be detected as early as one week after the onset of symptoms and persist for more than three years after an invasive amoebic episode. All classes of immunoglobulins are involved, but there is predominance of IgG. Humoral antibodies do not appear to be protective against *E. histolytica*.

Cell-mediated immune response probably has a role in limiting invasive amoebiasis and the rarity of recurrence of amoebic liver abscess. The existence of an effective cell-mediated immunity is supported by:

- the results of a few studies of passive transfer of immunity with cells; and
- the cytolytic effect of activated lymphocytes and macrophages against *E. histolytica*.

Cell-mediated immune response can be detected by delayed hypersensitivity to antigens of *E. histolytica*, macrophage migration inhibition and blast transformation.

Laboratory diagnosis

Intestinal amoebiasis

1. Stool examination

- In acute amoebiasis, stool or colonic scrapings from ulcerated areas are examined by macroscopic and microscopic examination. It should be carefully differentiated from bacillary dysentery (Table 3.1).

Table 3.1. Differences between amoebic and bacillary dysentery

Character	Amoebic dysentery	Bacillary dysentery
Macroscopic		
Number	6–8 motions a day	Over 10 motions a day
Amount	Copious	Small
Odour	Offensive	Odourless
Colour	Dark red	Bright red
Reaction	Acidic	Alkaline
Consistency	Not adherent to the container	Adherent to the container
Microscopic		
RBCs	In clumps	Discrete, sometimes in clumps due to rouleaux formation
Pus cells	Few	Numerous
Macrophages	Few	Numerous, many of them contain RBCs hence may be mistaken for *E. histolytica*
Eosinophils	Present	Scarce
Charcot–Leyden crystals	Present	Absent
Pyknotic bodies	Present	Absent
Ghost cells	Absent	Present
Parasites	Trophozoites of *E. histolytica*	Absent
Bacteria	Many motile bacteria	Few or absent

- For microscopic examination, stool is picked up with a matchstick or a platinum loop and emulsified in a drop of normal saline on a clean glass slide. A clean coverslip is placed over it and examined under microscope, first under low power and then under high power. This method is specially useful for the demonstration of the actively motile trophozoites of *E. histolytica*.
- Trophozoites may also be demonstrated by mixing a small amount of the specimen with the **eosin reagent**. Cover with a cover glass and see under microscope. Eosin does not stain the living amoebae but provides a pink background which can make the motile amoebae easier to detect.
- For the demonstration of cysts or dead trophozoites, stained preparation may be required for the study of the nuclear character. For this purpose iodine stained preparation is commonly employed. Stool is emulsified **in a drop of five times diluted solution of Lugol's iodine**, covered with a clean coverslip and examined under microscope. Both saline and iodine preparations may be prepared on the same slide.
- Trichrome stain is useful to demonstrate intracellular features of both trophozoites and cysts (Fig. 3.9).

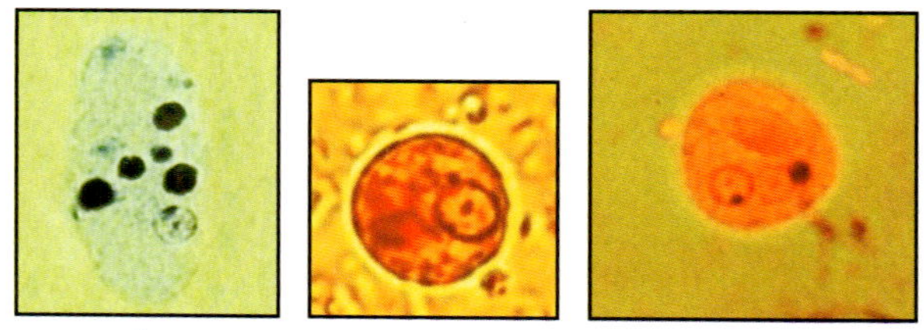

A B C

Fig. 3.9. Trichrome stain of trophozoite (A), and wet mount in iodine of uninucleate (B), and binucleate (C) cysts of *Entamoeba histolytica* in stool, (× 400).

Since excretion of cysts in the stool is often intermittent, at least three consecutive specimens should be examined.

Stool culture is useful especially in the cases of chronic and asymptomatic intestinal infections, excreting less number of cysts in the faeces.

Biopsy specimens should also be submitted for histopathologic studies.

DNA probe has been used to identify *E. histolytica* in the stool specimen and specific sequences can be amplified by **polymerase chain reaction (PCR)**.

E. histolytica must be differentiated from other intestinal protozoa including *E. coli*, *E. dispar*, *E. hartmanni*, *E. gingivalis*, *E. polecki*, *Endolimax nana*, and *Iodamoeba bütschlii*.

2. Blood examination

It shows moderate leucocytosis.

3. Serological tests

These are negative in early cases. However, in later stages of invasive intestinal amoebiasis antibodies appear and serological tests become positive. These tests include:

- Indirect haemagglutination (IHA)
- Indirect fluorescent antibody (IFA) test
- Enzyme-linked immunosorbent assay (ELISA).

Hepatic amoebiasis

1. Diagnostic aspiration

Trophozoites of *E. histolytica* may be demonstrated by microscopy of the pus aspirated by puncture of amoebic liver abscess in less than 15% cases.

2. Liver biopsy

Trophozoites of *E. histolytica* can be demonstrated in the specimens of liver biopsy from the cases of amoebic hepatitis or the wall of the liver abscess.

3. Blood examination

It shows leucocytosis with total leucocyte count of 15,000–30,000/µl of which 70–75% are polymorphonuclear leucocytes.

4. Stool examination

In less than 15% cases of amoebic hepatitis, cysts of *E. histolytica* can be demonstrated in the stool. This indicates persistence of intestinal infection.

5. Serological tests

Serological tests like IHA, IFA, and ELISA are of immense value in the diagnosis of hepatic amoebiasis. IHA and IFA tests have been reported positive with titres of $\geq$ 1 : 256 and $\geq$ 1 : 200 respectively, in almost 100% cases of amoebic liver abscess. ELISA is now replacing the IHA and is available commercially. The IgG ELISA has reported sensitivity of 99% and specificity of 90%. Amoebic antibodies persist for months to years even after clinical cure. Therefore, detection of serum antibodies is not useful to know whether the infection is recent or old, especially in individuals from endemic areas.

Amoebic antigen can be detected in the patient serum by ELISA and a simple and economical slide agglutination test, the **coagglutination test**. It is present in serum only in active infections, and disappear when the patient is cured of active amoebic disease. Therefore, demonstration of amoebic antigen in the serum indicates recent and active infection.

6. Histology

A histological diagnosis of amoebiasis can be made when the trophozoites within the tissue are identified. Organisms must be differentiated from host cells particularly histiocytes. Periodic acid–Schiff staining is often used to help locate the organisms. The organisms appear bright pink with a green-blue background (depending upon the counterstain used). Haematoxylin and eosin staining also allows the typical morphology to be seen, thus allowing accurate identification. As a result of sectioning, some organisms exhibit evenly arranged nuclear chromatin with central karyosome and some no longer contain nucleus.

7. Molecular methods

DNA probes and PCR are the recent molecular methods of promise for the detection of *E. histolytica* in stool and liver aspirates. The sensitivity is estimated at 87%.

Treatment

Very effective drug for the therapy of amoebiasis is metronidazole or its analogs tinidazole and ornidazole. Because metronidazole is so well absorbed in the gut, levels may not be therapeutic in the colonic lumen, and the drug is less effective against cysts. Hence patients with amoebic colitis also should receive a luminal agent to eradicate any *E. histolytica* trophozoites residing within the gut lumen. The nonabsorbed aminoglycoside *paromomycin* and the 8-hydroxyquinoline compound *iodoquinol* are effective luminal agents.

Prevention

The amoebic infection can be prevented by avoiding faecal contamination of food and water. There should be proper disposal of human faeces through proper drainage system. Contamination may result from discharge of sewage into rivers. Purified water should be distributed through pipelines to avoid contamination. Boiled water is safe. The amount of chlorine normally used to purify water is insufficient to kill cysts, higher levels of chlorine are effective but the water thus treated must be dechlorinated before use. Asymptomatic carriers passing large numbers of cysts in their stools are important source of infection. They should be removed from food-handling occupations and treated properly.

Using human excreta as fertilizer may lead to contamination of vegetables. Vegetables that are usually eaten raw should be cleaned with uncontaminated running water and treated with 5% acetic acid before consuming. Houseflies and cockroaches ingest cysts present in faeces and can pass them unharmed from their guts after periods as long as 24 hours. They may also carry cysts mechanically on their body. Therefore, food exposed to flies and cockroaches should not be consumed. One should wash hands before eating and after defecation. Homosexuals should avoid anal-oral sexual practices.

NONPATHOGENIC AMOEBAE

A number of species of the genus *Entamoeba* are of worldwide distribution but do not appear to cause disease. The knowledge of these species is of value in differentiating the harmless commensals from potentially pathogenic *E. histolytica.*

ENTAMOEBA DISPAR

Formerly a pathogenic invasive strain and a nonpathogenic strain of *E. histolytica* were thought to exist. Using isoenzyme-electrophoretic techniques, these two 'strains' have now been recognized as separate species based on antigenic differences, genomic DNA, and ribosomal RNA.

E. histolytica is the invasive pathogenic species and *E. dispar* (originally described by Brumpt in 1925) has been designated as noninvasive nonpathogenic species. The two species are morphologically identical. **Trophozoites containing ingested red cells can be identified as *E. histolytica* but the cysts of *E. histolytica* and *E. dispar* cannot be differentiated microscopically and should therefore be reported as *E. histolytica/E. dispar*.**

ENTAMOEBA HARTMANNI

E. hartmanni is cosmopolitan in distribution. It is morphologically similar to *E. histolytica,* but both its trophozoites and cysts are smaller and the former never contain ingested red blood cells. Earlier it was regarded as small race of *E. histolytica.* The trophozoites and the cysts of *E. hartmanni* range from 4–12 μm and 5–10 μm in diameter respectively. It is a **nonpathogenic amoeba**. It is acquired by ingestion of food or water contaminated with cyst-bearing faeces. Its life cycle is similar to that of *E. histolytica.* The diagnosis of *E. hartmanni* can be established by measurement of size of the trophozoites and cysts and the absence of red blood cells in the endoplasm of the trophozoite.

ENTAMOEBA COLI

It is a worldwide parasite. It lives freely in the lumen of large intestine of man and is nonpathogenic. Like *E. histolytica,* it exists in three stages – trophozoite, precyst and cyst (Table 3.2, Figs. 3.10 and 3.11). Life cycle of *E. coli* is similar to that of *E. histolytica*.

ENTAMOEBA POLECKI

E. polecki is a common parasite of the caecum and colon of pigs. It may rarely be found in human stool specimens, particularly in individuals who may have close association with pigs. The trophozoite resembles that of *E. coli* sharing the sluggish pattern of motility and the eccentricity of the nuclear karyosome. The cysts typically have only one nucleus (never more than two) with a small, eccentric karyosome and fine, even distribution of chromatin along the nuclear membrane. Small multiple, iodine-positive glycogen masses may be seen in the cytoplasm.

ENTAMOEBA GINGIVALIS

E. gingivalis is the **first parasitic amoeba to be recognized**. It was described by Gros in 1849 in the

Table 3.2. Trophozoites and cysts of *E. histolytica* and *E. coli*

	E. histolytica	***E. coli***
Trophozoite		
Size	20–30 μm	20–50 μm
Motility	Active, unidirectional, purposeful motility. They extend pseudopodia only along one plane.	Sluggish, nonpurposeful motility. They extend pseudopodia in multiple planes and "wander" aimlessly in one direction then the other.
Cytoplasm	Clearly defined into ectoplasm and endoplasm.	Not defined.
Cytoplasmic inclusions	Red blood cells, leucocytes and tissue debris but no bacteria.	Bacteria, yeasts and cellular debris, but very rarely erythrocytes.
Nucleus	Central karyosome, the nuclear membrane is delicate and is lined by fine chromatin granules. It is not visible in unstained preparations.	Eccentric karyosome, the nuclear membrane is thick and is lined by coarse chromatin granules. It is visible in unstained preparations.
Precyst	Oval with a blunt pseudopodium, 10–20 μm in diameter. Nucleus shows characteristics of that of its trophozoite.	20 μm in diameter, resembles in shape with that of *E. histolytica*. Nucleus shows characteristics of that of its trophozoite.
Cyst		
Size	Spherical, 10–15 μm in diameter.	Spherical, 15–20 μm in diameter.
Number of nuclei	1–4	1–8
Chromidial bars	Rounded	Filamentous

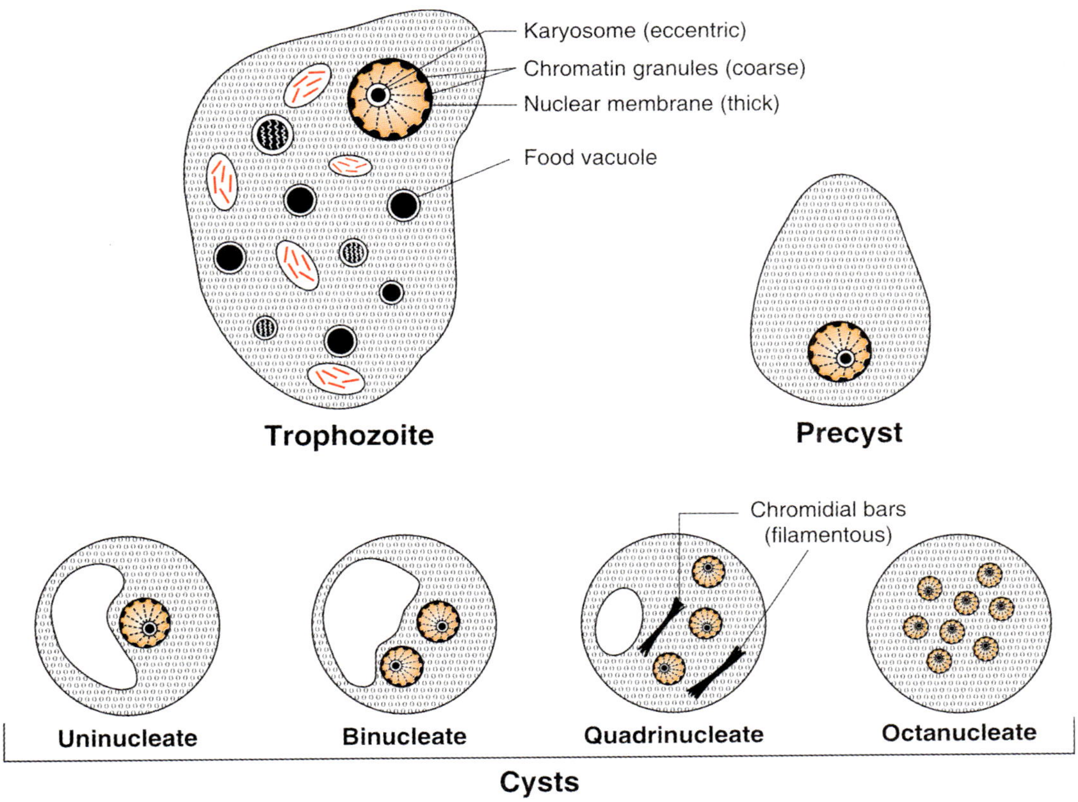

Fig. 3.10. Morphological forms of *Entamoeba coli*.

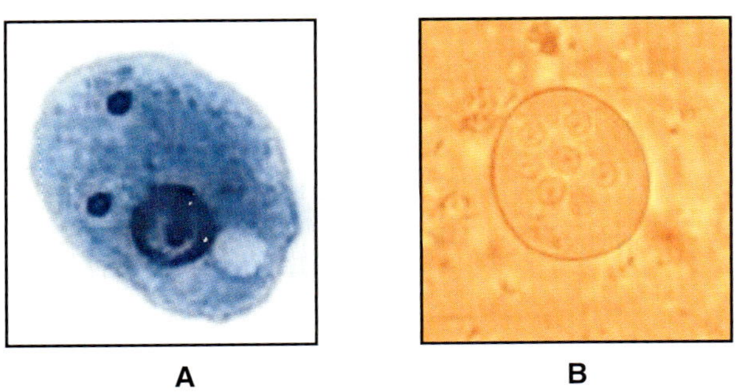

Fig. 3.11. Trichrome stain of trophozoite (A) and wet mount in iodine of cyst (B) of *Entamoeba coli* in stool, (× 400).

soft tartar between the teeth. It is unusual among the *Entamoeba* in two respects:

1. It inhabits the mouth rather than the large bowel.
2. No cyst of *E. gingivalis* has ever been found.

Morphology

Trophozoite

It measures 10–25 µm in diameter and is actively motile by multiple pseudopodia.

Cytoplasm

It is differentiated into clear ectoplasm and granular endoplasm in which digested leucocytes and epithelial cells are found within food vacuoles. At times bacteria and rarely red blood cells are also seen.

Nucleus

It is spherical, 2–4 µm in diameter. It has a central karyosome and nuclear membrane is lined with closely packed chromatin granules (Fig. 3.12).

Since morphologically *E. gingivalis* is very similar to the trophozoite of *E. histolytica*, it is important to make the correct identification from a sputum specimen, that is, *E. gingivalis*, which is considered to be a nonpathogen rather than *E. histolytica* from a pulmonary abscess.

Habitat

E. gingivalis occurs as a commensal in the gingival tissue around the teeth, particularly if there is suppuration, as in pyorrhoea alveolaris, but it also occurs in apparently hygienic mouth and on dental plates if they

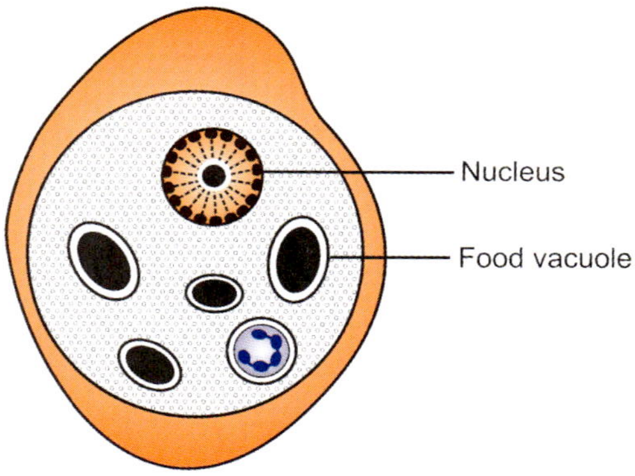

Fig. 3.12. Trophozoite of *Entamoeba gingivalis.*

are not kept clean. Occasionally, this amoeba has been identified from the crypts and in histologic sections of diseased tonsils and in vaginal and cervical smears from women using intrauterine devices. It is transmitted from person-to-person by close contact like kissing or from contaminated drinking utensils.

Laboratory diagnosis

It can be established by demonstration of trophozoites of *E. gingivalis* in the material removed from gingival margin of the gums, from between teeth or from denture.

ENDOLIMAX NANA

It is cosmopolitan, small (*nana*, small) amoeba found in the lumen of the large intestine of humans, primates and pigs. It has all the stages described for *E. histolytica* and *E. coli*, i.e., trophozoite, precyst and cyst.

Morphology

Trophozoite (Fig. 3.13)

It is small, measuring 6–15 μm (average 10 μm) in diameter. The cytoplasm has an inner finely granular endoplasm and a clear outer ectoplasm. It exhibits sluggish motility by means of short, blunt, hyaline pseudopodia. Cytoplasmic inclusions contain bacteria, small vegetable cells, and crystals but never red blood cells. Nucleus is minute spherical with a large irregular karyosome lying eccentrically from which several achromatic strands extend to the nuclear membrane. There is normally no peripheral chromatin on the nuclear membrane.

Cyst

It is oval measuring 8–10 μm in diameter. The number of nuclei varies from 1–4 but **mature cyst is quadrinucleate**. Chromidial bars and glycogen vacuole are absent.

Pathogenicity

E. nana is transmitted from man-to-man by ingestion of viable cysts in polluted water or food. It is normally regarded as nonpathogenic although there are isolated reports of gastrointestinal symptoms in AIDS patients for which no other cause could be found.

IODAMOEBA BÜTSCHLII

I. bütschlii is worldwide in its distribution. It lives as harmless commensal in the lumen of large intestine of man, monkeys and pigs.

Morphology

Trophozoite (Fig. 3.14)

It varies in size from 6–20 μm in diameter and is fairly active in freshly evacuated unformed stools and shows sluggish movement in older stools. The clear ectoplasm is not usually well differentiated from denser endoplasm that contains coarse and fine granules and has

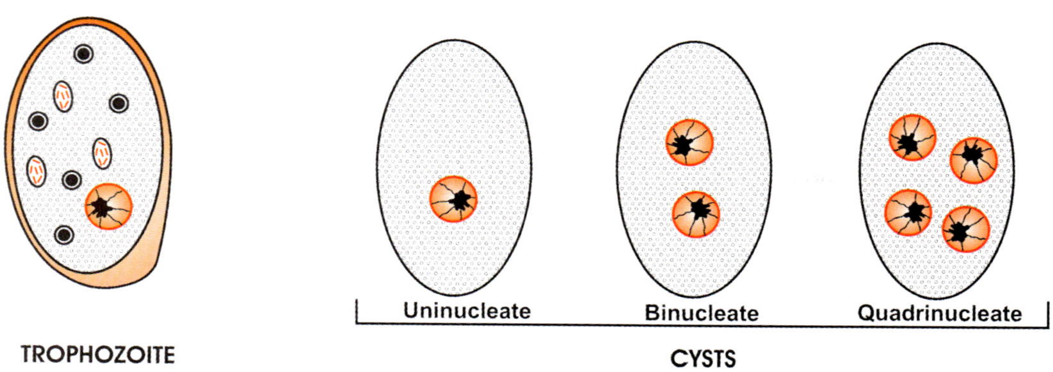

Fig. 3.13. Morphological forms of *Endolimax nana.*

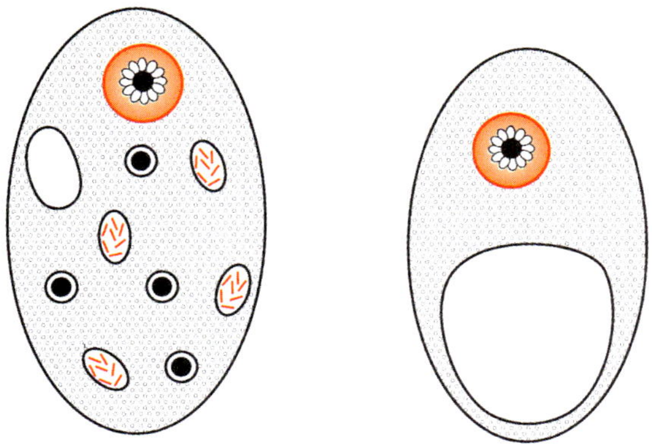

Fig. 3.14. Morphological forms of *Iodamoeba bütschlii.*

bacteria and yeast cells in food vacuoles. Occasionally, a discrete glycogen vacuole which stains golden brown with iodine may be demonstrated in the cytoplasm of the trophozoite.

Cyst

It is ovoid or irregularly pyriform in shape, uninucleate and measures 8–15 μm in longest diameter. The cytoplasm contains a large glycogen vacuole. Chromidial bars are absent (Figs. 3.14 and 3.15).

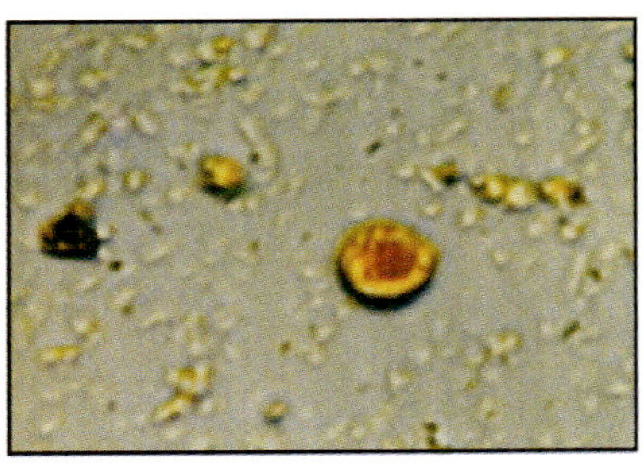

Fig. 3.15. Cyst of *Iodamoeba bütschlii* (iodine preparation), (× 400).

Nucleus

It is relatively large measuring 2.0–3.5 μm in diameter. The karyosome is a large circular mass, central in position and surrounded by refractile globules. Peripheral chromatin lining is absent.

Pathogenicity

The natural habitat of *I. bütschlii* is the lumen of large intestine. Here the trophozoite feeds on enteric bacteria. It is transmitted from man-to-man when the viable cysts are ingested in polluted water or food. It is non-pathogenic luminal parasite of large intestine.

OPPORTUNISTIC PROTOZOA

Free-living amoebae (phylum Amoebozoa) of the genera *Acanthamoeba* and *Balamuthia*, and flagellate of the genus *Naegleria* (phylum Percolozoa) are facultative parasites of man. They are ubiquitous in nature, found commonly in soil and water (swimming pools, tap water, and heating and air-conditioning units) where they feed on bacteria, but as opportunists, they may produce serious infection of the central nervous system and the eye. Therefore, they are known as opportunistic protozoa. Fowler and Carter in 1965, for the first time reported four fatal cases of human infection with free-living amoebae in Australia. Since then a number of similar infections have been reported from the USA, Europe, Asia, New Zealand and Africa.

These protozoa may be natural hosts for *Legionella* as well as for other bacteria such as *Listeria monocytogenes*, *Vibrio cholerae*, *Mycobacterium leprae*, *Burkholderia cepacia*, and *Pseudomonas aeruginosa*. Because of their well known resistance to chlorine, the protozoal cysts are considered to be vectors for these intracellular bacteria. This can have tremendous significance for any hospital where the water source is contaminated with free-living protozoa. These protozoa have also been found to be acceptable hosts for *Chlamydia pneumoniae*, echoviruses and polioviruses.

There is only one *Naegleria* species, *N. fowleri,* which is pathogenic to man. Several *Acanthamoeba* species are considered pathogenic to humans. These include *A. culbertsoni, A. castellanii, A. polyphaga, A. astronyxis, A. healyi* and *A. divionensis*. *Balamuthia mandrillaris* is newly described free-living protozoan.

The nuclei of these opportunistic protozoa possess a large central nucleolus or karyosome surrounded by a halo, and a nuclear membrane without chromatin granules. These features help to differentiate these opportunistic protozoa from *E. histolytica*.

NAEGLERIA FOWLERI

Morphology

N. fowleri has two stages – motile trophozoites and non-motile cysts (Fig. 3.16).

Trophozoites

These occur in two forms – amoeboid and flagellate. Amoeboid form is elongate. It is actively motile by means of eruptive, blunt pseudopodia called **lobo-**

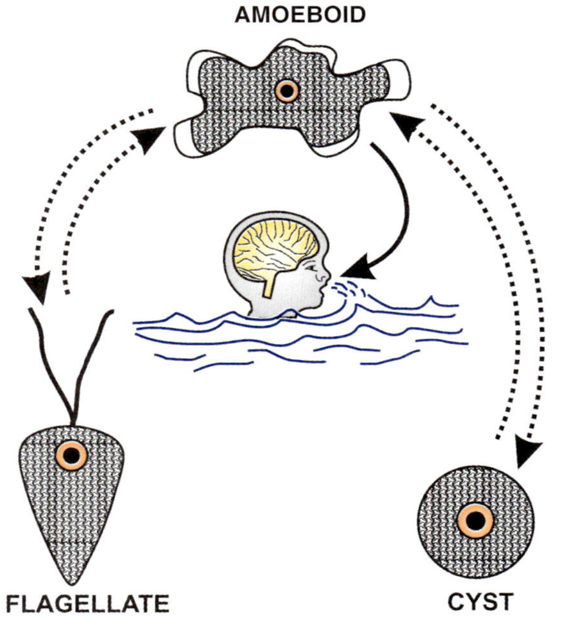

Fig. 3.16. Life cycle and pathogenicity of *Naegleria fowleri*.

podia. It measures 15–30 μm (average 22 μm) in length. It has distinctive phagocytic structures known as amoebostomes. They are used for engulfment and vary in number depending on the strain. With electron microscopy, they appear to be densely granular in contrast to the highly vacuolated body of the amoeba. With light microscopy, they appear as thick-walled vacuoles. In tissue, trophozoites ingest erythrocytes, leucocytes, and cause destruction of tissue. The nucleus is small, 3 μm in diameter, and has a large central karyosome surrounded by a halo and no peripheral nuclear chromatin. Reproduction in *Naegleria* is by simple binary fission of the trophozoite.

When amoeboid trophozoites are transferred to distilled water or non-nutrient buffer, from a culture or from teased tissue, and maintained at temperatures between 27° and 37°C, they transform into transient non-feeding, non-dividing flagellates, that after a time, revert back to amoeboid form. The flagellates are cigar- or pear-shaped with two flagella at the broader end. They move rapidly forward or spin slowly in circles.

Cysts

Cysts of *N. fowleri* are uninucleate, spherical, 7–15 μm in diameter and are surrounded by a **relatively thin cyst wall**, a feature that makes *N. fowleri* cysts susceptible to desiccation. Under electron microscopy they reveal 1–2 mucoid-plugged pores or ostioles. Trophozoites encyst when conditions are appropriate and, later, excyst in a favourable environment. Encystment is an adaptive mechanism that enables the organism to survive conditions that would kill trophozoite. Factors thought to induce cyst formation include starvation, drying and various chemicals. *Cysts and flagellate forms of N. fowleri have never been found in tissues or CSF*.

Life cycle and pathogenicity

The amoeboid form of *N. fowleri* is the invasive stage of the parasite. Man acquires infection by nasal contamination during swimming in freshwater lakes, ponds or swimming pools containing infective forms. Infection may also be acquired by inhalation of dust containing infective forms. It is likely that flagellate forms or cysts of *N. fowleri* could enter the nose. However, since the amoeboid form is the invasive stage of the parasite, therefore, it appears that flagellate forms revert to amoeboid forms and the amoeboid forms escape from the cysts in the nose.

The amoeboid forms invade the nasal mucosa, cribriform plate and travel along the olfactory nerves to brain. They first invade olfactory bulbs and then spread to the more posterior regions of the brain leading to a rapidly fatal infection known as **primary amoebic meningoencephalitis** (PAM). It occurs in healthy children and young adults with a recent history of swimming in freshwater. Patient develops severe frontal headache, fever (39°–40°C), anorexia, nausea, vomiting and signs of meningeal irritation, frequently evidenced by a positive Kernig's sign. Involvement of the olfactory lobes may lead to disturbances in smell or taste. Patient may also develop visual disturbances, confusion, irritability, seizures and coma. The disease usually results in death within 72 hours of the onset of symptoms. Although all cases were fatal before 1970, survival has been reported in a few cases in which the disease was rapidly diagnosed and treated.

The period between contact with the organism and onset of clinical symptoms vary from 2–3 days to as long as 7–15 days. PAM may resemble acute purulent bacterial meningitis, and these conditions may be difficult to differentiate particularly in the early stage.

PAM has been reported from the United States, Ireland, England, Belgium, Czechoslovakia, Australia, New Zealand, Brazil, Zambia and India. Clinical patient histories indicate exposure to the organism via fresh water lakes or swimming pools shortly before onset; patients had been previously healthy with no specific underlying problems. Pathogenic *Naegleria* organisms have also been isolated from nasal passages of individuals with no history of water exposure, thus suggesting the possibility of airborne exposure.

Laboratory diagnosis

Microscopy of CSF

The diagnosis of PAM can be made by microscopic identification of living or stained amoebae in CSF. Motile amoebae with characteristic morphology can be readily demonstrated in simple wet-mount preparation of fresh CSF specimen. *Refrigeration of CSF is not recommended because this may kill the amoebae.* When centrifuging the CSF, low speed (150 *g* for 5 minutes) should be used so that the trophozoites are not damaged. CSF smear may be stained with Wright or Giemsa stains. With these stains amoebae have considerable amount of sky-blue cytoplasm and relatively small, delicate pink nuclei. These can be differentiated from mononuclear leucocytes which have a small amount of sky-blue cytoplasm and large purplish nuclei.

In centrifuged deposit of CSF, the amoebae tend to be rounded and flattened without pseudopodia. Amoebae can also be demonstrated by fluorescent antibody staining of the CSF and in the histologic sections of the brain biopsied tissue by haematoxylin and eosin (Fig. 3.17), immunofluorescence and immunoperoxidase methods. The bacterial stain like Gram staining is of little value because heat fixing destroys the amoebae and causes them to stain poorly and appear as degenerating cells.

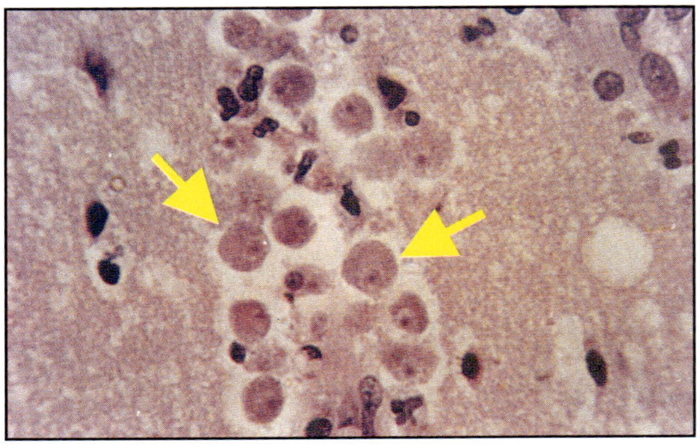

Fig. 3.17. *Naegleria fowleri* in brain (haematoxylin and eosin stain, × 400).

As in case of fulminating bacterial meningitis, the CSF is purulent or sanguinopurulent with leucocyte counts (predominantly neutrophils) varying from a few hundreds to >20,000 cells/µl. CSF protein content is generally increased and glucose level is low. No bacterium is detected by Gram staining or culture of CSF.

Culture

N. fowleri may be cultivated by placing some of the CSF on non-nutrient agar (1.5%) spread with a lawn of washed *Escherichia coli* or *Enterobacter aerogenes* and incubated at 37°C. The amoebae will grow on the moist agar surface and will use the bacteria as food, producing **plaques** as they clear the bacteria. As colonies grow and expand, cysts that survive moderate desiccation are formed; thus, strains can be maintained by transfer of either trophic or cystic forms.

Treatment

At present there is no satisfactory treatment for PAM. Antibacterial antibiotics and antiamoebic drugs are ineffective. Amphotericin B, a drug of considerable toxicity, is the antinaeglerial agent for which there is evidence of clinical effectiveness. In experimental infections, tetracycline acts synergistically with amphotericin B to protect mice.

ACANTHAMOEBA SPECIES

Although only one species of *Naegleria (N. fowleri)* is known to cause disease in man, several *Acanthamoeba* species including *A. culbertsoni, A. castellanii, A. polyphaga, A. astronyxis, A. healyi* and *A. divionensis* may do so.

Morphology

Acanthamoeba spp. exist as active trophozoites and resistant cysts. There is no flagellate form.

Trophozoites

Trophozoites of *Acanthamoeba* (Fig. 3.18) are larger than those of *Naegleria* and measure 24–56 µm in length. They have irregular appearance with spike-like pseudopodia known as **acanthopodia**; hence the name, *Acanthamoeba* (*acanth*, spine or thorn). It has a single nucleus with a large dense central prominent nucleolus surrounded by a halo.

Cysts

Cysts of *Acanthamoeba* are **double-walled** and, therefore, quite resistant in the environment. These are spherical, about 20 µm or more in diameter. The cyst

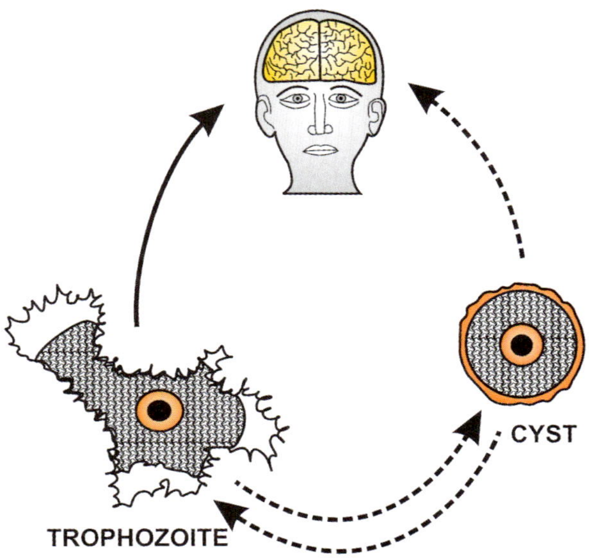

Fig. 3.18. Life cycle and pathogenicity of *Acanthamoeba* spp.

wall is made up of an outer wrinkled ectocyst and an inner endocyst.

Acanthamoeba differs from *Naegleria* in not having a flagellate stage and in forming cysts in tissues. Trophozoites of *Acanthamoeba* move slowly while those of *Naegleria* are actively motile. Differences between *N. fowleri* and *Acanthamoeba* spp. are given in Table 3.3.

Life cycle and pathogenicity

Man acquires infection by inhalation of aerosol or dust containing trophozoites and cysts. The trophozoites reach the lower respiratory tract and from there they invade central nervous system through the blood stream. The infection may also be acquired by direct invasion through broken or ulcerated skin or eye. Although *Acanthamoeba* is able to invade the nasal mucosa and cause fatal CNS disease in experimental animals, this is not thought to be the usual route of invasion in human infection. In contrast to *Naegleria,* cysts of *Acanthamoeba* are also formed in tissues.

Acanthamoeba causes **granulomatous amoebic encephalitis** (GAE) and single or multiple brain abscesses, primarily in persons who are debilitated or immunosuppressed including patients with AIDS and those undergoing immunosuppressive therapy. The disease is usually of gradual onset and takes a prolonged chronic course lasting weeks, months or years, and is characterized by focal granulomatous lesions. This is in sharp contrast to *Naegleria* infection.

In healthy persons, *Acanthamoeba* may cause **keratitis**. *Acanthamoeba* keratitis was described for the first time in 1974. Infection occurs by direct contact of the cornea with amoebae, which may be introduced through minor corneal trauma by exposure to contaminated water or contact lenses. Amoebae attach to the contact lenses stored in contaminated solutions and are transferred to the eye when lenses are placed over the cornea. Amoebae become established as part of the corneal flora and may invade the corneal stroma through a break in the epithelium or through the intact epithelium. They produce an infection that progresses to *Acanthamoeba* keratitis, which usually develops over a period of weeks to months. It causes severe ocular pain, affected vision and a stromal infiltrate that is frequently ring-shaped and composed predominantly of neutrophils. If not properly managed it may lead to loss of vision.

Laboratory diagnosis

Microscopy

Diagnosis of GAE is made by demonstration of trophozoites of *Acanthamoeba* in CSF or trophozoites and cysts in brain tissue (Fig. 3.19). Diagnosis of *Acanthamoeba* keratitis may be made by identifying trophozoites and cysts in corneal scrapings. Wet mount preparation of the corneal scraping shows motile trophozoites. Trophozoites and cysts can be demonstrated in histopathological preparations of corneal tissue stained

Table 3.3. Differences between *N. fowleri* and *Acanthamoeba* spp.

Characteristic	*N. fowleri*	*Acanthamoeba* spp.
Trophozoite	Two forms (amoeboid and flagellate), 15–30 μm in diameter; blunt pseudopodia; actively motile	Larger, no flagellate form; 24–56 μm in diameter with spike-like pseudopodia; move slowly
Cysts	Not present in tissue, small (7–15 μm in diameter), rounded, smooth relatively thin cyst wall	Present in tissue, large (≥ 20 μm in diameter) with double wall – outer wrinkled ectocyst and inner endocyst
Appearance in tissue	Smaller than *Acanthamoeba* spp.; dense endoplasm; less distinct nuclear staining	Large; rounded; less dense endoplasm; nucleus more distinct

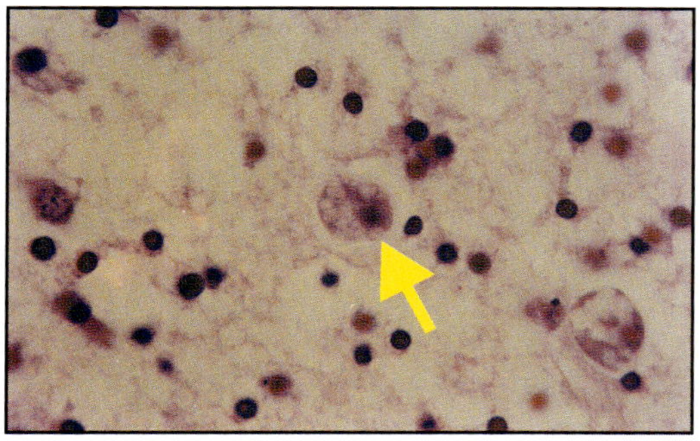

Fig. 3.19. *Acanthamoeba* in brain (haematoxylin and eosin stain, × 400).

with haematoxylin and eosin, Giemsa, Heidenhain's haematoxylin, Gomori's chromium haematoxylin, periodic acid-Schiff, Bauer chromic acid-Schiff, silver methenamine and indirect fluorescent antibody technique (IFAT). Rapid diagnosis of *Acanthamoeba* keratitis may be made by identifying amoebae or cysts in corneal scraping using procedures for Giemsa staining, calcofluor white staining and IFAT.

Culture

As in case of *N. fowleri, Acanthamoeba* may be cultured on non-nutrient agar spread with washed *E. coli* or *E. aerogenes* and incubated at 30°C instead of 37°C. *Acanthamoeba* does not have a flagellate stage but its trophozoites are identified by small spiky acanthopodia, and cysts are readily identified by their double-walled wrinkled appearance. Species identification may be made by IFAT.

Polymerase chain reaction (PCR)

PCR has also been applied for the diagnosis of *Acanthamoeba* infection.

Treatment

There is no satisfactory treatment for GAE. Total excision of the mass and treatment with ketoconazole, penicillin and chloramphenicol has been claimed to be useful. *Acanthamoeba* keratitis may be managed by use of combination of dibromopropamidine and propamidine isethionate ointment or drops, and neomycin drops. Topical miconazole and systemic ketoconazole; topical miconazole and neosporin with epithelial debridement; topical clotrimazole; oral itraconazole with topical miconazole and surgical debridement; and topical polyhexamethylene biguanide have also been claimed to be successful for the treatment of *Acanthamoeba* keratitis.

BALAMUTHIA MANDRILLARIS

B. mandrillaris is a newly described amoeba. Like *Acanthamoeba* spp. and unlike *N. fowleri,* it does not have a flagellate stage.

Morphology

Trophozoite

Trophozoites of *B. mandrillaris* (Fig. 3.20) are irregular or branching in shape. Their length ranges from 12–60 µm. They are sluggishly motile. In tissue culture, broad pseudopodia are usually seen; however, as the monolayer cells are destroyed, the trophozoites develop fingerlike pseudopodia.

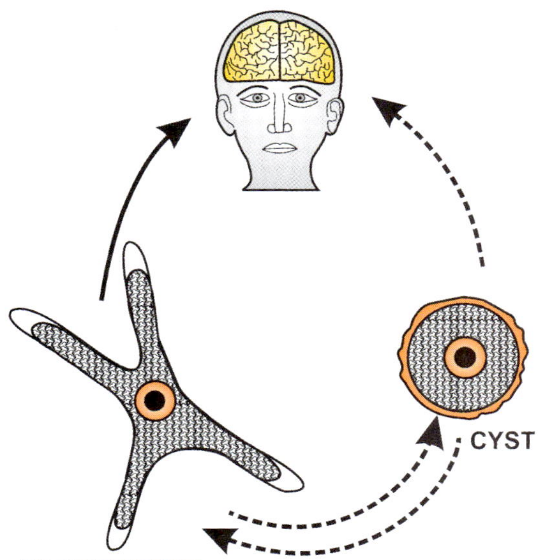

Fig. 3.20. Life cycle and pathogenicity of *B. mandrillaris.*

Cyst

It is spherical 6–30 µm in diameter with **two walls**. The inner wall is thin and spherical and the outer wall is thick and wrinkled much like the cysts of *Acanthamoeba*. Both trophozoites and cysts of *B. mandrillaris* are found in tissue.

Pathogenicity

Like *Acanthamoeba*, *B. mandrillaris* causes GAE and single or multiple brain abscesses, primarily in immunocompromised individuals. The portal of entry and spread of *B. mandrillaris* infection is believed to be the same as for *Acanthamoeba* spp. Incubation period is not known. *B. mandrillaris* can be grown in tissue culture, preferably Vero cell.

Laboratory diagnosis

It can be made by:

- Identifying trophozoites of *B. mandrillaris* in the CSF and trophozoites and cysts in brain tissue (Fig. 3.21).
- *Balamuthia* does not grow on agar plates used for *Naegleria* and *Acanthamoeba* but have been recovered in tissue culture preferably Vero cells.
- Most cases of *Balamuthia* infection are diagnosed by immunofluorescent antibody testing.
- PCR has also been used for the diagnosis of *Balamuthia* infection.

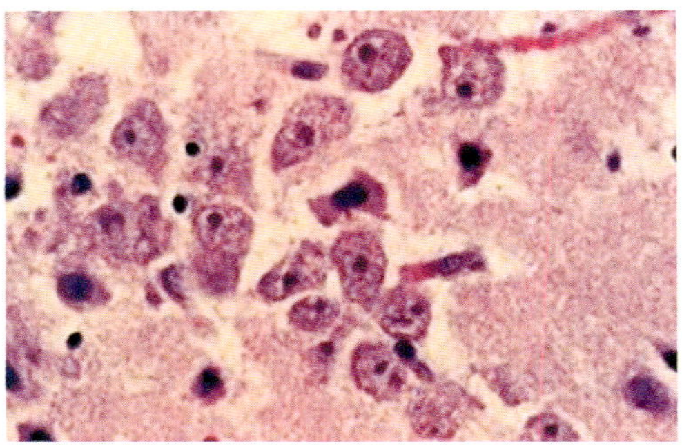

Fig. 3.21. *Balamuthia mandrillaris* in brain tissue (haematoxylin and eosin stain, × 400).

Further Reading

1. Anderson, K. and Jamieson, A. 1972. Primary amoebic meningoencephalitis. *Lancet*, **1**: 902–3.
2. Apley, J., Clark, S.K.R. et al. 1970. Primary amoebic meningoencephalitis in Britain. *Br. Med. J.*, **1**: 596–9.
3. Bier, J.W. and Sawyer, T.K. 1990. Amoebae isolated from laboratory eye wash stations. *Curr. Microbiol.*, **20**: 349–50.
4. Carter, R.F. 1968. Primary amoebic meningoencephalitis: Clinical, pathological and epidemiological features of six fatal cases. *J. Pathol. Bacteriol.*, **96**: 1–25.
5. Cox, F.E.G., Wakelin, D., Gillespie, S.H. and Despommier, D.D. 2005. Topley & Wilson's Microbiology & Microbial Infections: Parasitology, 10th ed. Hodder Arnold, ASM Press.
6. Garcia, L.S. 2001. *Diagnostic Medical Parasitology*, 4th ed. Washington D.C.: American Society for Microbiology Press.
7. Epstein, R.J., Wilson, L.A. et al. 1986. Rapid diagnosis of *Acanthamoeba* keratitis from corneal scraping using indirect fluorescent antibody staining. *Arch. Ophthalmol.*, **104**: 1318–21.
8. Fowler, M. and Carter, R.F. 1965. Acute pyogenic meningitis probably due to *Acanthamoeba* spp.: A preliminary report. *Br. Med. J.*, **2**: 740–2.
9. Haque, R., Neville et al. 1994. Detection of *Entamoeba histolytica* and *E. dispar* directly in stool. *Am. J. Trop. Med. Hyg.*, **50**: 595–6.
10. Yeoh, R., Warhurst, D.C. and Falcon, M.G. 1987. *Acanthamoeba* keratitis. *Br. J. Ophthalmol.*, **71**: 500–3.

Important Questions

1. Discuss geographical distribution, morphology, cultivation, life cycle, pathogenicity and laboratory diagnosis of *Entamoeba histolytica*.
2. Tabulate differences between:
   (a) Amoebic and bacillary dysentery.
   (b) *Entamoeba histolytica* and *Entamoeba coli*.
3. Name various nonpathogenic protozoa and describe morphology and life cycle of any one of them.
4. Name various opportunistic protozoa. Discuss their geographical distribution, morphology, life cycle, pathogenicity and laboratory diagnosis.
5. Tabulate differences between *Naegleria*, *Acanthamoeba* and *Balamuthia.*

Multiple Choice Questions

1. Mature cyst of *Entamoeba histolytica* is:
   (a) uninucleate.
   (b) binucleate.
   (c) quadrinucleate.
   (d) octanucleate.
2. Glycogen mass and chromidial bars are **absent** in the cysts of *Entamoeba histolytica* in:
   (a) uninucleate stage.
   (b) binucleate stage.
   (c) quadrinucleate stage.
   (d) octanucleate stage.
3. Cysts of *Entamoeba histolytica* are formed in:
   (a) the lumen of the intestine.
   (b) the tissues.
   (c) the soil.
   (d) All of the above.
4. Infective stage of *Entamoeba histolytica* is:
   (a) trophozoite.
   (b) binucleate cyst.
   (c) quadrinucleate cyst.
   (d) octanucleate cyst.

5. Superficial intestinal ulcers do not extend beyond:
   (a) muscularis mucosae.
   (b) submucosa.
   (c) muscular coat.
   (d) peritoneum.
6. Most common organ involved in extraintestinal amoebiasis is:
   (a) liver.
   (b) lung.
   (c) brain.
   (d) spleen.
7. All of the following characteristics are seen in the stools in amoebic dysentery **except**:
   (a) RBCs in clumps.
   (b) Charcot-Leyden crystals.
   (c) pyknotic bodies.
   (d) ghost cells.
8. Diagnostic titre of indirect haemagglutination test in hepatic amoebiasis is:
   (a) 1 : 16 or more.
   (b) 1 : 32 or more.
   (c) 1 : 64 or more.
   (d) 1 : 256 or more.
9. All are nonpathogenic *Entamoeba* **except**:
   (a) *Entamoeba coli.*
   (b) *Entamoeba histolytica.*
   (c) *Entamoeba hartmanni.*
   (d) *Entamoeba gingivalis.*
10. All nonpathogenic amoebae live in the lumen of large intestine **except**:
   (a) *Entamoeba coli.*
   (b) *Entamoeba hartmanni.*
   (c) *Entamoeba gingivalis.*
   (d) *Endolimax nana.*
11. Central karyosome surrounded by refractile globules is seen in:
   (a) *Entamoeba histolytica.*
   (b) *Entamoeba coli.*
   (c) *Iodamoeba bütschlii.*
   (d) *Endolimax nana.*
12. Following are the opportunistic protozoa **except**:
   (a) *Naegleria fowleri.*
   (b) *Acanthamoeba* spp.
   (c) *Balamuthia mandrillaris.*
   (d) *Entamoeba histolytica.*
13. Lobopodia are seen in trophozoites of:
   (a) *Naegleria fowleri.*
   (b) *Acanthamoeba* spp.
   (c) *Balamuthia mandrillaris.*
   (d) *Leishmania donovani.*
14. Infection with *Naegleria* can be acquired by:
   (a) swimming in lakes, ponds or pools containing infective forms.
   (b) blood transfusion.
   (c) sexual contact.
   (d) faecal-oral route.
15. *Naegleria fowleri* causes:
   (a) primary amoebic meningoencephalitis.
   (b) granulomatous amoebic encephalitis.
   (c) keratitis.
   (d) diarrhoea.
16. What is/are the characteristic/s of CSF in primary amoebic meningoencephalitis?
   (a) It is purulent.
   (b) Its leucocyte count varies from few hundreds to more than 20,000/μl.
   (c) It has high protein and low glucose content.
   (d) All of the above.
17. A 25-year-old patient with a recent history of swimming in fresh water developed severe frontal headache, fever, vomiting, signs of meningeal irritation, seizures and coma. The CSF examination revealed motile amoebae. Which of the following amoebae is the probable causative agent?
   (a) *Naegleria fowleri.*
   (b) *Acanthamoeba culbertsoni.*
   (c) *Balamuthia mandrillaris.*
   (d) *Entamoeba histolytica.*
18. Pseudopodia are the organelles of locomotion in:
   (a) *Giardia lamblia.*
   (b) *Trichomonas vaginalis.*
   (c) *Toxoplasma gondii.*
   (d) *Entamoeba histolytica.*
19. Amoebic ulcers are seen in:
   (a) duodenum.
   (b) jejunum.
   (c) ileum.
   (d) colon.
20. Reservoir host of *Entamoeba histolytica* is:
   (a) man.
   (b) pig.
   (c) dog.
   (d) sheep.

21. Red blood cells are seen in the endoplasm of trophozoites of:
    (a) *Entamoeba coli.*
    (b) *Entamoeba histolytica.*
    (c) *Entamoeba dispar.*
    (d) *Entamoeba hartmanni.*
22. Granulomatous amoebic encephalitis is caused by:
    (a) *Entamoeba histolytica.*
    (b) *Acanthamoeba culbertsoni.*
    (c) *Naegleria fowleri.*
    (d) *Leishmania donovani.*
23. Charcot-Leyden crystals are derived from:
    (a) neutrophils.
    (b) basophils.
    (c) eosinophils.
    (d) macrophages.
24. Cysts of which of the following intestinal parasites do not possess four or more nuclei?
    (a) *Entamoeba histolytica.*
    (b) *Entamoeba coli.*
    (c) *Entamoeba dispar.*
    (d) *Entamoeba polecki.*
25. Which of the following amoebae forms cysts in tissues?
    (a) *Acanthamoeba culbertsoni.*
    (b) *Naegleria fowleri.*
    (c) *Entamoeba histolytica.*
    (d) *Balantidium coli.*
26. Which of the following features characterize/s *Entamoeba histolytica/Entamoeba dispar* cysts?
    (a) Spherical measuring 10–15 μm in diameter.
    (b) Presence of four nuclei in mature cyst.
    (c) Presence of centrally located karyosome.
    (d) All of the above.
27. The maximum number of nuclei in the mature cysts of *Endolimax nana* is:
    (a) two.
    (b) four.
    (c) six.
    (d) eight.
28. Which of the following characteristics is satisfactory for distinguishing *Entamoeba histolytica* and *Entamoeba dispar* morphologically?
    (a) Progressive motility.
    (b) Fine peripheral chromatin.
    (c) Ingested red blood cells.
    (d) Ingested bacteria.
29. Amoebic cysts can be visualized with all of the following techniques **except**:
    (a) wet mount.
    (b) trichrome stain.
    (c) iron haematoxylin stain.
    (d) modified acid-fast stain.
30. Which of the following parasites causes keratitis?
    (a) *Naegleria fowleri.*
    (b) *Acanthamoeba culbertsoni.*
    (c) *Entamoeba histolytica.*
    (d) *Endolimax nana.*
31. Which of the following amoebae inhabits mouth rather than the large intestine?
    (a) *Entamoeba hartmanni.*
    (b) *Entamoeba polecki.*
    (c) *Entamoeba dispar.*
    (d) *Entamoeba gingivalis.*
32. Refrigeration of cerebrospinal fluid is **not** recommended because it may kill:
    (a) *Naegleria fowleri.*
    (b) *Haemophilus influenzae.*
    (c) Both of the above.
    (d) Neither of the above.
33. Which of the following is an important human pathogen?
    (a) *Entamoeba coli.*
    (b) *Entamoeba histolytica.*
    (c) *Entamoeba dispar.*
    (d) *Entamoeba hartmanni.*

ANSWERS TO MCQs

1 (c), 2 (c), 3 (a), 4 (c), 5(a), 6 (a), 7 (d), 8 (d), 9 (b), 10 (c), 11 (c), 12 (d), 13 (a), 14 (a), 15 (a), 16 (d), 17 (a), 18 (d), 19 (d), 20 (a), 21 (b), 22 (b), 23 (c), 24 (d), 25 (a), 26 (d), 27 (b), 28 (c), 29 (d), 30 (b), 31 (d), 32 (c), 33 (b).

4

Flagellates

Intestinal, Oral and Genital Flagellates
- *Giardia lamblia*
- *Trichomonas tenax*
- *Trichomonas hominis*
- *Trichomonas vaginalis*
- *Chilomastix mesnili*
- *Enteromonas hominis*
- *Retortamonas intestinalis*
- *Dientamoeba fragilis*

Blood and Tissue Flegellates

Old World Leishmaniasis
- *Leishmania donovani*
- *Leishmania infantum*
- *Leishmania tropica*
- *Leishmania major*
- *Leishmania aethiopica*

New World Leishmaniasis
- *Leishmania braziliensis* complex
- *Leishmania mexicana* complex
- *Leishmania peruviana*
- *Leishmania chagasi*

Trypanosomes
- *Trypanosoma brucei gambiense*
- *Trypanosoma brucei rhodesiense*
- *Trypanosoma cruzi*
- *Trypanosoma rangeli*

Flagellates are protozoa that bear one to several long, delicate, thread-like extensions of the cytoplasm. These are known as flagella (singular, flagellum). These arise from blepharoplasts and are organelles of locomotion. A central supporting rod, known as axostyle, and an undulating membrane supported at the base by a basal fibre are observed in some species. The nuclear characters are distinctive in every species.

Flagellates belong to kingdom Protozoa, and phyla Metamonada (*Giardia lamblia*, *Enteromonas hominis*, *Chilomastix mesnili* and *Retortamonas intestinalis*); Parabasala (*Dientamoeba fragilis*, *Trichomonas vaginalis*, *T. hominis* and *T. tenax*); Percolozoa (*Naegleria fowleri*); and Euglenozoa (*Leishmania donovani*, *L. infantum*, *L. major*, *L. tropica*, *L. braziliensis*, *L. mexicana*, *L. aethiopica*, *L. peruviana*, *L. chagasi*, *Trypanosoma brucei gambiense*, *T. b. rhodesiense*, *T. cruzi* and *T. rangeli*) (Table 1.5). *Dientamoeba fragilis* and *Naegleria fowleri* have already been described in previous chapter. According to their habitat, the flagellates are classified into two broad groups (Table 4.1):

1. Intestinal, oral and genital flagellates
2. Blood and tissue flagellates.

INTESTINAL, ORAL AND GENITAL FLAGELLATES

GIARDIA LAMBLIA (G. DUODENALIS; G. INTESTINALIS)

Giardia was discovered by Leeuwenhoek in 1681 in his own stool but was not described until 1859 by Lambl. The organism was named after Professor A. Giard of Paris and Professor F. Lambl of Prague.

Geographical distribution

Giardia lamblia is a cosmopolitan parasite. The highest prevalence of *G. lamblia* occurs in tropics and sub-

Group	Parasites	Habitat
Intestinal, oral and genital flagellates	*Giardia lamblia*	Duodenum and jejunum
	Trichomonas vaginalis	Vagina and urethra
	T. tenax	Mouth
	T. hominis	Caecum
	Chilomastix mesnili	Caecum
	Enteromonas hominis	Colon
	Retortamonas intestinalis	Colon
	Dientamoeba fragilis	Caecum and colon
Blood and tissue flagellates	*Leishmania* spp.	Reticuloendothelial cells
	Trypanosoma brucei gambiense and *T. b. rhodesiense*	Connective tissue, brain and blood
	T. cruzi	Reticuloendothelial cells and blood

Table 4.1. Flagellates

tropics where sanitation is poor. Travellers to tropical Africa, Mexico, Russia, Southeast Asia, and western South America are at a high risk of acquiring giardiasis. *Giardia* infects 200 million people worldwide and may produce symptoms in 500,000 individuals every year. Infections seem to be more common in children than adults.

Habitat

It inhabits duodenum and the upper part of jejunum of man.

Morphology

It exists in two forms:

1. Trophozoite
2. Cyst

Trophozoite

It is pear-shaped with rounded anterior and pointed posterior end (Figs. 4.1 and 4.2). It measures 10–20 μm in length and 5–15 μm in width. The dorsal surface is convex while on the ventral surface it has a shallow posteriorly notched concavity (sucking disc) that embraces anterior half of the organism. It acts as an organelle of attachment.

It is bilaterally symmetrical and has **one pair of nuclei**, one on each side of the midline, one pair of axostyles, one pair of parabasal bodies present on the axostyles, four pairs of flagella and probably four pairs of blepharoplasts from which the flagella arise.

- Two pairs of blepharoplasts (one lateral and one more median) are situated on each side of the midline,

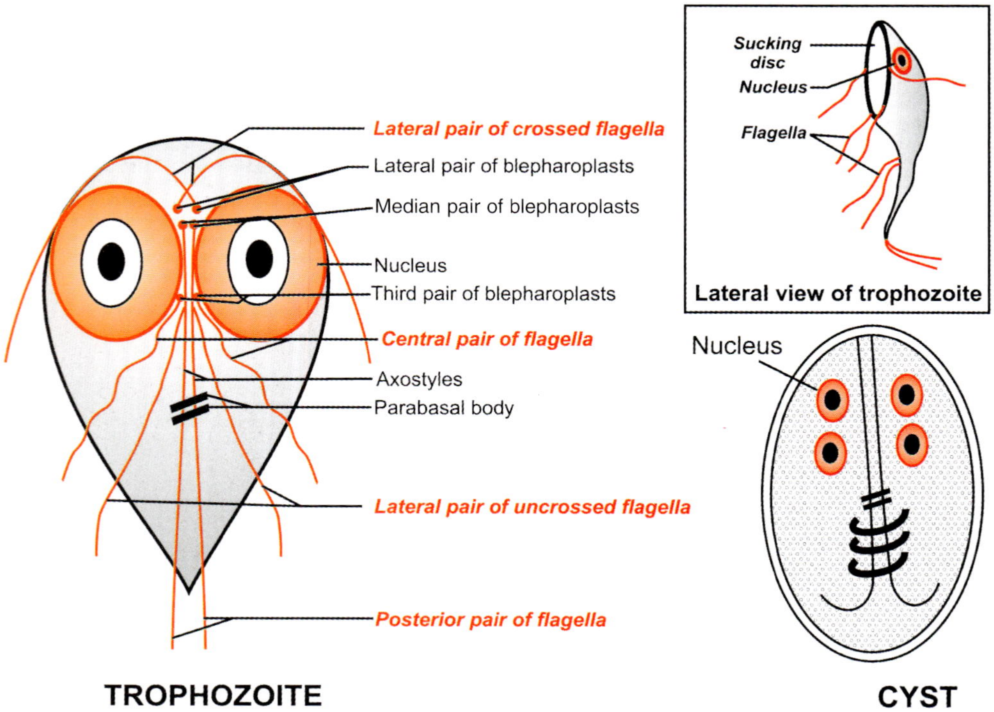

Fig. 4.1. Morphological forms of *Giardia lamblia*.

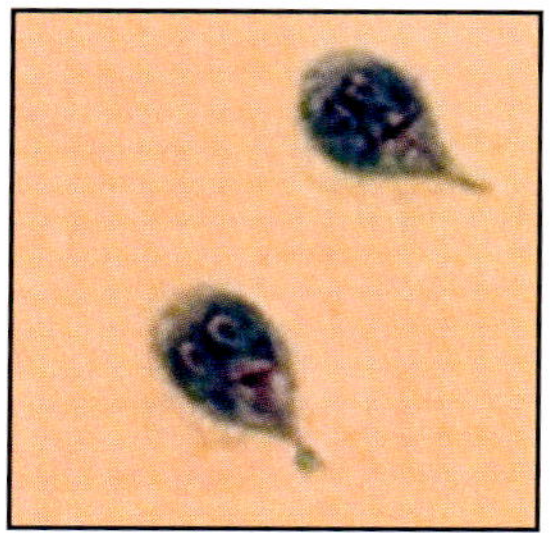

Fig. 4.2. Trophozoite of *Giardia lamblia* in stool (iron haematoxylin stain, × 400).

between and slightly anterior to the two nuclei. Two axonemes (also known as axostyles) arise from the median pair of blepharoplasts. These axonemes pass out from the posterior end of the body and give rise to posterior (caudal) pair of flagella.
- From the two lateral blepharoplasts there originate two axonemes that proceed forward in a curved course towards the midline, cross each other, then describe a wide arc and give rise to lateral pair of crossed flagella.
- Third pair of blepharoplasts lies near the centre of the sucking disc. They give rise to short axonemes and central pair of flagella.
- Fourth pair of blepharoplasts has not been located, but the axonemes that arise from them have been traced up to the notch of the sucking disc. This pair of blepharoplasts gives rise to lateral pair of uncrossed flagella. The trophozoites are motile by rapid movement of the flagella.

The **nuclei** are rounded and possess a central karyosome. The nuclear membrane is delicate and is not lined by chromatin material. By rapid movement of the flagella, the trophozoites move from place to place, and by applying their sucking discs to epithelial surfaces they become firmly attached.

Cyst

Mature cyst is oval in shape and measures 11–14 μm × 7–10 μm in size. It has **two pairs of nuclei** which may remain clustered at one end or lie in pairs at opposite poles. The remains of the flagella and margins of the sucking disc may be seen inside the cytoplasm of the cyst (Figs. 4.1 and 4.3).

Culture

G. lamblia can be grown axenically in Diamond's medium, the medium also used for axenic cultivation of *E. histolytica*.

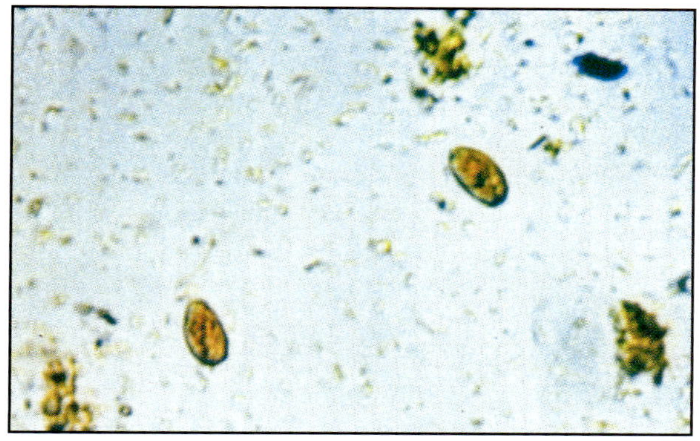

Fig. 4.3. Cysts of *Giardia lamblia* in stool (iodine preparation, × 400).

Life cycle

It passes its life cycle in a single host, the man. No intermediate host is required. Mature cyst is the infective form of the parasite. **Man acquires infection by ingestion of cysts in faecally contaminated water or food.** Infection may occur through ingestion of as few as 10–25 cysts. Infection may also be acquired by anal-oral sexual practices among male homosexuals. Within 30 minutes of ingestion **excystation** occurs in the duodenum. The cyst hatches out two trophozoites, which then multiply by binary fission to form enormous numbers and colonize in the duodenum and upper part of jejunum. To avoid acidity of duodenum, it may localize in biliary tract.

By means of the concavity on its ventral surface the trophozoite attaches to the mucosal surface of the duodenum and jejunum. In frankly diarrhoeic stools, it is usual to find only the trophozoites. **Encystation** occurs commonly in transit down the colon where the intestinal contents lose moisture and patient starts passing formed stools. The trophozoites retract the flagella into the axonemes, the cytoplasm becomes condensed and a thin tough hyaline cyst wall is secreted. As the cyst matures, the internal structures are doubled, so that when **excystation** occurs, the cytoplasm divides, thus producing two trophozoites.

Antigenic variation

G. lamblia is known to undergo surface antigenic variation. The antigens involved belong to a group of variant-specific surface proteins that are unique cysteine-rich zinc finger proteins. This may provide a mechanism enabling the organism to escape the host's immune response.

Pathogenicity

The presence of *G. lamblia* in the glandular crypts of duodenal-jejunal mucosa may not cause any pathology. These flagellates do not invade the tissues, but feed on mucous secretions. With the help of sucking disc the parasite attaches itself to the surface of the epithelial cells in the duodenum and jejunum, and in an appreciable number of cases it may cause duodenal and jejunal irritation leading to duodenitis and jejunitis. The incubation period, before symptomatic disease develops, ranges from 1–4 weeks (average, 10 days). Patient may complain of dull epigastric pain, flatulence and **chronic diarrhoea of steatorrhoea type**. The stool is voluminous, foul smelling and contains large amount of mucus and fat but no blood. This is due to malabsorption since the parasites are coated on the mucosa, thus absorption suffers. Patient loses weight. When the parasite localizes in the biliary tract, it may lead to chronic cholecystitis and jaundice.

Giardiasis is one of the more common causes of **traveller's diarrhoea**. Visitors to areas endemic for *Giardia* are more likely to present with symptoms than individuals who live in the area. This difference is probably due to the development of immunity from prior, and possibly continued, exposure to the organism. Although patients with HIV infection have also been found to have giardiasis, the infection does not appear to be more severe among this group, regardless of the $CD4^+$ cell count.

Immune response

Studies with humans and experimental animals have confirmed the presence of both humoral and cellular immune responses to *Giardia*. The majority of infected patients produce detectable levels of *Giardia*-specific antibodies; however, the biological role that these antibodies play in the host immune response to the infection is unclear. IgM anti-*Giardia* antibodies are short-lived and IgG antibodies may remain at high titres for many months after the patient has been treated and cured. *Giardia*-specific IgA may also be important in both defence against and clearance of the parasite. The degree of protection of breast-fed infants against *Giardia* infection has also been shown to depend on the level of IgA-specific antibodies in breast milk. In the intestine, IgA antibodies may influence the local immune response by inhibiting parasite adherence.

Experimental animal studies provide evidence that T lymphocytes and Peyer's patch helper T lymphocytes play a role in the host immune response. In athymic mice, which are deficient in both T lymphocytes and Peyer's patch helper T lymphocytes, inoculation with *G. muris* results in a chronic infection with large number of organisms. In contrast, immunocompetent mice clear the parasite and develop resistance to reinfection.

Laboratory diagnosis

Microscopy

Giardiasis can be diagnosed by identification of cysts of *G. lamblia* (Fig. 4.3) in the formed stools and the trophozoites of the parasite (Fig. 4.2) in diarrhoeal stools by normal saline and iodine preparation, and iron haematoxylin stain as in case of *E. histolytica*.

Because the parasites are attached firmly to the mucosa by means of sucking disc, a series of even five or six consecutive stool specimens may not show any parasite. These parasites also tend to be passed in the stool on a cyclic basis. Trophozoites of *G. lamblia* may be detected in the bile aspirated from duodenum by intubation and by duodenal capsule technique (**Enterotest**) (see Chapter 13). Motility of the trophozoites on wet preparations may be difficult to see because the organisms are caught up in mucus. It may be represented by nothing more than a slight flutter of flagella. For the detection of *G. lamblia* in faecal specimens, a fluorescent method using monoclonal antibodies is extremely sensitive and specific.

Biopsy

After multiple stool examinations, examination of bile aspirated from duodenum and Enterotest are negative, biopsy from multiple duodenal and jejunal sites may confirm the diagnosis of giardiasis. Touch preparations can be air dried, fixed in methanol, and stained with Giemsa stain. Trophozoites may be seen attached to the microvillous border within the crypts. They appear purple and epithelial cells appear pink. Routine histological procedures should also be performed, but trophozoites are very difficult to see and may be present in very few of the sections.

Immunologic tests

- ELISA test has been developed for the detection of *Giardia* antigen in faeces.
- Anti-*Giardia* antibodies, in the patient serum, may be detected by ELISA and indirect fluorescent antibody tests. However, these may indicate present or past infection. Axenically cultured *G. lamblia* trophozoites are used as antigens in these tests.

Treatment

Chemotherapy with a 5-day course of *metronidazole* usually is successful, although therapy may have to be repeated or prolonged in some instances. A single dose of *tinidazole* probably is superior to *metronidazole* for treatment of giardiasis. *Paromomycin* has been used to treat pregnant women to avoid any possible mutagenic effects of other drugs.

Prevention

Giardiasis can be prevented by:

- improved water supply,
- proper disposal of human faeces,
- improved personal hygiene,
- routine hand-washing,
- proper storage of food and water,
- control of insects which may come in contact with infected stools and then contaminate food or water, and
- treatment of symptomatic and asymptomatic individuals.

Prospects are poor for the development of a potential vaccine.

TRICHOMONAS

Genus *Trichomonas* contains three species which occur in humans:

1. *T. tenax*
2. *T. hominis*
3. *T. vaginalis*.

These flagellates **exist only in trophozoite stage**. Cystic stage is absent. They have four anterior flagella and one lateral flagellum which is attached to the surface of the parasite to form **undulating membrane**. The undulating membrane is supported at the base by a rod-like structure known as costa. The axostyle runs down the middle of the body and ends in the pointed tail-like extremity. A round nucleus is located in the anterior portion.

TRICHOMONAS TENAX

It is a pyriform flagellate. It measures 5–12 µm in length and 5–10 µm in width (Fig. 4.4). It is a **harmless commensal of the human mouth**, living in the tartar around the teeth, in cavities of carious teeth, in necrotic mucosal cells in the gingival margins of gums and in pus pockets in tonsillar follicles. It is transmitted by kissing, salivary droplets and fomites. Although *T. tenax* is considered to be harmless commensal in the mouth, there are reports of respiratory infections and thoracic abscesses. The majority of these cases have been reported from Western Europe.

Diagnosis can be made by demonstration of *T. tenax* in the tartar by microscopy, and no therapy is indicated. Better oral hygiene will rapidly eliminate the infection.

TRICHOMONAS HOMINIS

It is pyriform, measuring 5–14 µm in length and 7–10 µm in width (Fig. 4.4). **It inhabits the caecum of man** and several other primate species and feeds on enteric bacteria. It does not invade the intestinal mucosa. Though it has occasionally been found in the diarrhoeic stools, its pathogenicity is yet to be established.

In freshly passed specimens, particularly in unformed stools, the motility may be visible. In wet preparation, look for the flagellar movement, undulating membrane and the presence of the axostyle.

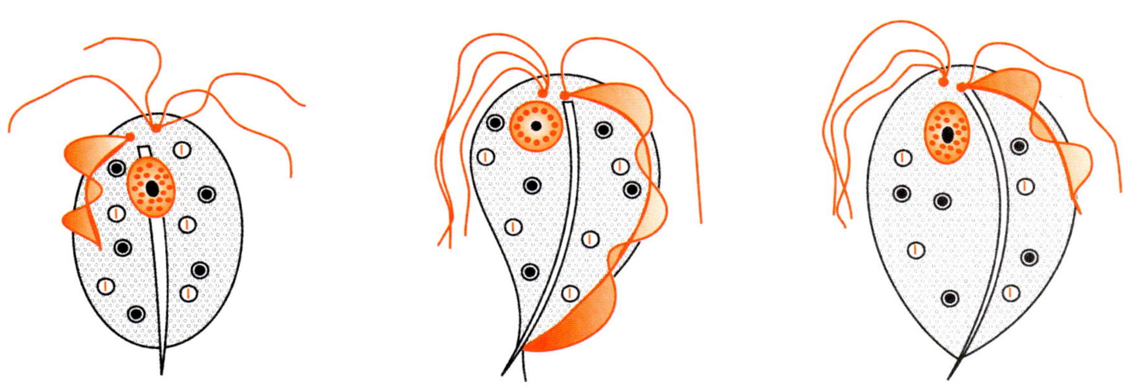

Fig. 4.4. Trophozoites of *Trichomonas* spp.

The undulating membrane extends the entire length of the body, in contrast to that seen in *T. vaginalis*, which extends along only half the body. Since there is no known cyst stage, transmission probably occurs in the trophic form. If ingested in a protected substance such as milk, these organisms can apparently survive passage through the stomach and small intestine in patients with achlorhydria.

TRICHOMONAS VAGINALIS

Trichomonas vaginalis was first observed by Donne in 1836. It has worldwide distribution with higher prevalence among persons with multiple sexual partners or other venereal diseases.

Morphology

It resembles *T. tenax* but it is larger than this. It measures 7–23 μm in length and 5–15 μm in width (Figs. 4.4 and 4.5). In a wet mount under the low-power objective the trophozoites show jerky movement. High-power examination may reveal the beating flagella and undulating membrane characteristic of the species.

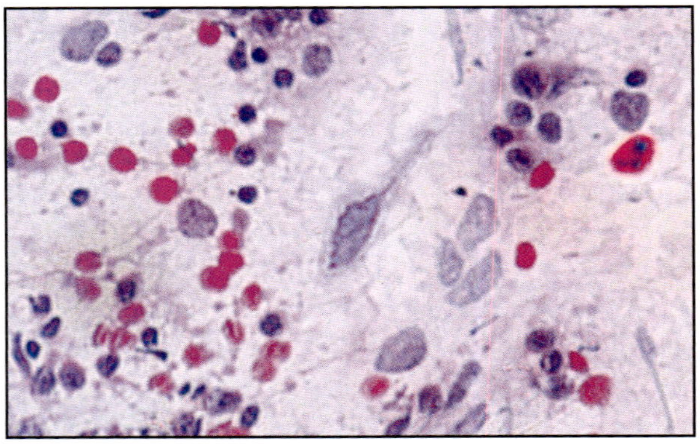

Fig. 4.5. Trophozoites of *Trichomonas vaginalis* in vaginal smear (Papanicolaou stain, × 400).

Habitat

The normal habitat of the parasite is the vagina and urethra of women, and the urethra, seminal vesicles and prostate of man. It may also be found in the Bartholin's glands and in urinary bladder in females.

Pathogenicity

The parasite lives on the mucosa feeding on bacteria and leucocytes. *T. vaginalis* is an **obligate parasite**. It cannot live without close association with the vaginal, urethral or prostatic tissues.

Human trichomoniasis is a **widely prevalent sexually transmitted disease of worldwide importance**. Approximately 10% of vulvovaginitis is due to infection with *T. vaginalis*. Asymptomatic infections have been observed in 50% of infected female patients.

The organism is responsible for a **mild vaginitis with discharge**. Vaginal discharge contains a large number of parasites and leucocytes and is liquid, greenish or yellow. It covers the mucosa down to the urethral orifice, vestibular glands and clitoris. Male patients usually have mild or asymptomatic infections. They may develop itching and discomfort inside penile urethra, especially during urination. The parasite is transmitted by sexual intercourse. It has been postulated that, in male patients, high concentration of zinc in prostatic fluid in urogenital tract may have lytic effect on the parasite.

The exact mechanism of pathogenesis is still not elucidated and appears to be multifactorial depending upon the inherent virulence of the parasite and host factors. The main mechanisms postulated seem to be mediated by cell to cell adhesion, haemolysis, excretion of soluble proteinases, pore-forming proteins and cell detaching factor. Presence of double-stranded RNA virus in few strains has been reported and the parasite is able to undergo phenotypic variation in its presence.

Laboratory diagnosis

Microscopy

The diagnosis can be made by demonstration of trophozoites of *T. vaginalis* in wet mounts of the sedimented urine, vaginal secretions or vaginal scrapings by bright-field, dark-field, or phase-contrast microscopy. In males it may be found in urine or prostatic secretions.

Fixed smears may be stained with Papanicolaou, Giemsa, Leishman and periodic acid-Schiff stain and seen under light microscope. The parasites may also be detected by fluorescence microscopy by staining with fluorescein-labelled monoclonal antibody (86% sensitivity).

Culture

T. vaginalis can be isolated from urethral and vaginal exudates on several commercially available media. Trussell and Johnson's medium is a simple medium that gives good growth. It consists of proteose peptone, sodium chloride, sodium thioglycollate and normal human serum. Simplified trypticase serum medium is also suitable for the isolation of *T. vaginalis*. It is also used to maintain bacteria-free cultures of the flagellate. It grows best at 35°–37°C under anaerobic conditions and less well aerobically. The optimal pH for growth is 5.5–6.0. Culture is very sensitive (95%) procedure for diagnosis of trichomoniasis. It is recommended when direct smear is negative.

Antibody and antigen detection

Several types of ELISA have been developed for *T. vaginalis*, either to measure antibodies or to detect antigen of *T. vaginalis* in clinical samples.

Molecular methods

- Nucleic acid hybridization methods for detection of *T. vaginalis* have sensitivity and specificity as good as culture methods.
- Polymerase chain reaction (PCR) for the diagnosis of trichomoniasis has also been developed.

Prevention

Since infection is contracted through sexual intercourse, therefore, the preventive measures include:

- detection and treatment of cases, both males and females;
- avoidance of sexual contact with infected persons; and
- use of condoms.

There is no vaccine currenty available for use against *T. vaginalis.*

Treatment

Metronidazole, 2 g oral single dose or *tinidazole*, 2 g oral single dose are highly effective against *T. vaginalis* infection.

CHILOMASTIX MESNILI

Chilomastix mesnili is a common flagellate living as a harmless commensal in the caecum and colon of man. Davaine (1854) observed this parasite for the first time in the stool. Wenyon (1910) provided the first accurate description of the parasite. It has a cosmopolitan distribution but is more prevalent in warm than in cool climates. It has well-defined trophozoite and cystic stages (Fig. 4.6).

Morphology

Trophozoite

It is pear-shaped measuring 6–20 μm in length and 3–10 μm in breadth. The posterior end of the trophozoite is drawn out into a long cone. The spherical nucleus,

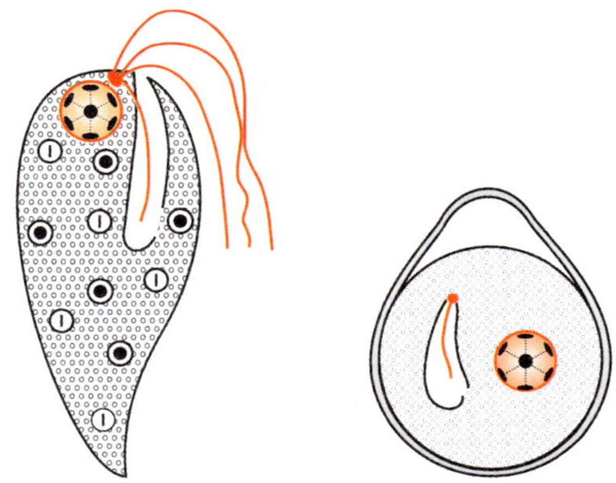

Fig. 4.6. Morphological forms of *Chilomastix mesnili*.

measuring 3–4 μm in diameter is situated anteriorly. It has a small distinct, central karyosome and a few achromatic fibrils extending to the nuclear membrane, and chromatin plaques lining the membrane. A large conspicuous cytostome (mouth) is seen on one side of the nucleus. It has three free anterior flagella and a delicate flagellum lying within the cytostome. The cytoplasm is finely granular and contains numerous food vacuoles.

Cyst

It is lemon-shaped with a small projection at the anterior end. It measures 7–10 μm in length and 4–6 μm in breadth and is surrounded by a thick tough cyst wall. The cytoplasm is densely granular and separated from the cyst wall at the narrower end of the cyst. The single nucleus lies near the centre. Remnants of the cytostome are also visible.

Habitat

C. mesnili is a normal inhabitant of the caecum and colon of man. The trophozoites live on enteric bacteria and multiply by binary fission. In freshly passed liquid stools, only trophozoites are seen, in semi-formed stools, both trophozoites and cysts may be observed, and in well-formed stools, only cysts are present. Transmission of the parasite, from one person to another, takes place by ingestion of food or water contaminated with cysts of *C. mesnili* in the stools of an infected individual.

Pathogenicity and laboratory diagnosis

C. mesnili is a harmless commensal and does not produce any symptom. The diagnosis can be made by detection of trophozoites and cysts of *C. mesnili* in the faecal smear.

ENTEROMONAS HOMINIS

Enteromonas hominis is a rare species living as a harmless commensal in the lumen of the caecum and other parts of the large intestine of humans and primates. It was first discovered by de Fonseca (1915) in diarrhoeic stool in Brazil. It has been reported from both warm and temperate climates.

Morphology

It exists in two forms – trophozoite and cyst (Fig. 4.7).

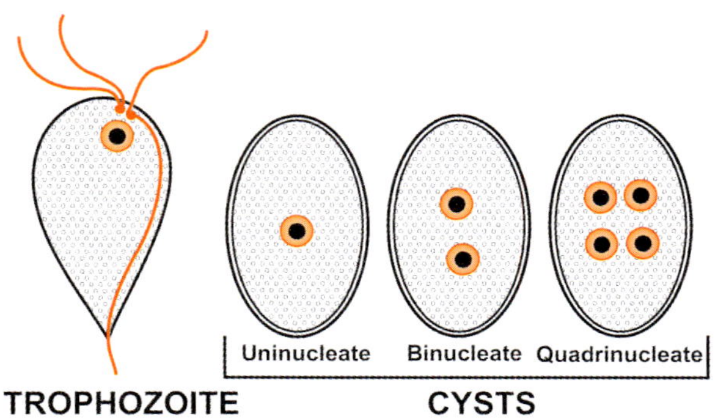

Fig. 4.7. Morphological forms of *Enteromonas hominis*.

Trophozoite

It is pear-shaped, rounded or ovoidal measuring 4–10 μm in length and 3–6 μm in width. It possesses four flagella. By means of its three anterior flagella it has jerky forward movement. The fourth flagellum is adherent to the body of the trophozoite and then extends posteriorly as free flagellum. The cytoplasm is finely vacuolated and contains numerous bacteria. The nucleus is situated at the anterior end. There is no cytostome.

Cyst

It is oval, 6–8 μm in length and 4–6 μm in breadth and contains one to four nuclei.

Pathogenicity and laboratory diagnosis

E. hominis is a harmless commensal. It does not produce any symptoms. It is transmitted by ingestion of food or water contaminated with cysts. Diagnosis is made by demonstration of trophozoites and cysts in fresh faecal films and haematoxylin-stained preparations.

RETORTAMONAS INTESTINALIS

Retortamonas intestinalis, also known as *Embadomonas intestinalis* is a rare harmless commensal in the caecum of man. Wenyon and O'Connor first observed this parasite in the stool in Egypt. It has been reported from both warm and temperate areas of the world.

Morphology

It exists in two forms – trophozoite and cyst (Fig. 4.8).

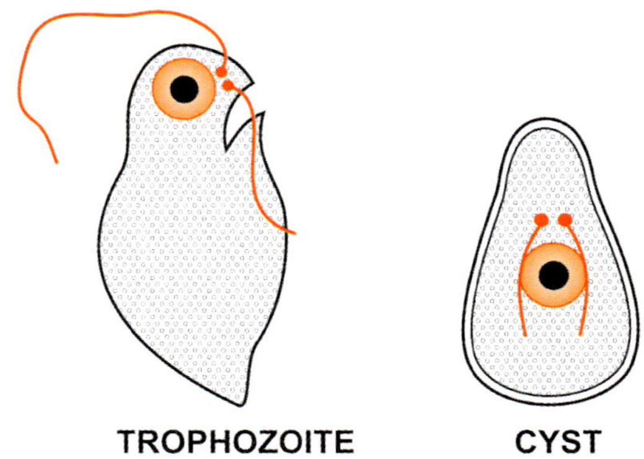

Fig. 4.8. Morphological forms of *Retortamonas intestinalis*.

Trophozoite

It is oval, small, measuring 6–9 μm in length and 3–4 μm in breadth. The cytoplasm is finely granular and vacuolated. The spherical nucleus with central karyosome is situated anteriorly and by its side lies the cleft-like cytostome. It has two flagella which originate from two minute blepharoplasts present near the nucleus. One of the flagella is longer and directed anteriorly and the other is slightly shorter, passes posteriorly through the cytostome before becoming free. The trophozoites multiply by longitudinal binary fission.

Cyst

It is pyriform, measures 4–7 μm in length and 3–4 μm in breadth. Like trophozoite, it also has single nucleus.

Pathogenicity and laboratory diagnosis

The infection is acquired by ingestion of food or water contaminated with cysts of *R. intestinalis* in the stools of an infected individual. It is nonpathogenic, although it is commonly discovered only in diarrhoeic stools. Diagnosis is made by demonstration of trophozoites and cysts in fresh faecal films and haematoxylin-stained preparations.

DIENTAMOEBA FRAGILIS

Dientamoeba fragilis was initially classified as an amoeba; however, the internal structures of the trophozoite are typical of a flagellate though flagella are not observed with light microscope. In practice, this organism may appear as an amoebic trophozoite, rather than as flagellate in microscopic mounts. The generic name is derived from the binucleate nature of the trophozoite and species name from the fragmented appearance of its nuclear chromatin. Wenyon (1909) first discovered this parasite. Jepps and Dobell (1918) described it. It is a cosmopolitan parasite.

Habitat

It lives in the lumen of human colon along with the true amoebae.

Morphology

Only the trophozoite stage is known (Fig. 4.9). The cyst stage has not been confirmed to date. It is small, varying from 6–12 μm in diameter. It is actively motile by means of hyaline pseudopodia that may be lobose or angular. Food vacuoles containing bacteria may be present. It can be easily differentiated from intestinal amoebae as it contains two and sometimes up to four nuclei. Flagellar structure can be demonstrated by electron microscopy. The karyosome is large and consists of four or more discrete granules. The nuclear membrane is not lined by chromatin.

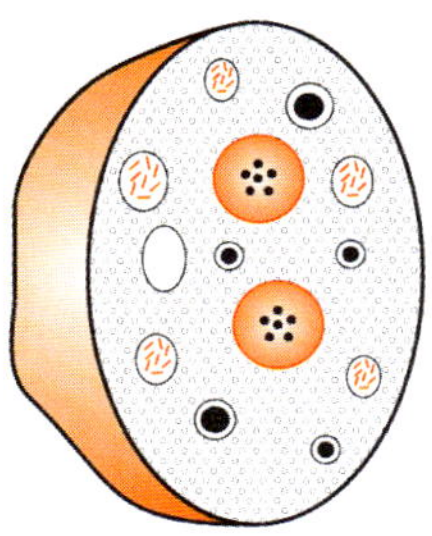

Fig. 4.9. *Dientamoeba fragilis.*

Life cycle

The life cycle of *D. fragilis* is not completely understood. Because *D. fragilis* does not have an identified cyst state and direct foodborne or waterborne transfer from host to host is less likely. The nine times higher incidence of *D. fragilis* in patients with pinworm infection suggests that the *Enterobius vermicularis* eggs may be infected with the flagellate and serve as the chief vector for transfer to humans. This possibility may also explain why almost 50% of reported cases of dientamoebiasis occur in patients under 20 years of age.

Pathogenicity

It is mildly pathogenic in about 25% of infected individuals, who may develop intermittent diarrhoea, abdominal pain, flatulence, nausea, vomiting, anorexia, malaise, weight loss, and unexplained eosinophilia.

Laboratory diagnosis and treatment

Infection can be diagnosed by detection of trophozoites in permanently stained smears (e.g., trichrome). The drugs of choice in the treatment of symptomatic cases include tetracycline and metronidazole.

Table 4.2. *Leishmania* species causing disease in man

Species	Form of disease	Geographical distribution
OLD WORLD LEISHMANIASIS		
Leishmania donovani	Visceral leishmaniasis, kala-azar, post kala-azar dermal leishmaniasis	Indian subcontinent, East Africa
L. infantum	Infantile visceral leishmaniasis	Mediterranean basin, Central and Western Asia
L. tropica	Urban, anthroponotic cutaneous leishmaniasis, Oriental sore	Central and Western Asia
L. major	Rural, zoonotic, cutaneous leishmaniasis, Oriental sore	North Africa, Sahel of Africa, Central and Western Asia
L. aethiopica	Cutaneous leishmaniasis, diffuse cutaneous leishmaniasis	Ethiopia, Kenya
NEW WORLD LEISHMANIASIS		
L. braziliensis complex	Mucocutaneous	Tropical South America
L. mexicana complex	Cutaneous	Central America
L. peruviana	Cutaneous	Western Peru
L. chagasi	American visceral leishmaniasis	Tropical South America

BLOOD AND TISSUE FLAGELLATES

Blood and tissue flagellates possess a single nucleus, a single kinetoplast and a single flagellum. The kinetoplast consists of parabasal body and an adjacent dot-like blepharoplast. The blepharoplast and parabasal body are connected by one or more delicate fibrils. The flagellum arises from the blepharoplast. The portion of the flagellum extending from the blepharoplast to the surface of the body of the parasite is known as axoneme. Family Trypanosomatidae consists of six genera, of which *Leishmania* and *Trypanosoma* are pathogenic to man. Species of this family may exist in two or more forms.

LEISHMANIA

The genus *Leishmania* is widely distributed in nature. It has a number of species (Table 4.2) that are nearly identical morphologically. Differentiation is, therefore, based on a number of biochemical and epidemiological criteria – use of monoclonal probes to detect specific antigens, promastigote growth patterns *in vitro* in the presence of antisera, and vectors and reservoir hosts. The parasites of the Old World leishmaniasis (*L. donovani*, *L. infantum*, *L. tropica, L. major* and *L. aethiopica*) are transmitted to humans by the bite of female sandflies of the genus *Phlebotomus*; while those of the New World leishmaniasis (*L. peruviana, L. chagasi, L. mexicana* complex and *L.braziliensis* complex) are carried by sandflies of the genera *Lutzomyia* and *Psychodopygus.* The term 'New World' refers to the Americas and the 'Old World' is used for the rest of the world.

Leishmanias pass their life cycle in two hosts – invertebrate hosts and vertebrate hosts. Former are the sandflies and the latter are mammals in which the parasites reside within the phagolysosomal system of mononuclear phagocytic cells, typically macrophages. However, in the invertebrate hosts, the parasites are extracellular, development occurs exclusively in the gut and transmission is via the mouthparts during blood feeding.

Leishmaniasis is a collection of diseases, each with its own clinical manifestations and epidemiology. It is mainly a **zoonosis**, although in certain areas of the world there is primarily human-vector-human transmission. The World Health Organization estimates that 1.5 million cases of cutaneous leishmaniasis and 500,000 cases of visceral leishmaniasis occur every year in 82 countries. Estimates indicate that there are approximately 350 million people at risk of acquiring leishmaniasis, with 12 million currently infected. In India, visceral leishmaniasis is a serious problem in Bihar, West Bengal, and eastern parts of Uttar Pradesh. Sporadic cases have been reported from Tamil Nadu, Pondicherry, Assam, Orissa and Gujarat.

Animal inoculation

The **hamster** is the laboratory animal of choice for the isolation of *Leishmania* spp. Young (2–4 months old) hamsters of either sex are inoculated intraperitoneally with aspirates or biopsy material obtained under sterile conditions from cutaneous ulcers, lymph nodes, spleen, liver, bone marrow, buffy coat cells or spinal fluid. It results in a generalized infection. Spleen impression smears should be examined for the presence of organisms. The infection develops slowly in hamsters. Several months may be required to produce a detectable infection. For this reason, culture procedures are usually selected as more rapid means of parasite recovery. Animals should be kept for 9–12 months before a negative report is given.

OLD WORLD LEISHMANIASIS

LEISHMANIA DONOVANI

Sir William Leishman in 1900 discovered this parasite in spleen smear of a soldier who had died of 'Dum Dum fever' or kala-azar contracted at Dum Dum, Calcutta now Kolkata. Leishman reported this finding from London in 1903, in which year Donovan also reported the same parasite in spleen smear of a patient from Madras now Chennai. The name *Leishmania donovani* was therefore given to this parasite.

Geographical distribution

L. donovani is endemic in Indian Subcontinent and East Africa.

Habitat

It is an **obligate intracellular parasite of reticulo-endothelial cells**, predominantly of liver, spleen, bone marrow and lymph nodes of man and other vertebrate hosts (dog and hamster) where it occurs in amastigote form.

Morphology

The parasite exists in two morphological forms:

1. Amastigote
2. Promastigote.

Amastigote

In the amastigote form the parasite resides in the cells of reticuloendothelial system (macrophages, monocytes, polymorphonuclear leucocytes, or endothelial cells) of vertebrate hosts. It is non-motile, round or oval body measuring 2–4 μm in length along the longitudinal axis (Figs. 4.10 and 4.11). Cell membrane is delicate and can be demonstrated in fresh specimens only. Nucleus is round or oval, less than 1 μm in diameter. It is situated in the middle of the cell or along the side of the cell wall. Kinetoplast consists of parabasal body and blepharoplast which are connected by one or more delicate fibrils. It lies tangentially or at right angle to the nucleus. The axoneme arises from the blepharoplast and extends to the margin of the body. It represents the intracellular portion of the flagellum. Alongside the axoneme lies a clear unstained space known as vacuole. In preparations stained with Giemsa or Wright stain, the cytoplasm appears pale blue, the nucleus red, parabasal body deep red and kinetoplast bright red.

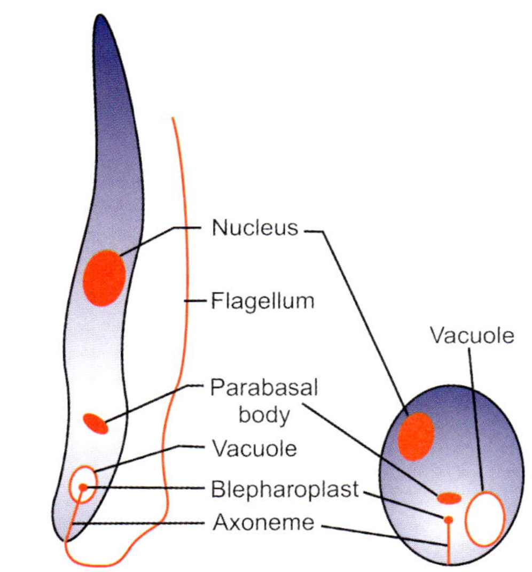

Fig. 4.10. Morphological forms of *Leishmania donovani.*

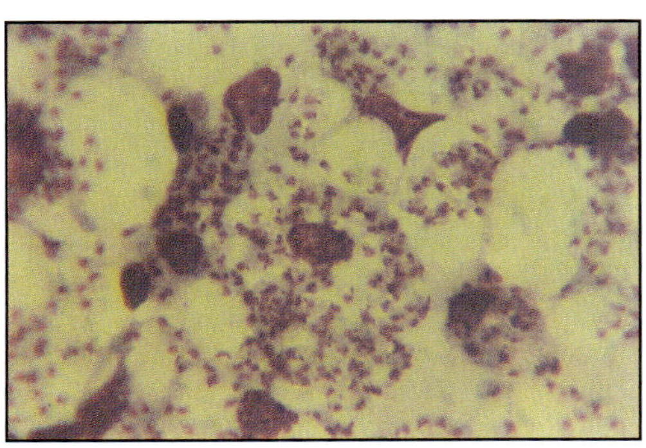

Fig. 4.11. Amastigote forms *of Leishmania donovani* in bone marrow (Giemsa stain, × 400).

Promastigote

Promastigotes are found in **the digestive tract of insect vector (sandfly) and in the culture media**. These are elongated, motile, extracellular stage of the parasite. Fully developed promastigotes measure 15–25 μm in length and 1.5–3.5 μm in breadth. Nucleus is situated centrally. Kinetoplast lies transversely near the anterior end. In front of the kinetoplast lies a pale staining vacuole. From the blepharoplast arises the axoneme which projects from the anterior end of the parasite as free flagellum. Flagellum may be of the same length as the body of the parasite or longer. It does not curve round the body of the parasite, therefore, there is **no undulating membrane** (Fig. 4.10).

Cultivation

NNN medium

L. donovani can be cultured on NNN medium which was first introduced by Novy and McNeal (1904), and later modified by Nicolle (1908). It consists of two parts of salt agar and one part of defibrinated rabbit blood. The tubed salt agar medium is melted and then cooled to 48° C. To each tube of medium one-third of its volume of sterile defibrinated rabbit blood is added and mixed thoroughly by rotating the tubes. The tubes are slanted and allowed to cool preferably on ice, as more water of condensation is obtained.

Blood, aspirates, or small biopsy samples from spleen, liver, or bone marrow obtained aseptically are inoculated into water of condensation of the medium and incubated at 22°–25° C. The amastigote form changes into promastigote form which then multiplies rapidly by longitudinal fission to produce a large number of flagellates, particularly in the water of condensation at the bottom of the tube (Fig. 4.12).

Hockmeyer's medium

This liquid medium consists of Schneider's commercially prepared insect cell culture medium, supple-

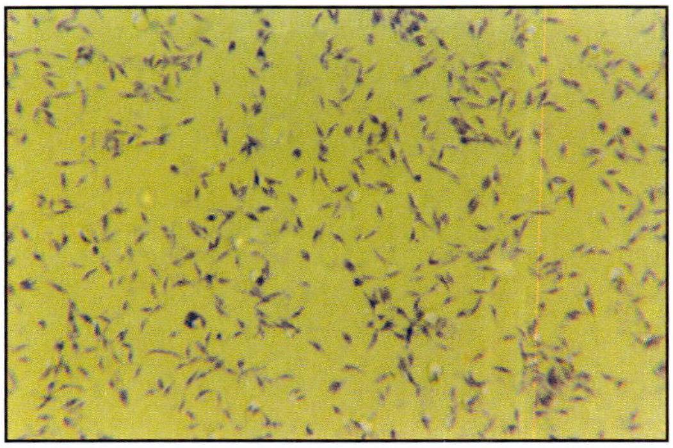

Fig. 4.12. Promastigote forms *of Leishmania donovani* in culture (Giemsa stain, × 400).

mented by the addition of 30% heat inactivated foetal calf serum and with 100 IU penicillin and 100 mg streptomycin per ml. The medium is inoculated with the specimen, incubated at 22°–25° C, and examined microscopically daily for the presence of promastigotes. The latter can usually be detected after 2–3 days of incubation but the cultures should be held for four weeks.

Life cycle

L. donovani passes its life cycle in two hosts – man and also dog in some areas are the vertebrate hosts, and female sandfly of the genus *Phlebotomus* is the invertebrate host. Indian kala-azar is considered to be a non-zoonotic infection with man as the sole reservoir. Important sandfly hosts include *P. argentipes, P. orientalis* and *P. martini*. Of these *P. argentipes* is the Indian vector.

Cycle in sandfly

Amastigotes of the parasite are present in the blood stream of the patient, both free as well as phagocytosed by polymorphonuclear leucocytes and monocytes. These are taken up by the sandfly in a blood meal and reach midgut of the insect. Here the parasite transforms into promastigotes and multiplies producing enormous numbers. The parasites then proceed forwards to the pharynx and buccal cavity which they block between the 6th and 9th day of its infective blood meal.

Cycle in man

Because of the blockage of pharynx and buccal cavity, the sandfly has difficulty in getting a blood meal, nevertheless, it pricks the skin of the victim and regurgitates the promastigotes in the wound caused by its proboscis. These are engulfed by nearby fixed macrophages and change into amastigotes within the cytoplasm of these host cells. Here the amastigotes multiply slowly and may remain more or less quiescent for weeks or months. Thereafter, parasitized macrophages are set free into the blood stream and are carried from the skin to spleen, liver, bone marrow, and other centres of reticuloendothelial activity. The amastigotes are now taken up by fixed macrophages such as Kupffer's cells in the liver, and multiply by simple binary fission till the cells become packed with the parasites (50–200 or more in the cytoplasm of the infected cell).

The infected cell ruptures and the parasites are liberated into the circulation. These are taken up by other reticuloendothelial cells followed by multiplication of the parasites and rupture of the cells. In this way the entire reticuloendothelial system becomes progressively infected. In the blood stream, some of the free amastigotes are phagocytosed by polymorphonuclear leucocytes and monocytes. A blood-sucking insect draws these free amastigotes, as well as those within the cells during its blood meal and the cycle is repeated.

Pathogenicity

L. donovani causes visceral leishmaniasis or kala-azar (*kala* meaning black and *azar* meaning disease), Dum Dum fever or tropical splenomegaly. In India, kala-azar has been known to occur in well defined areas in the eastern parts of the country mainly in Bihar, West Bengal, eastern districts of Uttar Pradesh, Assam, foothills of Sikkim, and to a lesser extent in Tamilnadu and Orissa.

Incubation period generally varies from 3–6 months, but it may be as short as 10 days or as long as 2 years. The parasite spreads from the site of inoculation to multiply in reticuloendothelial cells, especially in the spleen, liver, lymph nodes, and bone marrow. This leads to progressive enlargement of these organs. The host cellular and humoral defence mechanisms are stimulated. The former results in marked proliferation of macrophages. These cellular elements make up a large part of the bone marrow, compromising both the erythropoietic and granulocytic activity. The effect of this in the peripheral blood is leucopenia with granulocytopenia and relative monocytosis, anaemia (usually normocytic) and thrombocytopenia.

The spleen and liver become markedly enlarged, and hypersplenism contributes to the production of anaemia. It has been suggested that the erythrocytes adsorb immune complexes and become subject to enhanced phagocytosis by the macrophages of the liver and spleen. Lymphadenopathy is also produced. Production of globulin is greatly increased. This leads to reversal of the albumin: globulin ratio.

The disease is **reticuloendotheliosis** due to invasion of reticuloendothelial cells by *L. donovani.* Reticuloendothelial cells of various organs are proliferated and are packed with amastigote forms of the parasite. The disease manifests clinically with fever, malaise, headache, progressive enlargement of spleen, liver, and lymph nodes, anaemia, leucopenia and emaciation. Skin changes are often seen on the face, hands, feet, and abdomen, particularly in India, where patients acquire an earth-gray colour. If left untreated 75–95% patients die within 2 years. **Death in kala-azar is due to secondary infections.**

Visceral leishmaniasis and human immunodeficiency virus (HIV) together are synergistic infections because visceral leishmaniasis accelerates the development of acquired immunodeficiency syndrome (AIDS) and the presence of HIV infection enhances the spread of visceral disease. HIV may either activate subclinical leishmaniasis or make the patient susceptible to a new infection. *Visceral leishmaniasis has emerged as one of the most important opportunistic infections in HIV-infected patients.*

Immunity

In contrast to cutaneous leishmaniasis, cell-mediated immunity is impaired in active kala-azar patients who consequently lack a delayed type hypersensitivity response, but this can be demonstrated after cure.

Laboratory diagnosis

Various tests which can be carried out for the laboratory diagnosis of kala-azar are given in Flowchart 4.1.

Non-specific tests

These include:

1. ***Blood count:*** Total and differential leucocyte count reveals pancytopenia, mainly neutropenia and decreased erythrocyte count. The average total count of leucocytes is 3,000/µl of blood. During the course of the disease, the count may fall to 1,000/µl of blood or even below. Erythrocytes are also decreased in number.
2. ***Haemoglobin estimation:*** It reveals anaemia.
3. ***Estimation of serum proteins:*** It reveals raised serum proteins with reversal of the albumin: globulin ratio due to greatly raised IgG levels.

Parasitological diagnosis

Diagnosis of leishmaniasis can be confirmed by:

1. Peripheral blood film

Amastigote form of the parasite may be demonstrated

Flowchart 4.1. Laboratory diagnosis of kala-azar

Non-specific tests
- Blood count (pancytopenia mainly neutropenia and decreased erythrocyte count)
- Haemoglobin estimation (anaemia)
- Estimation of serum proteins (raised serum proteins with reversal of albumin:globulin ratio due to greatly increased IgG level)

Parasitological diagnosis
- Peripheral blood film by thick film method (amastigote form)
- Blood culture in NNN medium (promastigote form)
- Needle biopsy/aspiration
  - Lymph node / Bone marrow / Liver / Spleen
  - By touch preparation or smear stained with Giemsa stain (amastigote form)
  - Culture in NNN medium (promastigote form)
- Molecular methods
  - DNA probes
  - Polymerase chain reaction
- Animal inoculation

Immunological tests

Non-specific tests
- Aldehyde test
- Antimony test

(Indicate greatly increased serum proteins)
- Complement fixation test with WKK antigen

Specific tests
- Indirect fluorescent antibody test
- Indirect haem-agglutination test
- Enzyme-linked immunosorbent assay
- Direct agglutination test
- Leishmanin or Montenegro skin test

inside circulating monocytes and less often in neutrophils, in the stained peripheral blood film by thick film method. Owing to the small number of *Leishmania* parasites present in the peripheral blood, an examination of a thin film is often negative.

2. Needle biopsy/aspiration

Deeper tissues, e.g., lymph node, bone marrow, liver and spleen may be sampled by needle biopsy/aspiration. Amastigote forms of the parasite can be demonstrated, within reticuloendothelial cells, in touch preparations or smears stained with Giemsa stain. Spleen aspirate is the most reliable material for demonstrating parasites in kala-azar. However, bleeding might continue from the puncture wound in the soft and enlarged spleen, resulting in death. Therefore, spleen puncture should not be performed in a patient with haemorrhagic diathesis and leukaemia.

3. Culture

Whatever material is collected (blood and biopsy/aspiration material from various organs), it should be inoculated into the water of condensation of NNN medium and incubated at 22°–25° C and examined microscopically twice a week for first 2 weeks and once a week thereafter for up to 4 weeks before they are reported as negative. Promastigote stages can be detected microscopically in wet mounts taken from centrifuged culture fluid. The material can also be stained with Giemsa stain to facilitate observation at a higher magnification.

4. Molecular methods

A number of molecular methods have been developed for species identification of the promastigotes, including the use of DNA probes and polymerase chain reaction.

5. Animal inoculation

Aspirate or biopsy material obtained from lymph node, spleen, liver, bone marrow, etc. is inoculated intraperitoneally in young hamster 2–4 months old. The infection in hamsters develops slowly and may take several months to produce detectable infection. Splenic aspirate is collected. Smear of splenic aspirate, and impression smear of spleen are stained with Giemsa stain and examined under microscope for amastigote forms of *Leishmania donovani*.

Immunological tests

These include non-specific and specific tests:

1. Non-specific tests

- Aldehyde test
- Antimony test
- Complement fixation test with WKK antigen

1. ***Aldehyde test:*** A drop of full strength (40%) formalin is added to 1 ml of serum. A positive test is indicated by the rapid and complete coagulation of the serum. This serum test merely indicates greatly increased serum gamma globulin and thus is non-specific. This test is not positive till the disease is of at least three months duration. This test has also been found to be positive in infections with *Schistosoma japonicum* and *Trypanosoma brucei gambiense*, multiple myeloma and cirrhosis liver.
2. ***Antimony test:*** This test also depends upon a rise of serum gamma globulin. When a 4% urea stibamine solution in distilled water is mixed with serum from a patient with kala-azar, it leads to the formation of a profuse flocculent precipitate. It is less reliable than aldehyde test.
3. ***Complement fixation test with W.K.K. antigen:*** Complement fixation test may be carried out for detection of serum antibodies in visceral leishmaniasis. The antigen originally used was prepared from human tubercle bacillus by Witebsky, Kleingenstein and Kuhn hence known as W.K.K. antigen. Since the antigen is not prepared from *L. donovani*, therefore, this test is non-specific.

2. Specific tests

Complement fixation test with WKK antigen has been replaced with more specific tests such as indirect fluorescent antibody test (IFAT), indirect haemagglutination assay (IHA), and enzyme-linked immunosorbent assay (ELISA). These tests use the cultured promastigotes as antigen. These tests may often show cross-reactivity with sera of patients suffering from leprosy, malaria, schistosomiasis, Chagas' disease, and cutaneous leishmaniasis.

The direct agglutination test (DAT), using trypsin-treated Coomassie blue-stained promastigotes is a simple test for use in the diagnosis of kala-azar. This test detects specific IgM antibody at an early stage. It is useful in the detection of both clinical and subclinical infections.

Leishmanin or Montenegro test

It is a delayed hypersensitivity reaction to intradermal crude *Leishmania* antigen. It was first introduced in the South America by Montenegro. In this test, 0.2 ml of killed suspension of promastigotes of *L. donovani*, containing 6–10 million of the promastigotes per ml of 0.5% phenol saline, is injected intradermally. The test is read after 48–72 hours. A positive test shows an area of **erythema and induration 5 mm or more in diameter**. The test becomes positive 6–8 weeks after cure from kala-azar. Cell-mediated immunity is impaired in active kala-azar patients who consequently lack a delayed hypersensitivity response. Therefore, leishmanin test is negative in active cases of kala-azar. This test is of great value in epidemiological studies but is of little clinical use.

Diagnosis of visceral leishmaniasis in the presence of HIV infection is particularly difficult as the presentation may be very atypical and serological tests may be negative.

Differential diagnosis

Kala-azar must be differentiated from malaria, trypanosomiasis, schistosomiasis, liver abscess, tropical splenomegaly, histoplasmosis, brucellosis, tuberculosis, relapsing fever, myeloid leukaemia, lymphoma, cirrhosis of liver, thalassaemia and various gammopathies.

POST KALA-AZAR DERMAL LEISHMANIASIS

Post kala-azar dermal leishmaniasis (PKDL) was first described in patients with visceral leishmaniasis caused by *L. donovani* in India. It occurs in up to 20% of these patients. In India, skin lesions may appear 2–10 years after being partially treated, untreated or even those considered adequately treated for visceral leishmaniasis. In East Africa, lesions appear within a few months. It is caused by the reversal of *L. donovani* from viscerotropic to dermatotropic. It is not associated with *L. infantum* infection. PKDL is occasionally seen in patients with no history of visceral disease but only in places where *L. donovani* is transmitted, this is probably a sequel to subclinical infection.

Macules and papules usually appear first around the mouth and spread to the face and then to extensor surfaces of the arms, the trunk, and sometimes the legs. In the beginning they look like small hypopigmented patches; these then enlarge and may progress to nodules. The lesions are soft, painless, granulomatous of varying sizes and unless traumatized, do not ulcerate. When they are abundant, the clinical appearance may resemble that of lepromatous leprosy.

Laboratory diagnosis

Individuals with post kala-azar dermal leishmaniasis may be very important reservoirs for maintaining the infection in the population because of the high concentration of organisms in the skin.

Diagnosis of PKDL can be established by demonstration of amastigote form of *L. donovani* by a microscopical examination of Leishman-stained smear prepared from the biopsy material obtained from nodular lesions. Direct smear examination from the hypopigmented macules does not generally reveal any parasite.

LEISHMANIA INFANTUM

L. infantum is distributed in Mediterranean basin, and Central and Western Asia. Main vertebrate host is the domestic dog, which develops an acute or chronic disease. Canine visceral leishmaniasis presents abundant parasites in the skin available for transmission. Invertebrate hosts or vectors of *L. infantum* are *Phlebotomus ariasi* and *P. perniciosus*.

In man it causes **infantile visceral leishmaniasis classically restricted to children**, especially those below the age of 2 years. However, it may also involve adults, particularly those infected with HIV. **PKDL is not seen with *L. infantum* infection.**

LEISHMANIA TROPICA

Geographical distribution

The parasite is found in Central and Western Asia. In India, kala-azar is reported from eastern parts whereas *L. tropica* infection occurs in Central and Western India. It was first observed by Cunningham (1885) in Calcutta now Kolkata.

Habitat

It occurs inside reticuloendothelial cells (clasmatocytes) of the skin.

Morphology

The amastigote form occurs in man, whereas promastigote form is found in sandfly and in cultures. Morphologically, both these forms of *L. tropica* are indistinguishable from those of *L. donova*ni.

Cultivation

L. tropica, like *L. donovani*, can be cultured on NNN medium and Hockmeyer's medium.

Susceptible animal

As in case of *L. donovani*, hamster is susceptible to *L. tropica* infection.

Life cycle

The vertebrate host is man and invertebrate host is sandfly (*Phlebotomus sergenti*). The life cycle of *L. tropica*, in both vertebrate and invertebrate hosts, is similar to that of *L. donovani* except that in man amastigote form of the former resides in the reticuloendothelial cells of skin and not in the viscera. One factor restricting the parasites causing cutaneous leishmaniasis to the skin may simply be temperature, to which some species of *Leishmania* are particularly sensitive.

Pathogenicity

L. tropica causes urban anthroponotic **cutaneous leishmaniasis** or **Oriental sore** or **Delhi boil**. Infection is transmitted to man either by direct inoculation of promastigotes of *L. tropica* through the bite of the sandfly or by crushing of the infected sandfly into the punctured wound caused by the bite. At the site of inoculation, promastigotes are phagocytosed by reticuloendothelial cells of the skin and are transformed into amastigotes.

A cutaneous lesion or **leishmanioma** develops at the site of infective sandfly bite. It is characterized by a chronic infective granuloma with fibrosis. In the early stage, the lesion is due to the proliferation of reticuloendothelial cells of skin that contain a large number of amastigotes. Later, round cell infiltration (lymphocytes and plasma cells) associated with a marked reduction in the number of parasites and development of a delayed hypersensitivity skin reaction (leishmanin reaction) occur.

Incubation period varies from a few weeks to 6 months and in some cases it may be 1–2 years. Clinically, the lesion begins as a raised papule about 2.5 cm in diameter. In majority of cases, it ulcerates. The ulcer has clean-cut margin with a raised indurated edge, surrounded by red areola. At this stage, the parasite is found along the red margin and not on the floor of the ulcer. The ulcer heals spontaneously, in about 6 months, leaving a depressed scar and a **solid immunity**.

There is a marked development of cell-mediated immunity but a weak antibody response, although specific antibodies can be detected. The cell-mediated immunity is responsible for a marked delayed type hypersensitivity response to leishmanin in active and cured cases. The sores are distributed on the exposed parts of the body, particularly on the face and extremities. The average number of sores is around two. **Oriental sore is not associated with systemic manifestations although there may be enlargement of the draining lymph nodes.**

In contrast to *L. major* infection, *L. tropica* causes "dry" lesion. It is more swollen and less necrotic. The exudate is less profuse and accumulates as a thick crust.

Laboratory diagnosis

Microscopy

Diagnosis of *L. tropica* infection is made by the microscopic examination of material obtained by puncture of the indurated edge of the sore and stained with Giemsa or Wright stain. Amastigote form of the parasite will be seen in large numbers inside the macrophages. Smears made by scraping the floor of the ulcer are often negative because amastigote-infected macrophages are destroyed in the presence of secondary bacterial infection. If smears are negative, biopsy from the margin of the ulcer at times provides specific proof of infection.

Culture

Isolation of promastigote of *L. tropica* may be made from the aspirates of the ulcer by culture in NNN medium and Hockmeyer's medium. The specimen for culture is obtained by injecting a little volume of sterile physiological saline in the indurated margin of the ulcer and then aspirating it. A few drops of the aspirate are then inoculated into each medium.

Leishmanin skin test

Intradermal injection of leishmanin (killed promastigotes of *L. tropica* in 0.5% phenol saline) shows a marked delayed type hypersensitivity response.

LEISHMANIA MAJOR

Important mammalian hosts of *L. major* are great gerbil (*Rhombomys opimus*) and fat sand rat (*Psammomys obesus*), and important sandfly vectors are *Phlebotomus papatasi*, *P. dubosqi* and *P. salehi.*

L. major infection in humans occurs in epidemics in groups of people entering sparsely inhabited zoonotic foci. Major outbreaks have been reported in military groups and in workers on development projects. In sub-saharan Africa outbreaks are much less frequent and human cases occur sporadically. Transmission between humans without a mammalian reservoir host has not been well established.

L. major causes rural, zoonotic, **cutaneous leishmaniasis** or **Oriental sore**. It causes "wet" lesion which becomes necrotic and exudative, forming a loose crust above a granulomatous base that eventually produces the characteristic scar. The lesions may number more than 100. **Lymphatic spread may occur in *L. major* infections, with subcutaneous nodules in a linear distribution.** As in case of *L. tropica*, spontaneous cure of *L. major* infection usually results in a solid immunity and marked delayed type hypersensitivity response to intradermal inoculation of leishmanin. The latter may also be detected before healing.

Method of diagnosis of *L. major* infection is similar to that caused by *L. tropica*.

LEISHMANIA AETHIOPICA

Important mammalian hosts of this parasite are rock hyraxes (*Heterohyrax brucei* and *Procavia* spp.), and important sandfly hosts are *Phlebotomus longipes* and *P. pedifer*. In man it may cause **cutaneous leishmaniasis and diffuse cutaneous leishmaniasis (DCL)**. *L. aethiopica* lesions are more swollen and less necrotic than those of *L. tropica*. They are frequently barely exudative, with gradual scaling or exfoliation of the dermis at the centre. These lesions may last for years before healing.

DCL is a rare form of disease caused by *L. aethiopica*. The parasites are restricted to the skin, but become widely distributed over much of the surface, in large, swollen plaques and nodules. **This condition resembles lepromatous leprosy.** However, the abundant parasites in the nodules provide easy distinction. **In this condition, neither humoral nor cell-mediated immune responses are activated.** It is difficult to treat and this condition may last for the rest of the life of the patient.

NEW WORLD LEISHMANIASIS

LEISHMANIA BRAZILIENSIS COMPLEX AND LEISHMANIA MEXICANA COMPLEX

Geographical distribution

L. braziliensis complex and *L. mexicana* complex occur in tropical South America, and Central America respectively.

Habitat

These occur as intracellular parasites (amastigote form) inside the macrophages of the skin and mucous membrane of the nose and buccal cavity. These do not occur either in the internal organs or in the peripheral blood.

Morphology

These parasites are morphologically and culturally indistinguishable from other species of *Leishmania*.

Life cycle

The life cycle of *Leishmania* species causing the New World cutaneous and mucocutaneous leishmaniasis is similar to that of *L. donovani* and *L. tropica*, except that:

- amastigotes occur inside the macrophages of the skin and mucous membrane of the nose and buccal cavity but not in internal organs; and
- they are transmitted by sandflies of the genera *Lutzomyia* and *Psychodopygus*.

Pathogenicity

L. mexicana complex and *L. braziliensis* complex cause **chiclero's ulcer** and **espundia** respectively. These are zoonoses. The causative parasites are primarily those of wild animals. When the various sandfly vectors feed on humans these parasites may be transmitted. In this unnatural host they usually provoke an intense reaction and the eventual development of a skin lesion at the site of the bite. After about 7–10 days a tiny papule appears. In most cases it ulcerates, producing crater-like lesion with inflamed and elevated border.

The lesion may be single or multiple. The latter is due to the infected macrophages transporting the parasite to other parts of the body thus establishing secondary lesion. *L. braziliensis* tends to produce such metastatic lesions in the nasal, pharyngeal and laryngeal mucosae. These lesions may appear within a few months of the original skin lesion, or years later when the patient appears to have been cured of his initial infection.

The pathology of skin lesion is similar to that of *L. tropica*. *L. mexicana* complex may also cause **'anergic diffuse cutaneous leishmaniasis'** (**ADCL**). Histological examination of the skin and mucous lesion shows infiltration of lymphocytes, plasma cells and large mononuclear cells and necrosis of tissues. The parasites (amastigote forms) are found in large numbers inside the clasmatocytes and monocytes at the periphery of the lesion.

Laboratory diagnosis

Microscopy

The diagnosis is established by demonstration of amastigote forms of the parasites in the material obtained by puncture of the nodule or edge of the ulcer and stained with Giemsa or Wright stain.

Culture

L. mexicana complex and *L. braziliensis* complex can be isolated from clinical specimens by inoculation of NNN medium.

Animal inoculation

When inoculated into the skin of hamsters or mice *L. mexicana* complex causes large histiocytoma tumours containing abundant amastigotes, while *L. braziliensis* complex grows poorly in these animals.

Serology

- Antileishmanial antibodies may be detected in the patient serum by indirect fluorescent antibody (IFA) test using fixed amastigotes as antigens. It gives positive results in 89–95% of cases. IFA titre falls after successful chemotherapy.
- Enzyme-linked immunosorbent assay is also positive in 85% of cases.

Leishmanin or Montenegro skin test

This is positive in cutaneous and mucocutaneous leishmaniasis.

LEISHMANIA PERUVIANA

L. peruviana occurs in Western Peru. The dog, *Canis familiaris,* is the only known mammalian host other than humans, but this animal's role in the epidemiology of the human disease remains obscure. *Lutzomyia peruensis* and *L. verrucarum* are the vectors. This parasite causes simple cutaneous leishmaniasis without invasion of oro-nasal mucosa. It is particularly common in school children, commonly resulting in extensive facial scars. Ulcers are usually self-healing and impart a **solid immunity to reinfection** with the same parasite.

LEISHMANIA CHAGASI

Mammalian hosts include human and domestic dog, *Canis familiaris*. Among wild animals, the foxes (*Lycalopex vetulus* and *Cerdocyon thous*) seem to be important natural reservoirs. *Lutzomyia longipalpis* is the vector. It causes **visceral leishmaniasis** or **American visceral leishmaniasis (AVL). Unless treated it has a fatal outcome.**

Prophylaxis of Old and New World leishmaniasis

At present, no vaccine is available against the Old and New World leishmaniasis, although a number of vaccines are undergoing trials. Therefore, control of infection depends upon the following measures:

- Active case detection and treatment.
- Elimination of sandflies by spraying of inside walls of human dwellings and adjacent buildings with residual insecticides is an effective control measure. Spraying around the doors and windows is especially important.
- Insect repellents such as dimethylphthalate, when applied to exposed skin, protect for a few hours against the bites of sandfly.
- Use of fine mesh bed nets (45 holes in a square inch) or insecticide-impregnated bed nets and curtains.
- Sandfly is nocturnal and does not fly high above ground level, therefore, some interference with transmission of the disease may be achieved by sleeping at night on the roof or second floor of unsprayed houses.
- Destruction of desert rodents (natural reservoirs) colonies in inhabited areas.
- Elimination of dogs, where they act as reservoir hosts, as in China.
- Avoidance of areas of risk to military or other activities involving entry into areas where zoonotic *L. major* can be a serious risk.
- To prevent transmission to other persons the skin lesion should be protected from insects by a gauze bandage. This will also reduce the possibility of autotransmission.

Treatment of Old and New World leishmaniasis

The classic therapy for all cases of *Leishmania* is *pentavalent antimony* (sodium antimony gluconate; sodium stibogluconate). Resistance to this compound is widespread in India, although it remains useful in other parts of the world. As an alternative, *liposomal amphotericin B* is highly effective agent for visceral leishmaniasis, and it is currently the drug of choice for antimony-resistant disease. *Miltefosine* is the first orally active agent for the treatment of leishmaniasis.

TRYPANOSOMES

Trypanosomes are haemoflagellates that live in the blood and tissues of their human hosts. *Trypanosoma brucei* has three subspecies – *Trypanosoma brucei brucei, T. b. gambiense* and *T. b. rhodesiense*. The first one is an animal pathogen and the other two cause African trypanosomiasis or sleeping sickness in man. *T. cruzi* causes South American trypanosomiasis or Chagas' disease. *T. rangeli* infects humans without causing disease and must, therefore, be carefully distinguished from the pathogenic species.

T. brucei was first demonstrated by Bruce in horses and cattle suffering from 'nagana' during the year 1895. Forde, 1902 was first to demonstrate motile trypanosomes in the blood of a man suffering from fever. This parasite was subsequently named as *T. gambiense* by Dutton in 1902. Kleine, 1909 demonstrated the development of the parasite in the vector, tsetse fly.

TRYPANOSOMA BRUCEI GAMBIENSE

Geographical distribution

T. b. gambiense occurs in West and Central Africa.

Habitat

It inhabits:

- connective tissue spaces of the various organs;
- the reticular tissue of the lymph nodes and spleen;
- the intercellular spaces in the brain;
- lymph channels throughout the body;
- blood; and
- cerebrospinal fluid.

Morphology

In the blood of the vertebrate host, *T. b. gambiense* exists in trypomastigote form. It occurs in three forms – a long slender form having a flagellum, a short stumpy one without a flagellum, and an intermediate one. Because of these morphologic differences in the blood of the vertebrate host, this trypanosome is said to be **polymorphic**. The first form to appear is a long slender one and later when the infection is established, the short stumpy form together with the intermediate one appear.

In fresh blood the trypanosomes (Figs. 4.13 and 4.14) may be seen as motile, colourless, spindle-shaped bodies with a blunted posterior end and a finely pointed anterior end. The long slender and short stumpy forms measure 20 × 3 μm and 10 × 5 μm respectively. The nucleus is large, oval and central in position. Kinetoplast (parabasal body and blepharoplast) is situated on the posterior end. From the blepharoplast arises the flagellum. It curves round the body in the form of an undulating membrane and then continues beyond the anterior end as a free flagellum. The undulating membrane is thrown into 3 or 4 folds. The intracellular portion of the flagellum is known as axoneme. In Giemsa or Wright stained preparations, the cytoplasm and the undulating membrane appear pale blue, the nucleus reddish purple or red and the kinetoplast and the flagellum dark red.

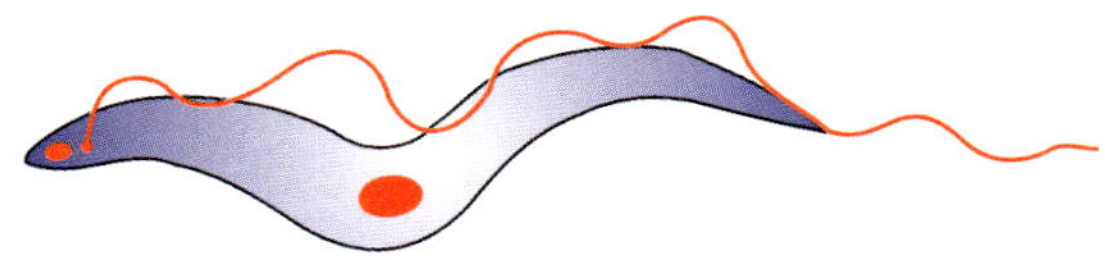

Fig. 4.13. *Trypanosoma brucei gambiense.*

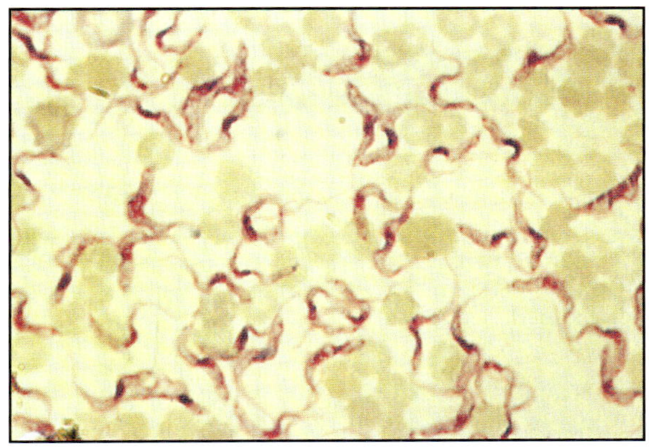

Fig. 4.14. *Trypanosoma brucei gambiense* in peripheral blood film (Giemsa stain, × 400).

Antigenic variation

One of the most interesting aspects of the trypanosomes is their ability to vary the antigenic nature of their surface coat. Within their genome, trypanosomes contain over 1,000 different genes coding for different variant surface glycoproteins (VSG). It appears that during the growth of trypanosomes new variant antigen types (VAT) are constantly being produced by mutations, additions, deletions and recombination. New surface coat variants appear at frequencies of 1 in 10^6 cells. Each wave of parasitaemia caused by a new variant emerges at 5–10 days' interval and is accompanied by fever and followed by monocytosis and production of antibody against the VSG.

This variant specific antibody is involved in the removal or clearance of majority of the trypanosomes from the blood and other body fluids. This process ends each wave of parasitaemia. However, there preexists within that population, a minor population of trypanosomes with a different VSG. This minor population then gives rise to the next wave of parasitaemia. **Antibody, therefore, acts as a selecting agent removing the major VSG population and allowing the other variant antigen types that exist in the population to develop.**

Cultivation

T. b. gambiense can be grown on NNN medium. It can also be grown in primary murine bone marrow culture in RPMI 1640 or Eagle's minimum essential medium supplemented with salts and 20% foetal calf serum.

Animal inoculation

In contrast to *T. b. rhodesiense,* laboratory animals such as mice, rats and guinea pigs are less susceptible to *T. b. gambiense* infection.

Life cycle

T. b. gambiense passes its life cycle in two hosts (Fig. 4.15). The vertebrate hosts are man, game and domestic animals, and invertebrate host is the tsetse fly of the genus *Glossina* (*G. palpalis*, *G. fuscipes* and *G. tachinoides*). *Both male and female flies bite man and may serve as vectors.*

Development in man and other vertebrate hosts

During the act of feeding, tsetse fly (*Glossina* spp.) introduces the metacyclic trypanosomal forms into the mammalian host in saliva injected into the puncture wound. They transform into long slender forms and multiply by binary fission at the site of inoculation. These then transform first into an intermediate stage and then into a non-dividing short stumpy form with no free flagellum. Subsequently, the parasites invade the blood stream, resulting in parasitaemia. The trypomastigote forms particularly the short stumpy forms are taken up by the tsetse fly along with its blood meal. It has been suggested that the short stumpy stage is the stage infective for the tsetse fly. The transition from the long slender form to short stumpy form may,

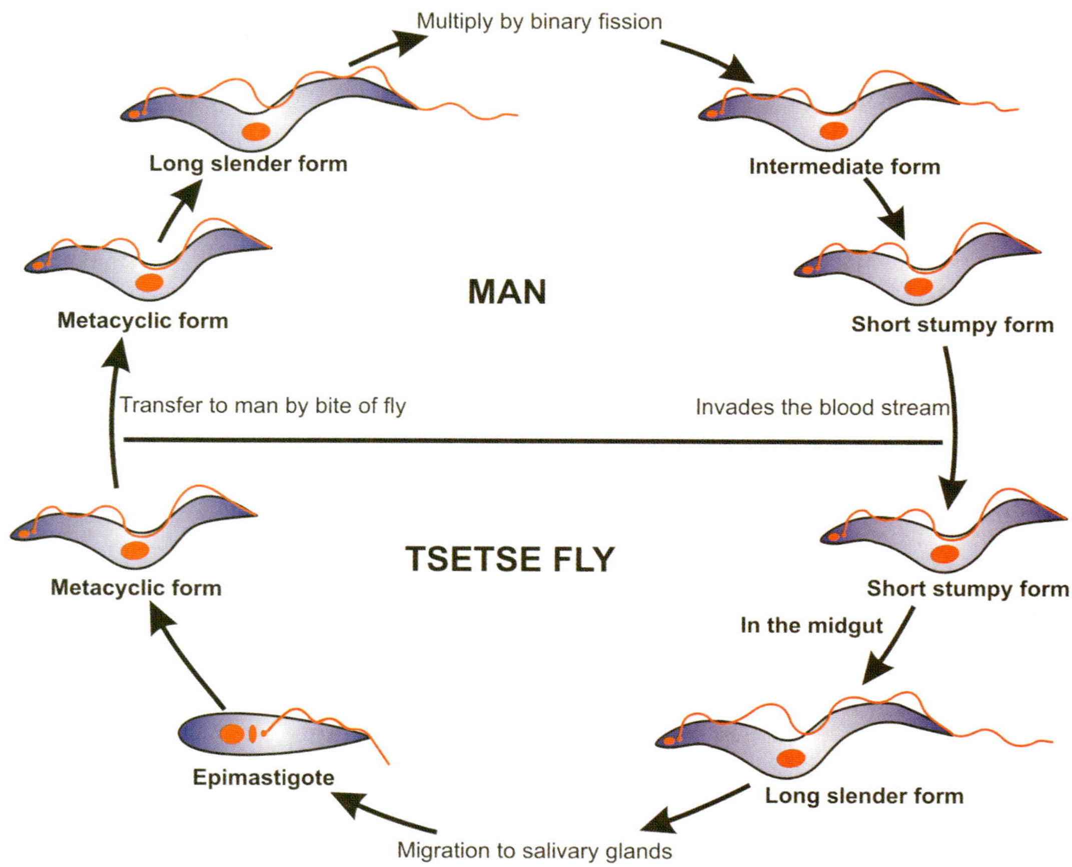

Fig. 4.15. Life cycle of *Trypanosoma brucei gambiense*.

therefore, be critical for the transmission of infection to the fly and the successful completion of the life cycle.

Development in invertebrate host

When an uninfected tsetse fly bites an infected vertebrate host the development in the vector is initiated. In the midgut of the insect short stumpy forms develop into long slender forms and multiply. These forms then pass to the posterior end of extraperitrophic space (a space between epithelial cells and peritrophic membrane), where they continue to multiply for some days. By the 15th day, they escape from the anterior end of the peritrophic space and enter the lumen of proventriculus. They then migrate forwards and gain access to the salivary glands via the hypopharynx and salivary ducts. In the salivary glands they develop into epimastigotes and attach to the cells of the glands. In the epimastigote forms, the nucleus is posterior to the kinetoplast, in contrast to the trypomastigote, in which the nucleus is anterior to the kinetoplast. They divide repeatedly and then transform into non-dividing metacyclic forms, which are highly motile, short and stumpy. When mature the metacyclic forms detach from the salivary gland cells and are infective to the vertebrate host. The time taken for the complete evolution of the infective forms (metacyclic forms) inside the tsetse fly is about 20 days.

Pathogenicity

T. b. gambiense causes **African trypanosomiasis** (**West African sleeping sickness**). It is chronic in nature lasting up to 4 years. The chronic nature of the disease can be attributed to antigenic variation in which waves of parasitaemia occur in the blood of infected person. Man develops infection by the bite of infected tsetse fly. *Both male and female tsetse flies suck blood and transmit infection. They bite during day, usually in the early morning and evening*. Metacyclic forms are injected into the subcutaneous tissue of man at the time of bite. Some of the parasites may enter directly into the blood stream but majority of them multiply locally. A **chancre** (3–4 cm) develops at the site of bite. It is hard and painful nodule and fluid withdrawn from it contains actively dividing trypomastigotes. It resolves spontaneously within 1–2 weeks.

Then the trypomastigotes spread throughout the entire body. They move through the blood and lymphatic vessels and multiply rapidly. Patients first experience intermittent recurring fever associated with lymphadenopathy. Lymph nodes in the posterior cervical region of the neck are frequently involved, producing a lesion known as **Winterbottom's sign**. Hepatosplenomegaly may also be evident during the early stage of infection.

If untreated, central nervous system is involved. Trypomastigotes enter the subarachnoid space and then the brain substance, with infiltration of plasma cells and lymphocytes, and perivascular proliferation of endothelial and neuroglial cells between the blood vessels and perivascular sheath. At this stage, patient develops severe headache and a wide array of behavioural changes ranging from aggressiveness to sleep-like states. Sleepiness becomes so pronounced that the patient falls asleep while eating, standing or sitting (sleeping sickness) and dies.

Laboratory diagnosis

Direct microscopy

The diagnosis of African trypanosomiasis depends upon **demonstration of the parasite** (trypomastigote forms) in blood, lymph node aspirates, sternal bone marrow, cerebrospinal fluid or fluid aspirated from the trypanosomal chancre by direct microscopic examination of unstained and stained films.

Concentration methods

If the parasites are scanty and cannot be detected in thin blood film, thick film or concentration methods such as miniature anion exchange columns, haematocrit tube centrifugation coupled with microscopic examination and acridine orange quantitative buffy coat technique may be employed. Trypomastigotes are present in largest numbers in the blood during febrile periods. Examination of multiple daily blood samples may be necessary to detect the parasite.

Culture

Trypanosomes in various clinical specimens can also be detected by cultivation in NNN medium.

Serologic techniques

A number of serological tests are available for the diagnosis of African trypanosomiasis. These include indirect fluorescent antibody test, indirect haem-agglutination test, enzyme-linked immunosorbent assay (ELISA) and card agglutination test for trypanosomes (CATT). These tests detect antibody in the sera of infected individuals and utilize antigens from blood stage trypanosomes.

Trypomastigotes are highly infectious, therefore, healthcare personnel must adhere to universal precautions when handling specimen from patients with suspected African trypanosomiasis.

Prophylaxis

- Destruction of tsetse habitats and elimination of reservoir hosts has given relief from trypanosomiasis but it is ecologically unsound.
- The use of fly traps and screens impregnated with insecticides is more economical than environmental spraying.

TRYPANOSOMA BRUCEI RHODESIENSE

Trypanosoma brucei rhodesiense occurs in East Africa. It was discovered by Stephans and Fanthan in 1910 in the blood of a patient in Rhodesia with symptoms consistent with "sleeping sickness". The habitat, antigenic variations and morphology of *T. b. rhodesiense*, both in man and in transmitting flies, are identical to those of *T. b. gambiense*. However, when it is inoculated into rats, mice or guinea pigs, posterior nucleate forms (Fig. 4.16) are more common in

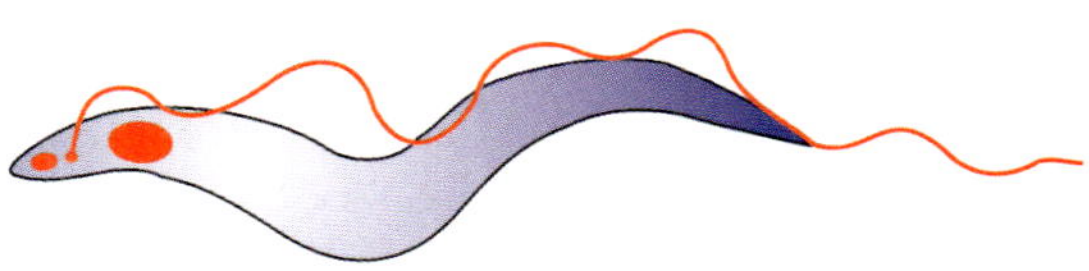

Fig. 4.16. Posterior nucleate form of *Trypanosoma brucei rhodesiense.*

T. b. rhodesiense than in *T. b. gambiense*. Like *T. b. gambiense*, it can also be cultured on NNN medium. Its life cycle is also similar to that of *T. b. gambiense*. However, the principal insect vectors are *G. morsitans*, *G. pallidipes* and *G. swynnertoni*. These flies inhabit low woodlands and thickets on lake shores. Antelopes and possibly other wild game and domestic cattle are reservoir hosts.

The disease produced by *T. b. rhodesiense* (**East African sleeping sickness**) is similar to that of *T. b. gambiense*. However, there are differences in the clinical manifestations of the disease they cause. The major difference between them is that the disease produced by *T. b. gambiense* is chronic in nature lasting up to 4 years, whereas the disease produced by *T. b. rhodesiense* is more acute, rarely lasting more than 9 months before death occurs.

In *T. b. rhodesiense* infection, febrile paroxysms are more frequent and oedema, weakness, rapid loss of weight, myocarditis and fever are striking symptoms, but lymph node enlargement is less pronounced. Mania and delusions are often noted, but the profound somnolence and other marked nervous symptoms of the 'sleeping sickness' stage are lacking or not so evident in this infection as in *T. b. gambiense* infection. *T. b. rhodesiense* is more resistant to treatment in advanced stage of the disease. The differences between *T. b. gambiense* and *T. b. rhodesiense* are given in Table 4.3.

Laboratory diagnosis, treatment and prophylaxis are same as for *T. b. gambiense* infection.

Table 4.3. Differences between *T. b. gambiense* and *T. b. rhodesiense*

	T. b. gambiense	***T. b. rhodesiense***
Geographical distribution	West and Central Africa	East Africa
Main tsetse vector	*G. palpalis, G. fuscipes* and *G. tachinoides*	*G. morsitans, G. pallidipes* and *G. swynnertoni*
Reservoir hosts	Mainly humans	Mainly animals
Virulence	Less	More
Number of trypomastigotes in blood	Less	More
Course of the disease	Chronic in nature, lasting up to 4 years	More acute, rarely lasting more than 9 months before death occurs
Febrile paroxysms	Less frequent	More frequent
Lymph node enlargement	More pronounced	Less pronounced
Profound somnolence and other marked nervous symptoms of the 'sleeping sickness' stage	Present	Lacking or not so evident
Posterior nucleate forms after inoculation into rats, mice or guinea pigs	Less common	More common
Resistance to treatment in advanced stage of the disease	Less	More

Treatment

Standard therapy for early-stage disease is *pentamidine* for *T. b. gambiense* and *suramin* for *T. b. rhodesiense*. Both compounds must be given parenterally over long periods and are not effective against late-stage disease. *Eflornithine* is used for the treatment of late-stage disease. It is ineffective as monotherapy for infections of *T. b. rhodesiense*. *Nifurtimox-eflornithine combination therapy* (NECT) allows a shorter exposure to eflornithine with good efficacy.

TRYPANOSOMA CRUZI

Geographical distribution

It occurs in Central and South America. Carlos Chagas, investigating malaria in Brazil in 1909, accidentally found this trypanosome in the faeces of a reduviid bug and in the blood of a monkey bitten by the infected bugs. It was only later that Chagas found the trypanosome in the blood of a sick child and showed that it was responsible for an endemic disease which came to be named after him. Chagas named the parasite *T. cruzi* after his mentor Oswaldo Cruz.

Habitat

It lives as trypomastigote in the blood and as an amastigote in reticuloendothelial cells and other tissue cells of man and many mammals. In man the most frequent locations of the parasites are reticuloendothelial cells of spleen, liver, lymph nodes, bone marrow, and myocardium. Parasites may also occur in cells of striated muscles, nervous system, histiocytes of cutaneous tissue, cells of the epidermis, and in the intestinal mucous membrane.

Morphology

Two main morphological forms are seen in human hosts.

1. Trypomastigote forms
2. Amastigote forms

Trypomastigote forms

These are present in the blood of the patient during the early acute stage and at intervals, thereafter in smaller numbers. In stained preparations, the parasite assumes a characteristic C-shape (Figs. 4.17 and 4.18). It measures 20 μm in length and 2–4 μm in width. It has a central nucleus and a large kinetoplast situated at the posterior end. Two forms occur in the blood, a long slender one and a short broad one.

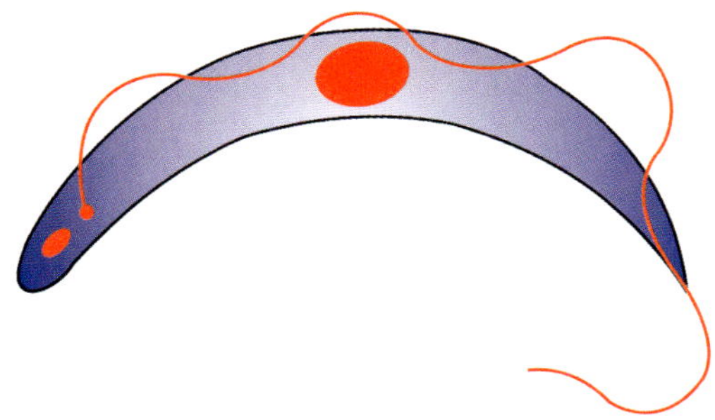

Fig. 4.17. Trypomastigote form of *Trypanosoma cruzi*.

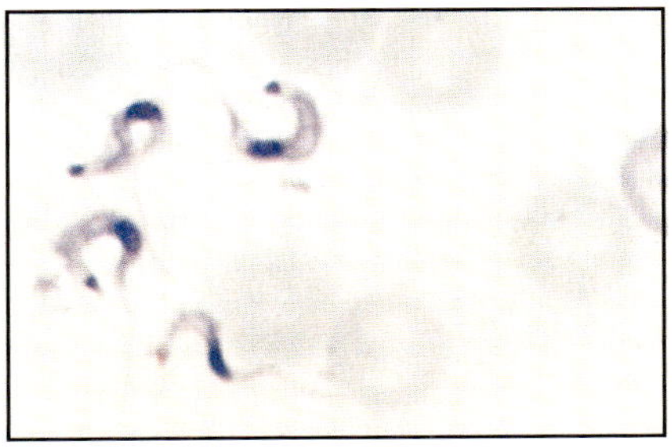

Fig. 4.18. *Trypanosoma cruzi* in peripheral blood film (Giemsa stain, × 400).

Amastigote forms

These are round or oval in shape, measure 1.5–4.0 μm in diameter, have a large nucleus and a kinetoplast. In fixed and wandering histiocytes, especially in spleen, liver, lymph nodes, and bone marrow, the amastigote is indistinguishable from that of *L. donovani*. In myocardium and neuroglial cells, the amastigote forms are collected within a cyst-like cavity in the invaded cells.

Staining reaction

It is the same as that of other trypanosomes.

Cultivation

It can be easily cultivated in the epimastigote form in NNN medium.

Life cycle

T. cruzi passes its life cycle in two hosts (Fig. 4.19) – one in man or the reservoir hosts such as armadillos, opossums, wood rats, and raccoons, the other in blood-sucking insect, the reduviid bug (*Panstrongylus megistus, Triatoma infestans* and *Rhodnius prolixus*).

Development in reduviid bug

Bugs acquire infection by feeding on an infected mammalian host. Trypomastigotes in the blood meal

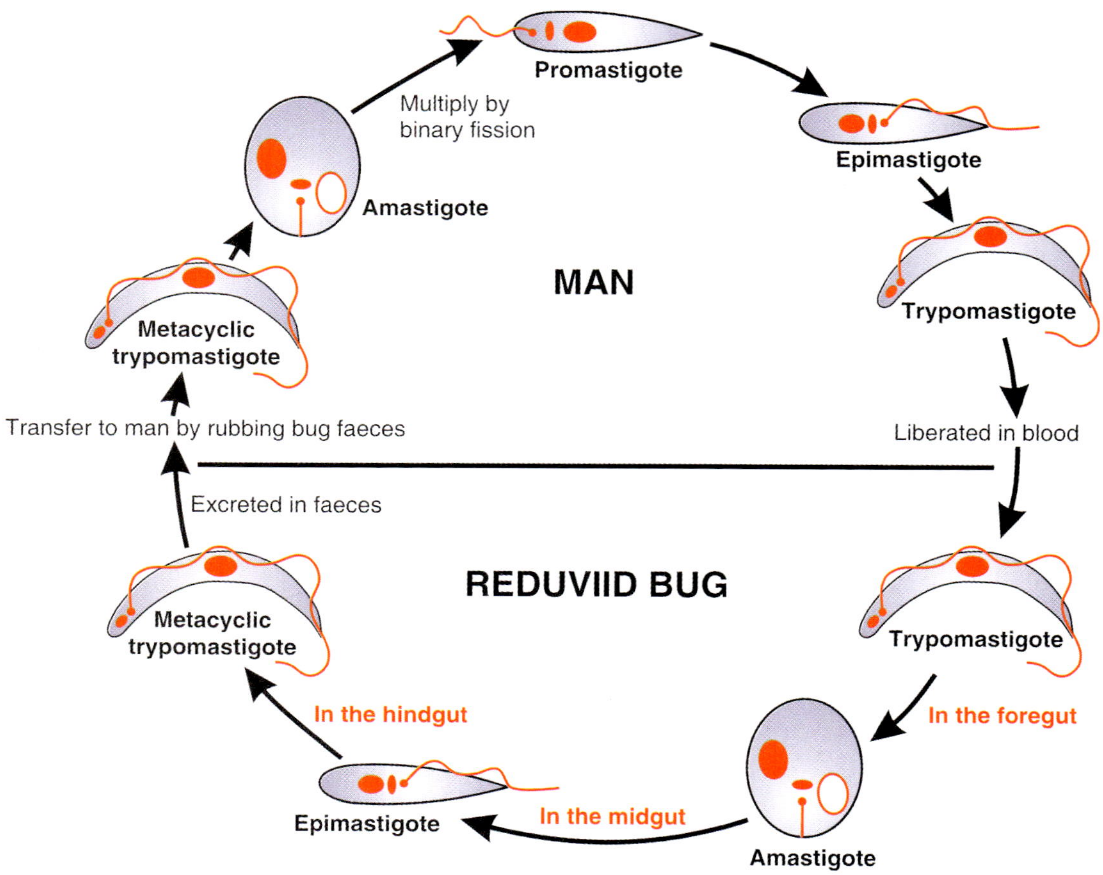

Fig. 4.19. Life cycle of *Trypanosoma cruzi.*

transform to amastigotes in the foregut and multiply by binary fission. In the midgut, they divide by binary fission in the epimastigote stage. In the hindgut, epimastigotes attach to the epithelium, transform to **metacyclic (infective) trypomastigotes** and are excreted in the faeces of the bug. The development of *T. cruzi* in the vector takes around 10–15 days.

Development in man

The infective forms of *T. cruzi* are found in bug's faeces. The bugs tend to defecate very soon after taking a blood meal. Since the bug's saliva contains an irritant, the person tends to scratch, thus scratching in the infective forms from the bug's faeces. Most reduviid bugs are nocturnal and feed on sleeping inhabitants of the house. They are attracted to the host by warmth, carbon dioxide, and odour.

The infection can also be transmitted by contamination of abraded skin and the conjunctiva, blood transfusion, organ transplantation, placental transfer, and accidental ingestion of parasitized reduviid bugs. The metacyclic trypomastigotes thus introduced, invade cells of reticuloendothelial system and other tissues particularly muscle and nervous tissue and are transformed into amastigote form. These multiply by binary fission and after passing through promastigote and epimastigote forms, are again transformed into trypomastigote forms which are liberated in the blood. This leads to dissemination of infection and infects fresh reduviid bugs when they next feed.

Pathogenicity

T. cruzi causes **South American trypanosomiasis** or **Chagas' disease**, a zoonotic disease that can be transmitted to humans by blood-sucking reduviid bug. **Incubation period** may be as short as two weeks, or several months if infection is acquired by blood transfusion. Prolonged incubation period in recipients given contaminated blood is thought to be due to the poor capacity of circulating broad blood forms to invade cells.

At the site of entry of *T. cruzi* a subcutaneous inflammatory nodule develops. It is known as **chagoma**. Rarely multiple chagomas have been described. When the entry is through conjunctiva, the patient develops painless, inflamed, periophthalmic, unilateral oedema and conjunctivitis. It is known as **Romana's sign**. The primary lesion is accompanied by fever, acute regional lymphadenitis and dissemination to blood and tissues. The parasites can usually be detected within 1–2 weeks as trypomastigotes in the blood.

Acute infections are more common and more severe in children. About 10% of children die during the acute stage. At this stage patient develops fever, hepatosplenomegaly, generalized lymphadenopathy, facial or generalized oedema, rash, vomiting, diarrhoea, anorexia and ECG changes like sinus tachycardia, increased P-R interval, T-wave changes and low QRS voltage, and patient may die of acute myocarditis. It may also lead to meningoencephalitis mainly in infants and AIDS patients.

Patients surviving the acute infection, develop chronic disease in which cardiac changes are most common with arrhythmias, palpitations, chest pain, oedema, dizziness, syncope and dyspnoea. Patient may also develop dilatation of oesophagus (megaoesophagus) and colon (megacolon), loss of peristalsis, regurgitation, dysphagia, and severe constipation.

Congenital transmission can occur in both the acute and chronic stages of the disease. Common clinical findings of congenital infection are stillbirth, low birth weight, myocarditis, neurologic alterations, and death shortly after birth. Infants of seropositive mothers should be monitored for up to 1 year after birth. Monitoring should include examination of blood for parasites and serologic tests.

Immune response

Shortly after infection, both humans and animals develop an immune response to the presence of the parasite. Both antibody-mediated and cell-mediated mechanisms are involved. During initial phase of infection, IgM is predominant, whereas later, IgG and IgA become major antibody classes. **Antigenic variation, which is characteristic of infections with African trypanosomes, is less common in *T. cruzi* infection.** In spite of humoral and cellular immunity against *T. cruzi*, the infection is able to persist in the host. Cell-mediated immunity has also been implicated as a cause of tissue destruction, including cardiomyopathy and megacolon, seen in Chagas' disease.

Laboratory diagnosis

The definitive diagnosis depends on demonstration of trypomastigotes in the blood, amastigote stages in tissues, positive polymerase chain reaction (PCR) and serological tests.

Microscopic examination

- Aspirates from chagomas and enlarged lymph nodes can be examined for amastigotes and trypomastigotes.
- In acute infection *T. cruzi* may be found transiently in the peripheral blood by direct microscopy of Giemsa stained and unstained, wet blood film. If the parasites are scanty and cannot be detected in thin stained and unstained film, thick film or concentration methods may be employed. The latter include:
  - Haematocrit centrifugation followed by searching for trypomastigotes in or immediately above the buffy coat layer.
  - Allowing the blood to coagulate and searching for trypomastigotes in centrifuged serum.
  - Lysis of red cells with 0.85% ammonium chloride and centrifugation to sediment trypomastigotes.
- In chronic disease trypomastigote stage is rare or absent, except during febrile episodes.

Laboratory workers should use bloodborne-pathogen precautions when examining blood films from Chagas' disease patients because the trypomastigotes are infective.

Culture

Blood and other specimens are inoculated in NNN medium and incubated at 25°C. The cultures are examined for epimastigote stages twice weekly during the first 2 weeks and once every week thereafter for up to 4 weeks before they are considered negative.

Polymerase chain reaction (PCR)

PCR may be very useful for the diagnosis of patients with chronic Chagas' disease because of the lack of sensitivity and specificity of serologic tests and the lack of sensitivity with xenodiagnosis.

Animal inoculation

Blood or CSF of the patient is inoculated intraperitoneally into mice. After 10 days, tail blood is collected and examined for motile trypanosomes.

Xenodiagnosis

In the indeterminate and chronic phases of the infection, *T. cruzi* is present in such low numbers in the peripheral blood that parasitemia may not be detectable by microscopy even after the concentration methods. In xenodiagnosis, colony-bred uninfected reduviid bugs are fed on a suspect host and dissected about 20–25 days later to detect epimastigotes in the faeces, hemolymph, hindgut, and salivary glands. Xenodiagnosis is generally favoured because, unlike blood culture, it does not require stringent aseptic precautions. Colonies of reduviid bugs are usually maintained by feeding on chicken blood, as birds are not susceptible to *T. cruzi* infection.

Serodiagnosis

Serology detects exposure to infection rather than an active infection. Antibodies against *T. cruzi* may be detected in patient serum by complement fixation test, indirect fluorescent antibody test, enzyme-linked immunosorbent assay and indirect haemagglutination test. In *T. cruzi* infection, seropositivity is generally maintained for life unless specific anti-parasite chemotherapy has been given. Depending on the antigens used cross-reactions have been noted to occur in patients with *T. rangeli* infection, leishmaniasis, syphilis, toxoplasmosis, hepatitis, leprosy, schistosomiasis, infectious mononucleosis, systemic lupus erythematosus, and rheumatoid arthritis. The Western blot method has been recommended for confirmatory serologic diagnosis of Chagas' disease.

Intradermal test

After intradermal inoculation of extract of *T. cruzi* culture (cruzin), a delayed hypersensitivity reaction is obtained.

Biopsy

Biopsy of involved lymph node or muscle may reveal amastigote forms of *T. cruzi*.

Treatment

Nifurtimox and *benznidazole* may be used for the treatment of American trypanosomiasis. Both these agents suppress parasitemia and can cure acute phase of Chagas' disease in 60–80% of cases.

Prophylaxis

Since no effective treatment is available, it is, therefore, important to control the vector with residual insecticides, health education and housing improvement.

TRYPANOSOMA RANGELI

T. rangeli infects humans and other vertebrates in both Central and South America. It is often found in areas where *T. cruzi* is also present. Human infections are asymptomatic, and trypomastigotes have been noted to persist in the blood for longer than a year. *T. rangeli* and *T. cruzi* use the same reduviid bug to transmit infections. *T. rangeli* infections can be transmitted by inoculation of bug saliva during feeding or by vector's faeces.

Trypomastigotes can be detected in the blood of infected patients using thin and thick smears and buffy coat concentration techniques. The parasites can be stained with Giemsa stain. Differences between *T. cruzi* and *T. rangeli* are given in Table 4.4. Blood can be cultured in NNN medium or injected into laboratory animals (mice) and examined for epimastigotes and trypomastigotes respectively. Polymerase chain reaction has been used to detect infections in humans and vectors.

Table 4.4. Differences between *T. cruzi* and *T. rangeli*

Characteristic	*T. cruzi*	*T. rangeli*
Size of trypomastigote	20 μm	30 μm
Shape	Often C-shaped in fixed preparations	Rarely C-shaped
Posterior kinetoplast	Large and terminal	Small and subterminal
Parasites in salivary gland or proboscis or both of reduviid bug	Always absent	Usually present, therefore, non-pathogenic *T. rangeli* pass to humans by the bite of reduviid bug

Further Reading

1. Adam, R.D. 2001. Biology of *Giardia lamblia*. *Clin. Microbiol. Rev.*, **14**: 447–75.
2. Agbo, E.E.C., Majiwa, P.A., et al. 2002. Molecular variation of *Trypanosoma brucei* subspecies as revealed by AFLP finger printing. *Parasitology*, **124**: 349–58.
3. Altar, Z.T., Chance, M.L., et al. 2001. Latex agglutination test for the detection of urinary antigens in visceral leishmaniasis. *Acta. Trop.*, **78**: 11–16.
4. Beard, C.B., Pye, G., et al. 2003. Chagas' disease in a domestic transmission cycle, southern Texas, USA. *Emerg. Infect. Dis.*, **9**: 103–5.
5. Black, S.J., Seed, J.R., et al. 2001. Innate and acquired resistance to African trypanosomiasis. *J. Parasitol.*, **87**: 1–9.
6. Brandao-Filho, S.P., Brito, M.E., et al. 2003. Wild and synanthropic hosts of *Leishmania* (*Viannia*) *braziliensis* in the endemic cutaneous leishmaniasis locality of Amaraji, Pernambuco State, Brazil. *Trans. R. Soc. Trop. Med. Hyg.*, **97**: 291–6.
7. Costa, C.H.N., Gomes, R.B.B., et al. 2000. Competence of human host as a reservoir for *Leishmania chagasi*. *J. Infect. Dis.*, **182**: 997–1000.
8. Cu-uvin, S., Ko, H., et al. 2002. Prevalence, incidence, and persistence or recurrence of trichomoniasis among human immunodeficiency virus (HIV)-positive women and among HIV-negative women at high risk for HIV infection. *Clin. Infect. Dis.*, **34**: 1406–11.
9. Garcia, L.S. 2001. *Diagnostic Medical Parasitology*, 4th edn. Washington DC: American Society for Microbiology Press.
10. Handman, E. 2001. Leishmaniasis: current status of vaccine development. *Clin. Microbiol. Rev.*, **14**: 229–43.
11. Lainson, R., Ishikawa, E.A.Y., et al. 2002. American visceral leishmaniasis, wild animal hosts. *Trans. R. Soc. Trop. Med. Hyg.*, **96**: 630–1.
12. Myler, P.J. and Stuart K.D. 2000. Recent developments from the *Leishmania* genome project. *Curr. Opin. Microbiol.*, **3**: 412–16.
13. Schijman, A.G., Vigliano, C.A., et al. 2004. *Trypanosoma cruzi* DNA in cardiac lesions of Argentinian patients with end-stage chronic Chagas' heart disease. *Am. J. Trop. Med. Hyg.*, **70**: 210–20.
14. Traub, R.J., Morris, P.T., et al. 2004. Epidemiological and molecular evidence supports the zoonotic transmission of *Giardia* among humans and dogs living in the same community. *Parasitology*, **128**: 253–62.
15. Wendel, K.A., Erbelding, E.J., et al. 2002. *Trichomonas vaginalis* polymerase chain reaction compared with standard diagnostic and therapeutic protocols for detection and treatment of vaginal trichomoniasis. *Clin. Infect. Dis.*, **35**: 576–80.

Important Questions

1. Discuss geographical distribution, morphology, life cycle, pathogenicity, laboratory diagnosis and treatment of *Giardia lamblia*.
2. Discuss in detail geographical distribution, habitat, morphology, life cycle and pathogenicity of *Leishmania donovani*.
3. Discuss laboratory diagnosis of kala-azar.
4. Write short notes on:
   (a) *Trichomonas vaginalis*
   (b) *Leishmania infantum*
   (c) *Leishmania tropica*
   (d) *Leishmania major*
   (e) *Leishmania aethiopica*
   (f) Post kala-azar dermal leishmaniasis
   (g) Leishmanin test
5. Discuss geographical distribution, habitat, morphology, life cycle, pathogenicity and laboratory diagnosis of *Leishmania braziliensis* complex and *Leishmania mexicana* complex.
6. Tabulate differences between *Trypanosoma brucei gambiense* and *Trypanosoma brucei rhodesiense*.
7. Write short notes on:
   (a) *Leishmania peruviana*
   (b) *Leishmania chagasi*
8. Discuss geographical distribution, habitat, morphology, life cycle, pathogenicity and laboratory diagnosis of:
   (a) *Trypanosoma brucei gambiense*
   (b) *Trypanosoma brucei rhodesiense*
   (c) *Trypanosoma cruzi*

Multiple Choice Questions

1. How many pairs of flagella are present in the trophozoite of *Giardia lamblia*?
   (a) One pair.
   (b) Two pairs.
   (c) Three pairs.
   (d) Four pairs.
2. Which is the infective form of *Giardia lamblia*?
   (a) Trophozoite.
   (b) Cyst.
   (c) Precyst.
   (d) Pseudocyst.

3. *Giardia lamblia* resides in:
   (a) duodenum and upper part of jejunum.
   (b) caecum.
   (c) colon.
   (d) rectum.
4. *Trichomonas tenax* resides in:
   (a) vagina.
   (b) mouth.
   (c) duodenum.
   (d) caecum.
5. Trussell and Johnson's medium is employed for the cultivation of:
   (a) *Giardia lamblia*.
   (b) *Trichomonas vaginalis*.
   (c) *Entamoeba histolytica*.
   (d) *Leishmania donovani*.
6. Diagnosis of *Trichomonas vaginalis* infection can be established by:
   (a) demonstration of trophozoites in wet mounts.
   (b) cultivation.
   (c) nucleic acid hybridization techniques.
   (d) All of the above.
7. *Chilomastix mesnili* lives in:
   (a) duodenum.
   (b) mouth.
   (c) vagina.
   (d) caecum.
8. All of the following are characteristics of trophozoites of *Enteromonas hominis* **except**:
   (a) four flagella.
   (b) nucleus at the anterior end.
   (c) pear-shaped structure.
   (d) cytostome.
9. *Dientamoeba fragilis* is classified under:
   (a) amoebae.
   (b) flagellates.
   (c) sporozoa.
   (d) ciliata.
10. *Dientamoeba fragilis* can be differentiated from the amoebae by the presence of:
    (a) two and sometimes up to four nuclei.
    (b) cytostome.
    (c) cyst stage.
    (d) food vacuoles containing RBCs.
11. Old World leishmaniasis is caused by:
    (a) *Leishmania donovani*.
    (b) *Leishmania infantum*.
    (c) *Leishmania tropica*.
    (d) All of the above.
12. New World leishmaniasis is caused by:
    (a) *Leishmania donovani*.
    (b) *Leishmania aethiopica*.
    (c) *Leishmania tropica*.
    (d) *Leishmania braziliensis* complex.
13. Amastigote form of *Leishmania donovani* resides in the:
    (a) cells of reticuloendothelial system.
    (b) culture media.
    (c) digestive tract of insect vector.
    (d) All of the above.
14. Promastigote form of *Leishmania donovani* is seen in the:
    (a) red blood cells.
    (b) culture media.
    (c) hepatocytes.
    (d) cells of reticuloendothelial system.
15. *Leishmania donovani* can be cultivated in:
    (a) Lowenstein-Jensen medium.
    (b) Hockmeyer's medium.
    (c) Boeck and Drbohlav's diphasic medium.
    (d) Trussell and Johnson's medium.
16. Which is the most susceptible experimental animal used for inoculation of *Leishmania donovani*?
    (a) Guinea pig.
    (b) Hamster.
    (c) Rabbit.
    (d) Mouse.
17. Kala-azar must be differentiated from:
    (a) malaria.
    (b) tuberculosis.
    (c) histoplasmosis.
    (d) All of the above.
18. Patients of post kala-azar dermal leishmaniasis present with:
    (a) hypopigmented macules.
    (b) erythematous patches.
    (c) yellowish-pink nodules.
    (d) All of the above.
19. Post kala-azar dermal leishmaniasis is probably a sequel to infection with:
    (a) *Leishmania donovani*.
    (b) *Leishmania infantum*.
    (c) *Leishmania tropica*.
    (d) *Leishmania major*.

20. Invertebrate host for *Leishmania tropica* is:
    (a) *Phlebotomus argentipes*.
    (b) *Phlebotomus orientalis*.
    (c) *Phlebotomus sergenti*.
    (d) *Phlebotomus papatasi*.
21. In *Leishmania tropica* infection amastigote form resides in:
    (a) clasmatocytes of skin.
    (b) reticuloendothelial cells of viscera.
    (c) sandfly vector.
    (d) artificial culture medium.
22. *Leishmania tropica* causes:
    (a) kala-azar.
    (b) oriental sore.
    (c) espundia.
    (d) chiclero's ulcer.
23. *Leishmania braziliensis* complex resides inside the macrophages of:
    (a) skin and mucous membrane of nose and buccal cavity.
    (b) in the internal organs.
    (c) in the peripheral blood.
    (d) All of the above.
24. Espundia is caused by:
    (a) *Leishmania mexicana* complex.
    (b) *Leishmania braziliensis* complex.
    (c) *Leishmania peruviana*.
    (d) *Leishmania chagasi*.
25. American visceral leishmaniasis is caused by:
    (a) *Leishmania mexicana* complex.
    (b) *Leishmania peruviana*.
    (c) *Leishmania chagasi*.
    (d) *Leishmania tropica*.
26. Which of the following trypanosomes is nonpathogenic?
    (a) *Trypanosoma brucei gambiense*.
    (b) *Trypanosoma brucei rhodesiense*.
    (c) *Trypanosoma cruzi*.
    (d) *Trypanosoma rangeli*.
27. Chagas' disease is caused by:
    (a) *Trypanosoma brucei gambiense*.
    (b) *Trypanosoma brucei rhodesiense*.
    (c) *Trypanosoma cruzi*.
    (d) *Trypanosoma rangeli*.
28. *Trypanosoma brucei gambiense* infection is transmitted by:
    (a) female anopheles mosquito.
    (b) tsetse fly.
    (c) triatomine bug.
    (d) female sandfly.
29. Which stage of *Trypanosoma brucei gambiense* is infective for mammalian host?
    (a) Metacyclic trypomastigote.
    (b) Long slender form.
    (c) Short stumpy form.
    (d) Intermediate form.
30. Which form of *Trypanosoma brucei gambiense* is infective to tsetse fly?
    (a) Long slender form.
    (b) Intermediate form.
    (c) Short stumpy form.
    (d) Metacyclic trypomastigotes.
31. Which of the following drugs is used to treat early-stage disease caused by *Trypanosoma brucei gambiense*?
    (a) Suramin.
    (b) Pentamidine.
    (c) Melarsoprol.
    (d) Amphotericin B.
32. Chagoma is seen in infection with:
    (a) *Trypanosoma brucei gambiense*.
    (b) *Trypanosoma brucei rhodesiense*.
    (c) *Trypanosoma cruzi*.
    (d) *Trypanosoma rangeli*.
33. Which animal is used for xenodiagnosis of American trypanosomiasis?
    (a) Guinea pig.
    (b) Mouse.
    (c) Reduviid bug.
    (d) Hamster.
34. Commonest cause of steatorrhoea is:
    (a) *Giardia lamblia*.
    (b) *Entamoeba histolytica*.
    (c) *Toxoplasma gondii*.
    (d) *Naeglaria fowleri*.
35. *Giardia lamblia* was discovered by:
    (a) Giard.
    (b) Lambl.
    (c) Leeuwenhoek.
    (d) Robert Koch.
36. Enterotest is useful for the identification of which of the following parasites?
    (a) *Entamoeba histolytica*.
    (b) *Giardia lamblia*.

(c) *Trichomonas hominis.*
(d) *Cryptosporidium parvum.*

37. In *Trypanosoma cruzi* infection the parasitic form present in fixed and wandering histiocytes is:
(a) amastigote.
(b) promastigote.
(c) trypomastigote.
(d) epimastigote.

38. Non-ulcerated nodules are characteristic of:
(a) oriental sore.
(b) espundia.
(c) post kala-azar dermal leishmaniasis.
(d) kala-azar.

39. *Trypanosoma brucei gambiense* is transmitted by:
(a) housefly.
(b) sandfly.
(c) tsetse fly.
(d) reduviid bug.

40. *Trypanosoma cruzi* is transmitted by:
(a) sandfly.
(b) tsetse fly.
(c) housefly.
(d) reduviid bug.

41. Sandfly is the vector of:
(a) *Leishmania donovani.*
(b) *Plasmodium falciparum.*
(c) *Wuchereria bancrofti.*
(d) *Brugia malayi.*

42. Romana's sign is positive in:
(a) malaria.
(b) filariasis.
(c) Chagas' disease.
(d) kala-azar.

43. Chiclero's ulcer is caused by:
(a) *Leishmania mexicana* complex.
(b) *Leishmania braziliensis* complex.
(c) *Leishmania tropica.*
(d) *Leishmania infantum.*

44. Oriental sore is caused by:
(a) *Leishmania donovani.*
(b) *Leishmania infantum.*
(c) *Leishmania aethiopica.*
(d) *Leishmania tropica.*

45. Which of the following parasites attaches to the mucosa of the duodenum and the upper part of the jejunum with sucking disc?
(a) *Entamoeba histolytica.*
(b) *Balantidium coli.*
(c) *Giardia lamblia.*
(d) *Balamuthia mandrillaris.*

46. Which of the following is **not** true about *Trichomonas vaginalis*?
(a) It is a pyriform flagellate.
(b) It has four anterior and one posterior flagella.
(c) Cyst of the parasite is the infective stage.
(d) It causes vaginitis with discharge.

47. Which of the following parasites is **not** intracellular in human beings?
(a) *Trypanosoma brucei gambiense.*
(b) *Plasmodium vivax.*
(c) *Leishmania donovani.*
(d) *Toxoplasma gondii.*

48. How many nuclei does a mature cyst of *Giardia lamblia* possess?
(a) One.
(b) Two.
(c) Three.
(d) Four.

49. Montenegro test is used for the diagnosis of which of the following diseases?
(a) Kala-azar.
(b) Cysticercosis.
(c) Toxoplasmosis.
(d) Echinococcosis.

50. Enterotest is used for sampling:
(a) alveolar lavage specimen.
(b) urogenital specimen.
(c) duodenal contents.
(d) rectal specimen.

51. Dum Dum fever is the name given to:
(a) hepatic amoebasis.
(b) visceral leishmaniasis.
(c) cerebral malaria.
(d) neurocysticercosis.

52. Romana's sign refers to:
(a) unilateral oedema and conjunctivitis.
(b) ileo-caecal amoebiasis.
(c) greenish or yellow vaginal discharge.
(d) sleeping sickness.

53. Which of the following parasites possesses ability to vary the antigenic nature of their surface coat?
(a) *Trypanosoma brucei gambiense.*
(b) *Trypanosoma rangeli.*

(c) *Leishmania donovani*.
(d) *Leishmania tropica*.

54. Which of the following acts as a vector for *Trypanosoma cruzi*?
(a) Reduviid bug.
(b) Tsetse fly.
(c) Dearfly.
(d) Blackfly.

55. West African sleeping sickness is caused by:
(a) *Trypanosoma brucei gambiense*.
(b) *Trypanosoma brucei brucei*.
(c) *Trypanosoma cruzi*.
(d) *Trypanosoma rangeli*.

56. Which morphological form of *Trypanosoma brucei gambiense* is seen in humans?
(a) Amastigote.
(b) Promastigote.
(c) Epimastigote.
(d) Trypomastigote.

57. In which of the following parasites both amastigote and trypomastigote forms are seen in humans?
(a) *Trypanosoma brucei gambiense*.
(b) *Trypanosoma brucei rhodesiense*.
(c) *Trypanosoma cruzi*.
(d) *Trypanosoma rangeli*.

58. *Trypanosoma brucei gambiense* can be grown in:
(a) NNN medium.
(b) Diamond's medium.
(c) chocolate agar medium.
(d) Boeck and Drbohlav's diphasic medium.

59. *Trypanosoma cruzi* can be grown in:
(a) Trussell and Johnson's medium.
(b) Diamond's medium.
(c) NNN medium.
(d) Boeck and Drbohlav's diphasic medium.

60. Which of the following protozoan parasites inhibits the absorption of fats in the intestine?
(a) *Giardia lamblia*.
(b) *Cryptosporidium parvum*.
(c) *Isospora belli*.
(d) *Entamoeba histolytica*.

ANSWERS TO MCQs

1 (d), 2 (b), 3 (a), 4 (b), 5 (b), 6 (d), 7 (d), 8 (d), 9 (b), 10 (a), 11 (d), 12 (d), 13 (a), 14 (b), 15 (b), 16 (b), 17 (d), 18 (d), 19 (a), 20 (c), 21 (a), 22 (b), 23 (a), 24 (b), 25 (c), 26 (d), 27 (c), 28 (b), 29 (a), 30 (c), 31 (b), 32 (c), 33 (c), 34 (a), 35 (c), 36 (b), 37 (a), 38 (c), 39 (c), 40 (d), 41(a), 42 (c), 43 (a), 44 (d), 45 (c), 46 (c), 47 (a), 48 (d), 49 (a), 50 (c), 51 (b), 52 (a), 53 (a), 54 (a), 55 (a), 56 (d), 57 (c), 58 (a), 59 (c), 60 (a).

5

Sporozoa

Sporozoa belong to the kingdom Protozoa, phylum Sporozoa, class Coccidia, and orders Eimeriida, Piroplasmida and Haemosporida (Table 1.5). These organisms have a system of organelles at their apical end that produces substances to help the organism to penetrate host cells and thus become intracellular parasites.

MALARIA PARASITES

In 1880, a French army surgeon, Charles Laveran found and described the malaria parasite. Romanowsky developed a staining method of malaria parasites in 1891. The life cycle of malaria parasite was described by the Italian scientists Amico Bignami, Battista Grassi, and Giovanni Bastianelli in 1898. Ronald Ross, an army surgeon in Indian Medical Service, while in India, demonstrated that mosquitoes of *Anopheles* species act as vectors of malaria parasites. For this monumental discovery he was awarded Nobel Prize in 1902. In 1976, Trager and Jensen cultured malaria parasites *in vitro* for the first time.

There are approximately 172 named species of *Plasmodium* which infect various species of vertebrates. Five species are known to infect humans – *P. falciparum*, *P. vivax*, *P. malariae*, *P. ovale*, and *P. knowlesi*, a species of monkeys, can also infect humans. Malaria continues to be an important vector-borne disease. Infection with *Plasmodium* spp. accounts for 1–5 billion febrile episodes and 1–3 million deaths annually, 85% of which are in Africa. The incidence of malaria is increasing due to resistance of vectors to insecticides and drug resistant parasites.

P. vivax and *P. falciparum* account for 95% of infections. *P. vivax* has widest distribution, extending throughout the tropics, subtropics, and temperate zones. *P. falciparum* is generally confined to the tropics, *P. malariae* is sporadically distributed, and *P. ovale* is rare in much of the world but relatively common in western Africa. In India, *P. vivax* and *P. falciparum* are very common, a few cases of *P. malariae* and *P. ovale* have also been reported. Human *P. knowlesi* infections have been described in high numbers only in Malaysia.

Life cycle

Malaria parasites exhibit a complex life cycle (Figs. 5.1 and 5.2) involving alternating cycles of asexual division (schizogony) occurring in man (intermediate host) and sexual development (sporogony) occurring in female *Anopheles* mosquito (definitive host). Therefore, **malaria parasites exhibit alternation of generations and alternation of hosts**.

Human cycle

The sporozoites are the infective form of the parasite. They are present in the salivary glands of female Anopheles mosquito. Man gets infection by the bite of infected mosquito. It usually bites at night or during the twilight hours, either right after sunset or before sunrise. During the act of biting, the proboscis of the mosquito pierces the skin and saliva containing sporozoites is injected directly into the blood stream. The cycle in man comprises of following stages:

- Primary exo-erythrocytic or pre-erythrocytic schizogony
- Erythrocytic schizogony
- Gametogony
- Secondary exo-erythrocytic or dormant schizogony

Primary exo-erythrocytic or pre-erythrocytic schizogony

Within one hour all the **sporozoites** leave the blood stream and enter into liver parenchyma cells. The sporozoites which are elongated, spindle-shaped bodies become rounded inside the liver cells. They undergo a process of multiple nuclear division, followed by cytoplasmic division and develop into **primary exo-erythrocytic schizont** or **pre-erythrocytic schizont**. In different species it varies in size from 24–60 μm in diameter and contains 2,000–30,000 merozoites (Fig. 5.3). Primary exoerythrocytic schizogony consists of **only one generation**. The duration of this cycle of *P. falciparum, P. vivax, P. ovale* and *P. malariae* is 6, 8, 9 and 13–16 days, respectively. When primary exo-erythrocytic schizogony is complete, the liver cell ruptures and releases several thousand individual parasites (merozoites) into blood stream.

Erythrocytic schizogony

The **merozoites** liberated from primary exo-erythrocytic schizogony enter the blood stream, attach to specific receptors on the surface of erythrocytes and enter the cells where they multiply at the expense of the host cells thus initiating erythrocytic schizogony. Here they pass through the stages of trophozoites, schizonts and merozoites (Table 5.1, Figs. 5.1, 5.2, 5.4–5.7). Depending on the species, 6–32 nuclei are produced followed by cytoplasmic division, and the red cell ruptures to release the individual merozoites, which then infect fresh red blood cells.

The parasitic multiplication during the erythrocytic phase is responsible for bringing on a clinical attack of malaria. Erythrocytic schizogony may be continued for a considerable period, but in the course of time the infection tends to die out. *P. falciparum* differs from the other malaria parasites in that developing erythrocytic schizonts aggregate in the capillaries of the brain and other internal organs, so that only young ring forms are found in peripheral blood.

The metabolism of the malaria parasite is largely dependent on the digestion of red cell haemoglobin, which is transformed into malaria pigment. Pigment is absent in the ring stage and becomes detectable only in late trophozoite and the schizont stage. The malaria pigment may be yellowish-brown or dark brown in colour (Table 5.1).

Gametogony: After malaria parasites have undergone erythrocytic schizogony for certain period, some merozoites develop within red cells into male and female gametocytes known as **microgametocytes** and **macrogametocytes** respectively (Figs. 5.1, 5.2 and 5.8). All merozoites emerging from a single schizont transform into gametocytes of the same sex and in most *Plasmodium* species the process of gametocytogenesis leads to a female-biased ratio.

Mature gametocytes of *P. vivax*, *P. malariae* and *P. ovale* are round, but the gametocytes of *P. falciparum* are elongated or crescent-shaped (Figs. 5.2 and 5.8). They develop in the red blood cells of the capillaries of internal organs like spleen and bone marrow. Only mature gametocytes are found in the peripheral blood. They do not cause any febrile condition in human host. These are produced for the propagation and continuance of the species.

A variety of factors have been shown to stimulate gametocytogenesis, including hyperparasitaemia, anaemia, and antimalarial drug treatment and it appears as though the parasite is capable of sensing hostile conditions, and by transforming into gametocytes, prepares to escape into a new host.

The host carrying gametocytes is known as **carrier**. The microgametocytes of all the species of

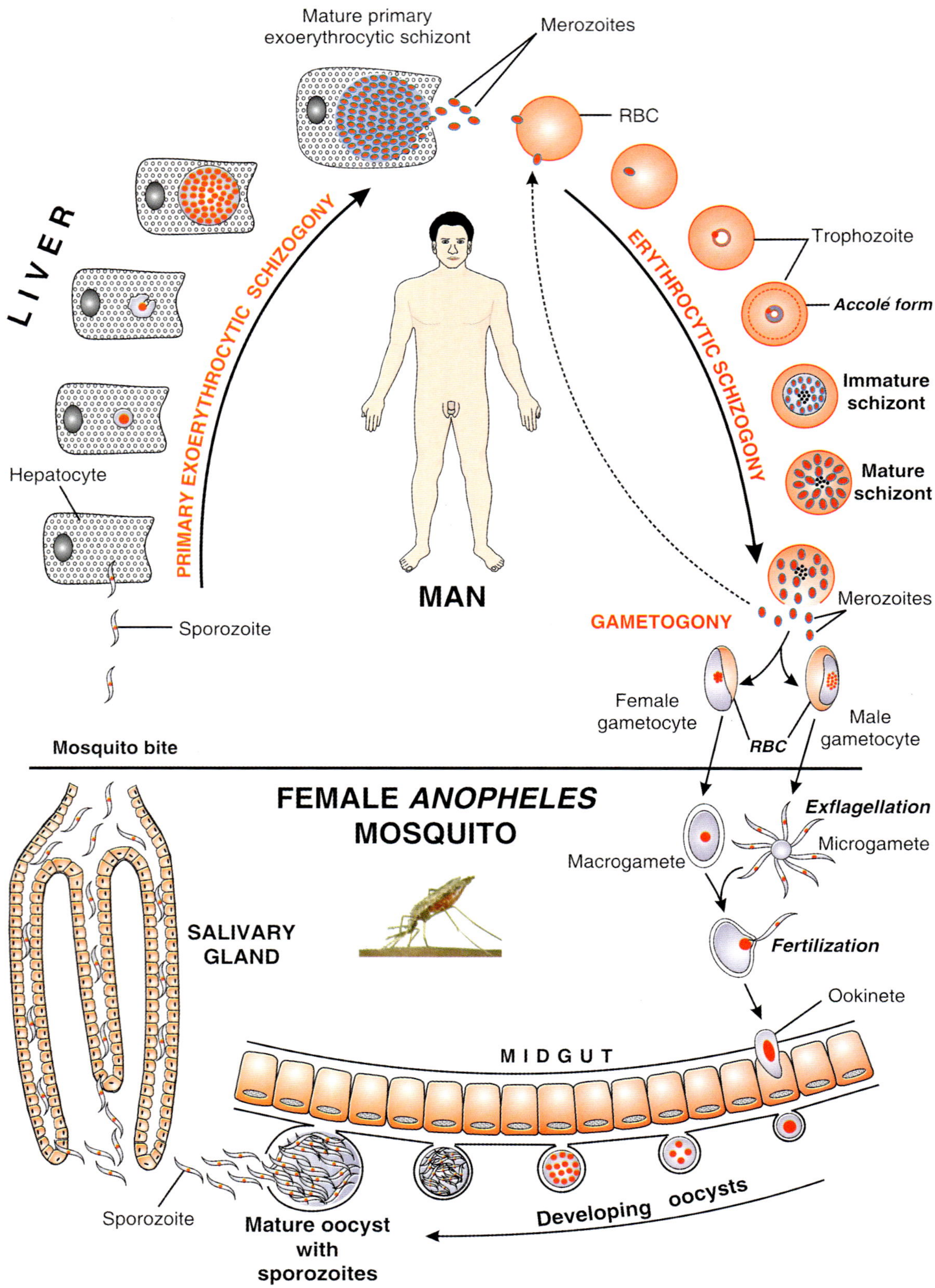

Fig. 5.1. Life cycle of malaria parasite.

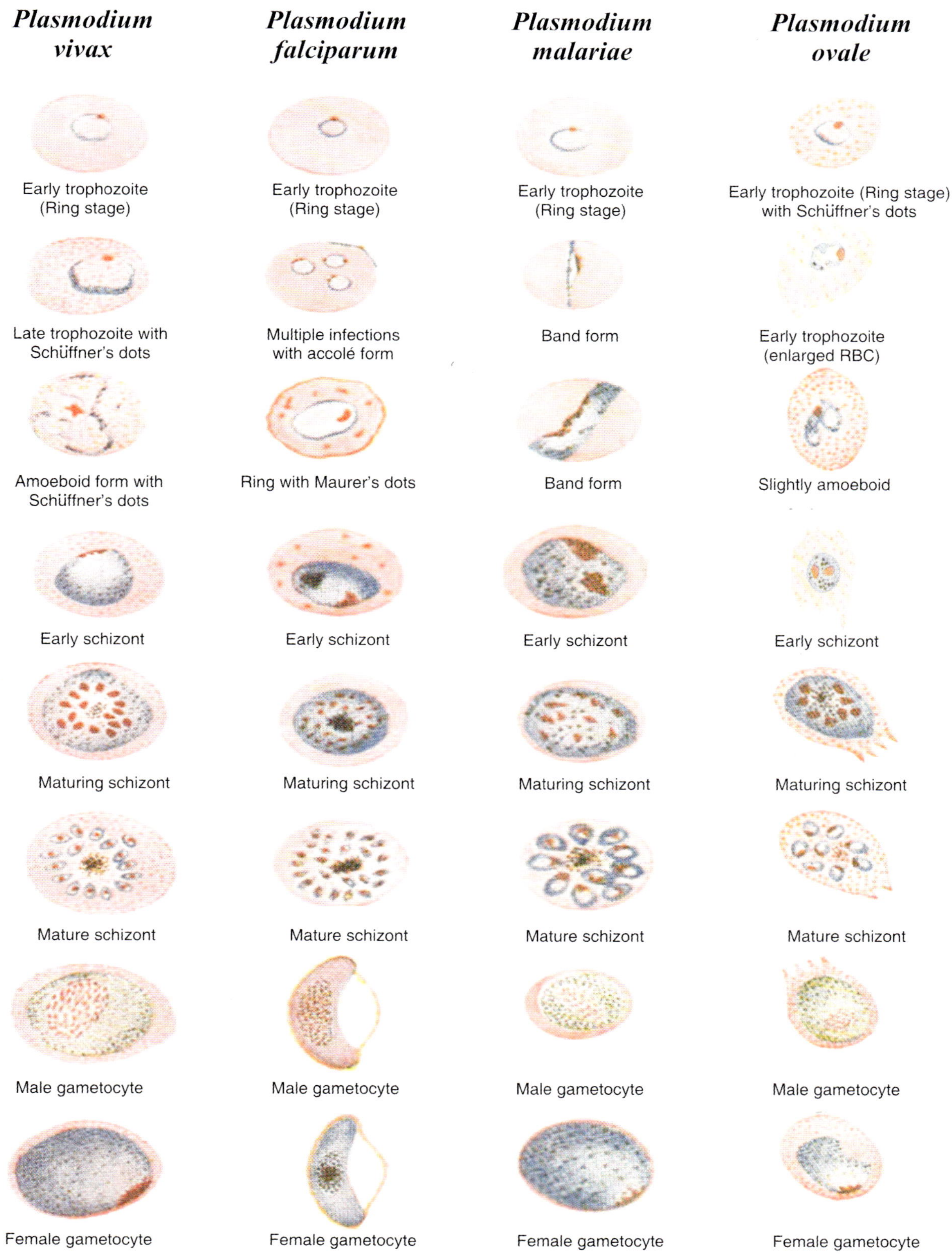

Fig. 5.2. Morphological forms of malaria parasites.

Table 5.1. Differential characters of erythrocytic phase of plasmodia of man

	P. vivax	*P. falciparum*	*P. malariae*	*P. ovale*
1. Forms in peripheral blood	Trophozoites, schizonts and gametocytes.	Rings and crescents (gametocytes).	Trophozoites, schizonts and gametocytes.	Trophozoites, schizonts and gametocytes.
2. Early trophozoite or ring stage	Large, 2.5 μm in diameter, usually one prominent chromatin dot, sometimes two, cytoplasm opposite the chromatin dot thicker, usually one and occasionally two rings in one red blood cell.	Small, delicate, 1.25–1.5 μm in diameter, often with two chromatin dots, two rings in one red blood cell common. Some parasites lie along the red cell membrane. These are known as accolé forms.	Similar to that of *P. vivax.*	Similar to that of *P. vivax.*
3. Late trophozoite	Large, markedly amoeboid, prominent vacuole.	Medium-sized, compact and rounded.	Small, compact, band-shaped, slightly amoeboid, vacuole disappears early.	Slightly amoeboid.
4. Schizont	Large, 9–10 μm in diameter, almost fills an enlarged red cell.	Small, 4.5–5.0 μm in diameter, fills two-thirds of normal-sized red blood cell which is not enlarged.	Small, 6.5–7.0 μm in diameter, almost fills a normal-sized red blood cell.	Small, 6.2 μm in diameter, fills about three quarters of slightly enlarged red blood cell.
5. Number of merozoites	12–24	14–32	6–12	8–12
6. Microgametocytes	Spherical, 9–10 μm in diameter, compact, no vacuole, diffuse chromatin, cytoplasm stains light blue or reddish.	Crescent-shaped (banana-shaped), 8–10 μm × 2–3 μm, chromatin diffuse.	Similar to that of *P. vivax* but smaller.	Similar to that of *P. vivax* but smaller.
7. Macrogametocytes	Spherical, 10–12 μm in diameter, compact, larger than microgametocyte, compact chromatin, cytoplasm stains dark blue.	Crescent-shaped, longer and more slender, 10–12 μm × 2–3 μm, chromatin compact, cytoplasm stains dark blue.	Similar to that of *P. vivax* but smaller.	Similar to that of *P. vivax* but smaller.
8. Malaria pigment	Yellowish-brown; fine granules	Dark brown; one or two solid blocks	Dark brown coarse granules	Dark yellowish-brown, coarser than those of *P. vivax*
9. Age of red blood cells invaded	Young	All ages (young and old)	Old	Young
10. Alterations in infected red cell	Enlarged, pale and the portion of the cytoplasm not occupied by the parasite shows a dotted or stippled appearance, called Schüffner's dots. With Leishman stain they appear as fine pink granules.	Normal size and possesses 6–12 Maurer's dots which stain brick-red with Leishman stain.	Normal size and occasionally show fine stippling (Ziemann's dots) on prolonged staining.	Enlarged, pale, James's dots resembling Schüffner's dots appear early and infected cell may be oval.
11. Duration of erythrocytic schizogony	48 hours	36–48 hours	72 hours	48 hours
12. Presence of secondary exoerythrocytic cycle	Yes	No	No	Yes

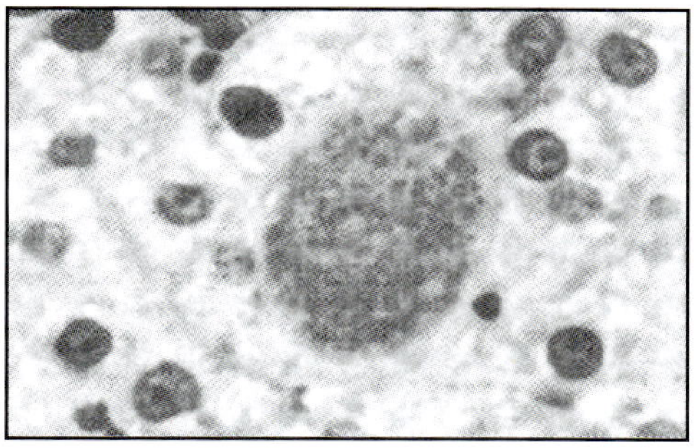

Fig. 5.3. Primary exo-erythrocytic schizont in the liver (Giemsa stain, × 400).

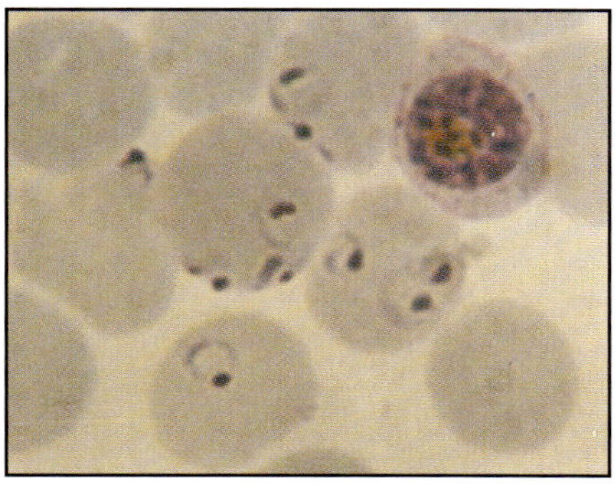

Fig. 5.4. Early trophozoites (ring forms) of *Plasmodium falciparum* (Giemsa stain, × 1000).

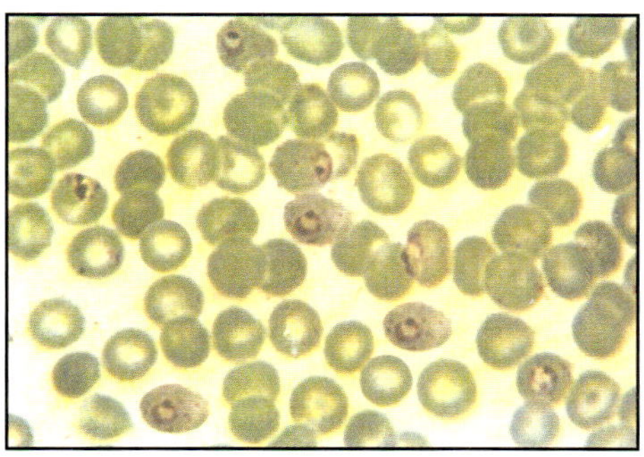

Fig. 5.5. Early trophozoites (ring forms) of *Plasmodium vivax* (Giemsa stain, × 1000).

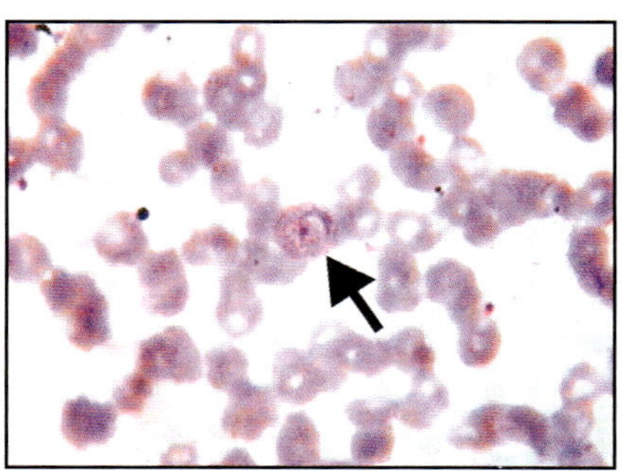

Fig. 5.6. Late trophozoite of *Plasmodium vivax* (Giemsa stain, × 1000).

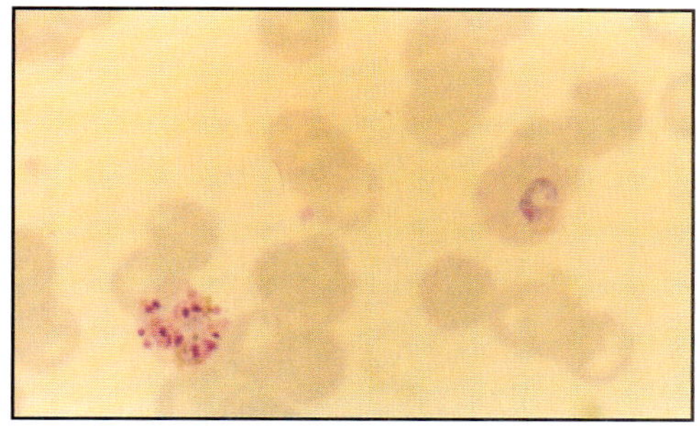

Fig. 5.7. Late trophozoite and mature schizont of *Plasmodium vivax* (Giemsa stain, × 1000).

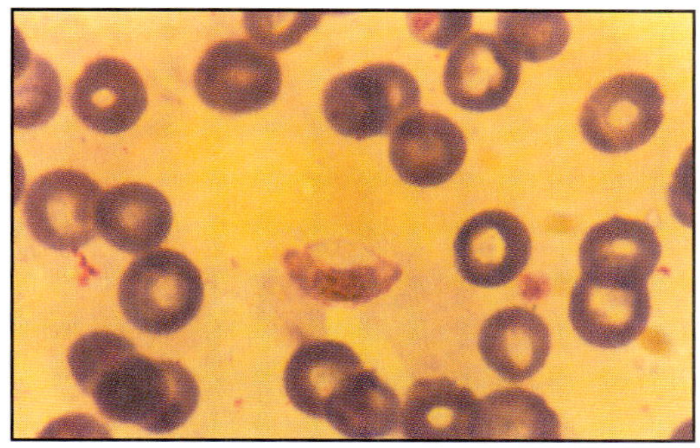

Fig. 5.8. Gametocyte (crescent) of *Plasmodium falciparum* in peripheral blood (Giemsa stain, × 1000).

Plasmodium are smaller in size. Cytoplasm stains light blue and the nucleus (chromatin) is diffuse and large. On the other hand the macrogametocytes are larger, the cytoplasm stains deep blue and the nucleus is compact and small (Table 5.1).

Although the longevity of mature gametocytes may exceed several weeks, their half-life in the blood stream may be only 2 or 3 days, while waiting for the mosquito to take them up.

Secondary exo-erythrocytic or dormant schizogony: In case of *P. vivax* and *P. ovale,* some sporozoites on entering into hepatocytes enter into a resting (dormant) stage before undergoing asexual multiplication while others undergo multiplication without delay. The resting stage of the parasite is rounded, 4–6 μm in diameter, uninucleate and is known as **hypnozoite** or **sleeping form**. After a period of weeks, months or years (usually up to 2 years) hypnozoites are reactivated to become secondary exo-erythrocytic schizonts and release merozoites which infect red blood cells producing **relapse** of malaria. The relapse, therefore, is the situation in which the erythrocytic infection is eliminated and a relapse occurs later because of a new invasion of the RBCs from liver merozoites.

Hypnozoites are not formed in case of *P. falciparum* and *P. malariae,* therefore, relapse does not occur in disease caused by these species. On the other hand, the situation in which the RBC infection is not eliminated by the immune system or by therapy and the numbers in the RBCs begin to increase again with subsequent clinical symptoms is called a **recrudescence**. Drug resistance creates a situation in which the initial peak of parasitaemia is only partially controlled and a recrudescence of resistant parasites occurs shortly after. All species of *Plasmodium* may cause a recrudescence. *P. malariae* can survive in the peripheral blood at a very low level of parasitaemia for a considerable time (10 years or more), occasionally producing detectable peaks with a recrudescence of clinical symptoms.

Mosquito cycle

Sexual cycle actually starts in the human host itself by the formation of gametocytes which are present in the peripheral blood. Both asexual and sexual forms of the parasite are ingested by female *Anopheles* mosquito during its blood meal from the patient. *The female Anopheles mosquito has a stout proboscis which can pierce the human skin like a needle. On the other hand the proboscis of the male is not stout, it is flexible; hence it cannot pierce through the skin.* In the mosquito, only the mature sexual forms are capable of further development and rest die. In order to infect a mosquito, **the blood of human carrier must contain at least 12 gametocytes/µl and the number of female gametocytes must be in excess of the number of males**.

In the stomach of the mosquito (Fig. 5.1) from one microgametocyte eight thread-like filamentous structures called **microgametes** are formed by the process of exflagellation. The macrogametocyte does not show any exflagellation. It develops into a **macrogamete**, its nucleus shifts to the surface, where a projection is formed. **Fertilization** occurs when a microgamete penetrates this projection. The fertilized macrogamete is known as **zygote**. This occurs in 20 minutes to 2 hours. In next 24 hours, the zygote lengthens and matures into **ookinete**, a motile vermiculate stage. It penetrates the epithelial lining of the stomach of the mosquito and comes to lie between the external border of the epithelial cell and peritrophic membrane.

Here it develops into **oocyst**. It is rounded, 6–12 µm in diameter with a single vesicular nucleus. It increases in size to reach a diameter of 40–50 µm. Inside this develop sporozoites. The number of sporozoites in each oocyst varies from a few hundreds to a few thousands and number of oocysts in the stomach wall varies from a few to more than a hundred. On about 10th day the oocyst is fully mature, ruptures and releases sporozoites in the body cavity of the mosquito. Through the body fluid the sporozoites are distributed to various organs of the body except the ovaries. They have special predilection for salivary glands and ultimately reach in maximum numbers in the salivary ducts. At this stage the mosquito is capable of transmitting infection to man.

Only the sporozoite, merozoite and ookinete, which are designed for invasion of the hepatocyte, erythrocyte or midgut epithelial cell of the mosquito respectively, possess a surface coat and the specialized apical end characteristic of Coccidia. Other stages of the life cycle, which are designed for growth and development within the host cell, lack these invasion organelles.

Culture

Trager and Jensen (1976), successfully cultivated and maintained *P. falciparum in vitro*, in human red blood cells. They used medium RPMI 1640 in a continuous-flow system in which human erythrocytes were in a shallow stationary layer covered by a shallow layer of medium. The medium was made to flow slowly and continuously over the layer of settled red cells, under an atmosphere with 7% carbon dioxide and 1–5% oxygen. This culture system is now widely used for the production of antigen.

Pathogenicity

Man develops infection by the bite of infected female *Anopheles* mosquito. However, infection may also be transmitted by:

- Transfusion of blood from a patient of malaria. This is known as **transfusion malaria**. Plasmodia can remain viable in refrigerated blood for up to 10 days.
- Transmission of infection to foetus in utero through some placental defect. This is known as **congenital malaria**.
- By the use of contaminated syringes particularly in drug addicts. This is known as **"mainline" malaria**.

The above conditions are also known as **trophozoite-induced malaria**. In these conditions there is no primary and secondary exoerythrocytic schizogony, incubation period is short and there is no relapse.

After an **incubation period** of 12 days for *P. falciparum*, 13–17 days for *P. vivax* and *P. ovale,* and

28–30 days for *P. malariae* patient develops malaria. However, in case of *P. vivax* and *P. ovale*, if all sporozoites that invaded hepatocytes transformed into hypnozoites, the first symptoms may occur months to as many as 3 years after exposure. The typical picture of malaria consists of febrile paroxysm, anaemia and splenomegaly.

Febrile paroxysm

It generally begins in the early afternoon and comprises of three successive stages – cold stage, hot stage and sweating stage. In the cold stage, lasting for 15–60 minutes, the patient experiences intense cold and shivering. This is followed by hot stage, lasting for 2–6 hours, when the patient feels intense hot. Patient develops high fever (40°–40.6°C), severe headache, nausea and vomiting. Thereafter, fever ends by crisis accompanied by profuse sweating.

The periodicity of the attack varies with the species of the infecting parasite. The periodicity is 48 hours in *P. vivax* (**benign tertian**) and *P. ovale* (**ovale tertian**), and 72 hours in *P. malariae* (**quartan**). However, with *P. falciparum*, the cycles of different broods of parasite do not become synchronized as they do in other species. Therefore, typical tertian fever is not usual in falciparum (**malignant tertian**) malaria. **Quotidian periodicity** with the fever occurring at 24 hour intervals may be due to two broods of tertian parasites maturing on successive days or due to mixed infection. The periodicity of paroxysms in *P. knowlesi* is 24 hours.

Mixed infection with more than one species of *Plasmodium* is more common than previously suspected. Febrile paroxysms follow the completion of erythrocytic schizogony when the mature schizont ruptures releasing merozoites, malarial pigment and other parasitic debris. Macrophages and polymorphs phagocytose these and release endogenous pyrogens leading to pyrexia. Primary as well as secondary exo-erythrocytic schizogony and gametogony do not contribute to clinical illness.

Anaemia

After a few paroxysms, anaemia of a microcytic or a normocytic hypochromic type develops as a result of:

- Direct RBC lysis as a result of life cycle of the parasite.
- Splenic removal of both infected and uninfected RBCs (coated with immune complexes).
- Autoimmune lysis of coated infected and uninfected RBCs.
- Decreased incorporation of iron into heme.
- Increased fragility of RBCs.
- Decreased RBC production from bone marrow suppression.

Since *P. vivax* and *P. ovale* infect only young RBCs, therefore, the parasitaemia is usually limited to around 2–5% of available RBCs. *P. malariae* invades primarily the older RBCs, so that the number of infected cells is somewhat limited. *P. falciparum* tends to invade all ages of RBCs, and the proportion of infected cells may exceed 50%.

Splenomegaly

After a few paroxysms, spleen gets enlarged and becomes palpable (Fig. 5.9). Splenomegaly is due to **massive proliferation of macrophages** which phagocytose both parasitized and non-parasitized red blood cells.

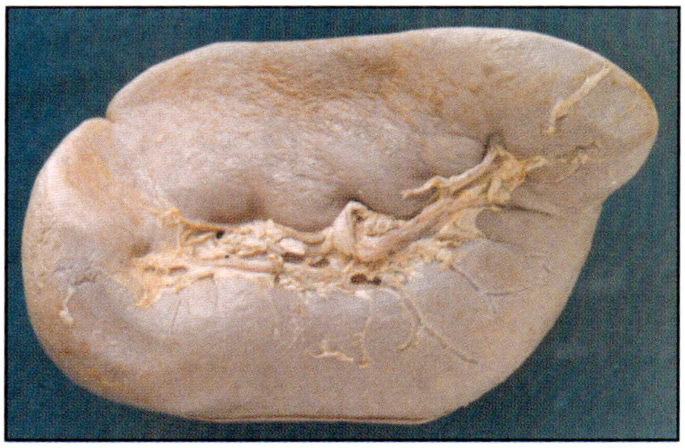

Fig. 5.9. Enlarged malarial spleen.

Non-immune pregnant women are susceptible to all the usual manifestations of malaria. Moreover, they have an increased risk of abortion, stillbirth, premature delivery and of low birth weight of their infants. Pregnant women are particularly prone to hypoglycaemia and pulmonary oedema.

The characteristic lesions of falciparum malaria are due to blockade of small vessels by **sticky parasitized erythrocytes**. This leads to tissue hypoxia.

Pernicious malaria

Pernicious malaria is a complex of **life-threatening complications** that sometimes supervene in acute falciparum malaria. It is due to heavy parasitization and is of three types:

1. Cerebral malaria
2. Algid malaria
3. Septicaemic malaria

Cerebral malaria

Cerebral malaria is a severe complication of falciparum malaria and frequently leads to death, even when appropriate therapy has been given. It is characterized by **hyperpyrexia**, **coma** and **paralysis**. Capillaries of the brain are plugged with parasitized red blood cells, each cell containing malaria pigment (Fig. 5.10). In holoendemic areas of malaria, cerebral malaria occurs in children between 6 months and 5 years, most commonly in children aged 3–4 years.

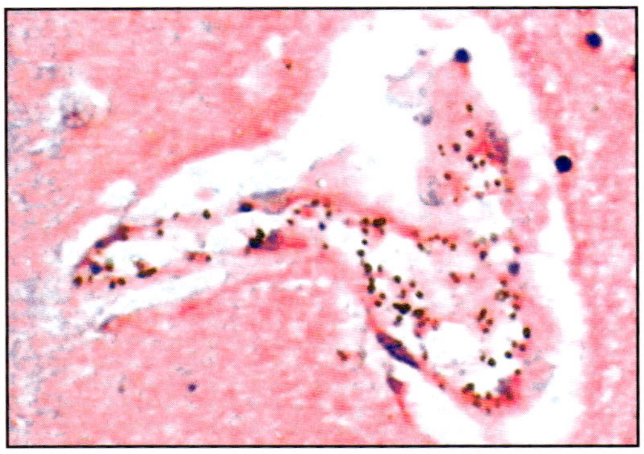

Fig. 5.10. Cerebral malaria. The malaria pigment inside the erythrocytes is clearly visible (haematoxin and eosin stain, × 400).

Algid malaria

It resembles surgical shock with cold clammy skin, peripheral circulatory failure and profound shock. Patient may also develop vomiting and diarrhoea or dysentery.

Septicaemic malaria

It is characterized by a high degree of prostration, there is high continuous fever with involvement of various organs.

Blackwater fever

It is a manifestation of repeated infections with *P. falciparum* which were inadequately treated with quinine. Sometimes resumption of quinine therapy for new attack is followed by massive destruction of RBCs, fever, haemoglobinuria and renal failure.

The exact mechanism of haemolysis in blackwater fever is not known. An **autoimmune mechanism** has been suggested. Parasitized and quininized red blood cells, during previous infection, act as antigen against which antibodies are formed. With subsequent infection and treatment with quinine, there is massive destruction of both infected and uninfected red blood cells. As other antimalarials have replaced quinine, blackwater fever has now become rare.

Characteristics of *Plasmodium falciparum*

Of all the human malaria parasites *P. falciparum* is the most pathogenic and responsible for '**malignant tertian malaria**', a form of the disease which runs an acute course in nonimmune patients and is frequently fatal if untreated. It is generally confined to tropical or subtropical areas because its development in the mosquito is greatly retarded when the temperature falls below 20°C. Characteristic biological features of *P. falciparum* are as follows:

- It infects **erythrocytes of all ages** (young and old).
- Membrane protuberances (knobs) appear on the surface of the erythrocytes infected with late-stage trophozoites or schizonts, so they stick to endothelial cells in various tissues. This cytoadherence is responsible for the sequestration of the parasite.
- The ability of *P. falciparum* to remain sequestered by cytoadherence to the capillary lining of certain tissues is regarded as a selective advantage as such parasites can avoid frequent passage through spleen and thus exposure to immune effector mechanisms.
- The duration of primary exo-erythrocytic or pre-erythrocytic schizogony is short (6 days).
- It **does not produce hypnozoites**, therefore, relapses do not occur.
- Primary exo-erythrocytic or pre-erythrocytic schizogony produces upto 30,000 merozoites; erythrocytic schizogony produces 14–32 merozoites and sporogony produces upto 20,000 sporozoites which may be the cause of its virulence.
- In the peripheral blood rings and gametocytes (crescents) are seen, whereas late trophozoites and schizonts are only seen exceptionally.
- The level of parasitemia may be high and **multiple infection** in a single erythrocyte is common.
- Some parasites lie along the erythrocyte membrane, these are known as **accolé forms**.

Host immunity

Immunity in malaria is of two types:

1. Innate immunity
2. Acquired immunity

Innate immunity

This refers to inherent, non-immune mechanisms of

host defence against malaria. This is due to age of red blood cells, nature of haemoglobin, enzyme content of red blood cells and presence or absence of certain factors.

Age of red blood cells

P. falciparum infects both young and old red blood cells while *P. vivax* and *P. ovale* infect only young erythrocytes, and *P. malariae* only old erythrocytes.

Nature of haemoglobin

Presence of abnormal haemoglobin like thalassemia haemoglobin and foetal haemoglobin confers resistance against all *Plasmodium* spp., while sickle cell anaemia trait and haemoglobin E protect against *P. falciparum* and *P. vivax* respectively.

Enzyme content of red blood cells

A genetic deficiency known as glucose-6-phosphate dehydrogenase (G6PD) trait confers some protection against *P. falciparum* infection. This enzyme is essential for respiratory process of the parasite.

Presence or absence of certain factors

The presence of the Duffy factor increases the susceptibility to malaria. It is believed that Duffy factor present on the surface of erythrocytes acts as receptor for attachment of malaria parasite.

Acquired immunity

Acquired immunity in malaria involves both humoral and cellular immunity. Antibodies against sporozoites and asexual and sexual blood stages develop in malaria patients. Antibodies (IgM, IgG and IgA) against asexual blood stages may protect by inhibiting red cell invasion and antibodies against sexual stages are believed to reduce malaria transmission. A variety of cellular mechanisms may play a role in conferring protection against malaria. These include natural killer activity and activated macrophages. The latter phagocytose and induce extracellular killing of target cells. T cells are crucial for malaria immunity. Their major function seems to provide help for the production of antibodies and to activate macrophages.

Immunity produced following infection with malaria parasites is species-specific, stage-specific and strain-specific and the immunity lasts only till original infection remains active. This is known as **concomitant immunity** (previously called **premunition** or **infection-immunity**).

Malaria parasites like many other microorganisms, are **capable of periodically changing the expression of their antigens**. This provides the parasite with a powerful means for evading host immunity.

Laboratory diagnosis

Malaria is one of the few parasitic infections considered to be **immediately life-threatening**, and a patient with the diagnosis of ***P. falciparum* malaria should be considered a medical emergency because the disease can be rapidly fatal**.

Microscopy

Diagnosis of malaria can be established by demonstration of malaria parasites in the blood (Figs. 5.4–5.8). Thick and thin smears of the blood are prepared on the same or different slides. Blood is taken by pricking a finger or ear lobule before starting treatment with antimalarials. For preparation of thick smear take a large drop of blood on the slide. Spread it in an area of 12 mm square. Dehaemoglobinization of thick smear is done by keeping the slide in distilled water in Koplin's jar in vertical position for 5–10 minutes till the slide becomes white and then it is dried in air. Both thick and thin smears are stained with Leishman stain. The smears are then examined under oil-immersion lens.

The parasites are most abundant in peripheral blood late in the febrile paroxysm (a few hours after the height of paroxysm). Therefore, blood for smear should be collected at this period. All asexual erythrocytic stages, as well as gametocytes can be seen in peripheral blood in infection with *P. vivax, P. malariae* and *P. ovale,* but in *P. falciparum* infection, only the ring forms and crescent-shaped gametocytes can be seen. Late trophozoite and schizont stages of *P. falciparum* are usually confined to the internal organs and appear in peripheral blood only in severe or pernicious malaria.

The occurrence of **multiple rings** in an individual red blood cell with **accolé forms** is diagnostic of *P. falciparum* infection. Malaria pigment may be demonstrated inside the monocytes and polymorphonuclear leucocytes. The presence of malaria pigment only, in the absence of malaria parasites, suggests *P.*

falciparum infection. Schüffner's, Maurer's, Ziemann's and James's dots can be seen in the red blood cells infected with *P. vivax*, *P. falciparum*, *P. malariae* and *P. ovale* respectively. Red blood cells are enlarged in *P. vivax* infection.

Thin film is examined first and if parasites are found, there is no need for examining the thick film. If parasites are not seen in thin film in a few minutes the thick film should be examined. If parasites are seen in thick film but identity is not clear, the thin film is re-examined more thoroughly to determine the identity of the species. The parasites are more along **the upper and lower margins of the "tail" of the film**. Examination of thin film usually takes 15–20 minutes ($\geq$ 300 oil-immersion fields), and examination of thick film usually requires 5–10 minutes (at least 100 oil-immersion fields).

The staining of films with acridine orange, which can be examined either under a flourescence microscope or a microscope equipped with an interference filter system, allows quicker screening of films, because parasites are more readily recognized and a lower power lens may be used.

Conventional light microscopy is the established method for the laboratory confirmation of malaria.

Advantages

- It is sensitive. When used by skilled and careful technicians, microscopy can detect densities as low as 5–10 parasites per µl of blood.
- It is informative. When parasites are found, they can be characterized in terms of their species and of the circulating stage.
- It is relatively inexpensive.
- It can provide permanent record (the smears) of the diagnostic findings.

Disadvantages

Microscopy suffers from three main disadvantages:

1. It is labour-intensive and time-consuming, normally requiring 60–120 minutes from specimen collection to result.
2. It is exacting and depends absolutely on good techniques, reagents, microscopes and most importantly well-trained and well-supervised technicians.
3. There are often long delays in providing the microscopy results to the clinician so that decisions on treatment are often taken without the benefit of the results.

RAPID DIAGNOSTIC TESTS (RDTs)

RDTs are based on the detection of malaria antigens in lysed blood, using immunochromatographic methods. Most frequently they employ a dipstick or test strip bearing monoclonal antibodies directed against the target parasite antigens. The tests can be performed in about 15 minutes. Several commercial test kits are currently available.

Antigens targeted by currently available RDTs

- Histidine-rich protein II (HRP-II) is water-soluble protein produced by trophozoites and young (but not mature) gametocytes of *P. falciparum*. Commercial kits currently available detect HRP-II from *P. falciparum* only.
- Parasite lactate dehydrogenase (pLDH) is produced by asexual and sexual stages (gametocytes) of malaria parasites. Test kits currently available detect pLDH from all four important *Plasmodium* species that infect humans. They can distinguish *P. falciparum* from the non-*falciparum* species, but cannot distinguish between *P. vivax*, *P. ovale* and *P. malariae*.
- Other antigen(s) that is/are present in all four important species are also targeted in kits that combine detection of the HRP-II antigen of *P. falciparum* together with that of an, as yet unspecified, "pan-malarial" antigen of other species.

General test procedure

- Test strip (most often nitrocellulose) (Fig. 5.11) consists of a sample pad, three detection lines containing capture antibodies specific for *P. falciparum*, all *Plasmodium* spp. and control antibody respectively and an absorbent pad.
- Depending on the kit, 2–50 µl of finger prick blood specimen is collected. Some manufacturers state that anticoagulated blood or plasma can also be used.
- The blood specimen is mixed in a separate test tube or a well, or on a sample pad with a buffer solution that contains a haemolysing compound as well as specific antibody that is labelled with a visually detectable marker such as colloidal gold. If the malaria antigen is present, an antigen-antibody complex is formed.
- The labelled antigen-antibody complex migrates up the test strip by capillary action towards the detection lines containing capture antibodies that have been pre-deposited during manufacture.

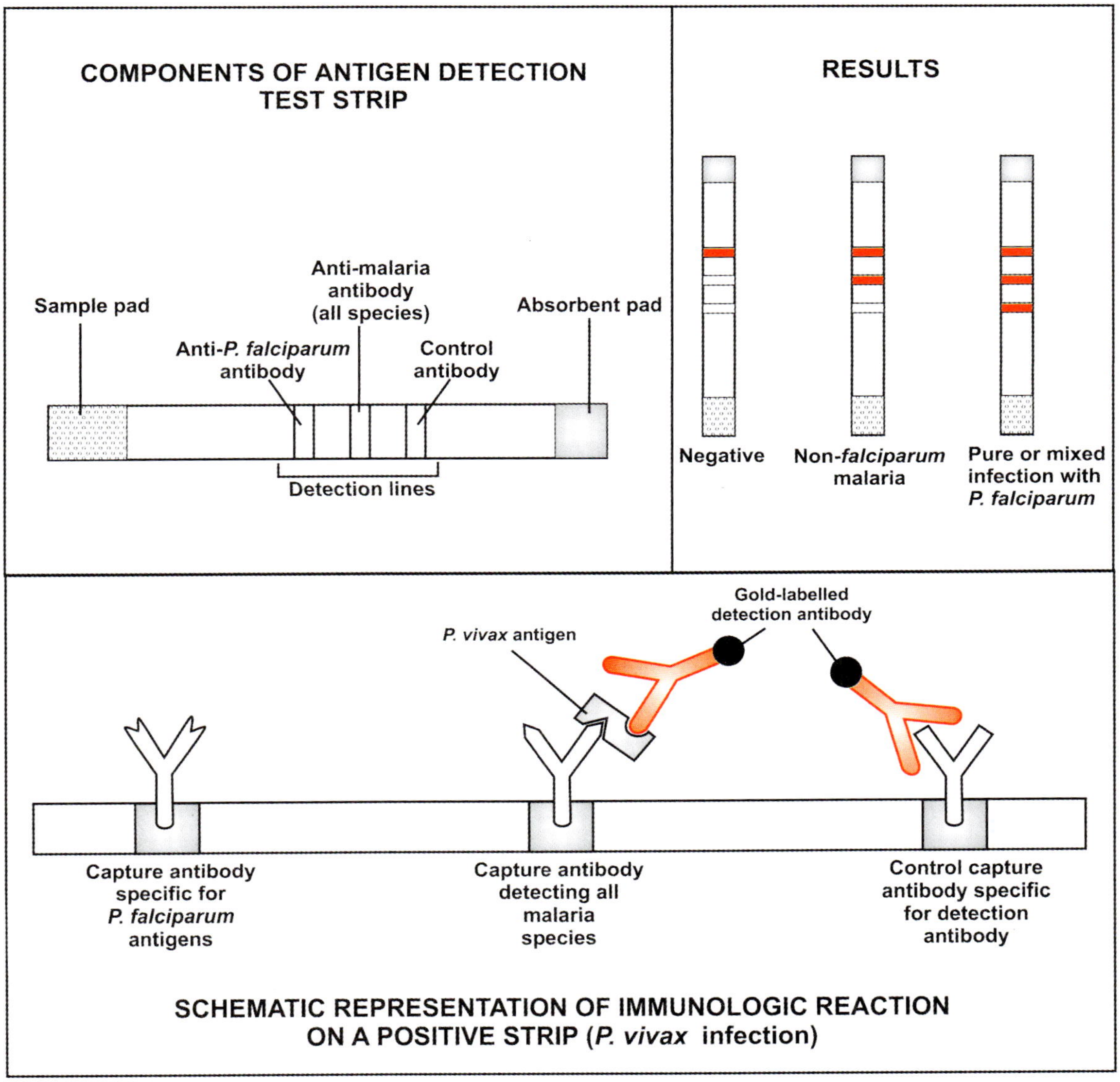

Fig. 5.11. General test procedure of rapid diagnostic test for the diagnosis of malaria.

- A washing buffer is then added to remove the haemoglobin and permit visualization of any coloured line on the strip.
- If the blood contains malaria antigen (*P. falciparum* or all *Plasmodium* spp.), the labelled antigen-antibody complex will be immobilized at the corresponding pre-deposited line of capture antibody and will be visually detectable. The complete test run time varies from 5–15 minutes.

Some RDTs detect the four *Plasmodium* spp. that infect humans, depending on the antigens on which they are based. Some RDTs detect *P. falciparum* only, while others detect *P. falciparum* and the other malaria parasites on two separate bands. No commercial RDT has been reported to differentiate reliably between *P. vivax*, *P. ovale* and *P. malariae*, although research to develop such a test is continuing.

The sensitivity of the RDTs has been most studied for *P. falciparum*, since the *P. falciparum* kits, targeting mostly *P. falciparum* HRP-II, have been available for a longer time. RDTs for *P. falciparum* generally achieve a sensitivity of > 90% at parasite densities above 100 parasites per μl of blood. Below the level of 100 parasites per μl of blood, sensitivity decreases markedly. RDT sensitivity for non-*falciparum* spp. has been less extensively studied. The specificity of RDTs is also > 90%. The predictive values, both positive and negative, vary with parasite prevalence and are often found to be acceptable.

Advantages of RDTs over microscopy

- RDTs are simple to perform and to interpret.
- They do not require electricity, special equipment or training in microscopy.
- Health workers with minimal skill can be trained in RDT techniques in periods varying from three hours to one day.
- Since RDTs detect circulating antigens, they may detect *P. falciparum* infection even when the parasites are sequestered in the deep vascular compartment and thus undetectable by microscopic examination of a peripheral blood smear.

Disadvantages of RDTs

- RDTs are more expensive than microscopy.
- Kits cannot differentiate between *P. vivax*, *P. ovale* and *P. malariae* nor can they distinguish pure *P. falciparum* infections from mixed infections that include *P. falciparum*.
- RDTs that detect antigens produced by gametocytes (such as pLDH) can give positive results in infections where only gametocytes are present. Gametocytes do not cause any febrile condition, and those of *P. falciparum* are not affected by schizonticidal drugs. Such positive RDT results can thus lead to erroneous interpretations and unnecessary treatment.

QUANTITATIVE BUFFY COAT (QBC) TEST

The QBC test developed by Becton and Dickenson Inc. is a new method for identifying the malaria parasite in the peripheral blood. It involves staining of the centrifuged and compressed red cell layer with acridine orange and its examination under UV light source. It is fast, easy and claimed to be more sensitive than the traditional thick smear examination.

Method

The QBC tube is a high-precision glass hematocrit tube, pre-coated internally with acridine orange stain and potassium oxalate. It is filled with 60 µl of blood from a finger, ear or heel puncture. A clear plastic closure is then attached. A precisely made cylindrical float, designed to be suspended in the packed red blood cells, is inserted. The tube is centrifuged at 12,000 rpm for 5 minutes. The components of the buffy coat separate according to their densities, forming discrete bands (Fig. 5.12A). Because the float occupies 90% of the internal lumen of the tube, the leucocyte and the thrombocyte cell band widths and the top-most area of red cells are enlarged to 10 times normal. The QBC tube is placed on the tube holder (Fig. 5.12B) and examined using a standard white light microscope equipped with the UV microscope adapter, and epi-illuminated microscope objective. Fluorescing parasites are then observed at the red blood cell/white blood cell interface.

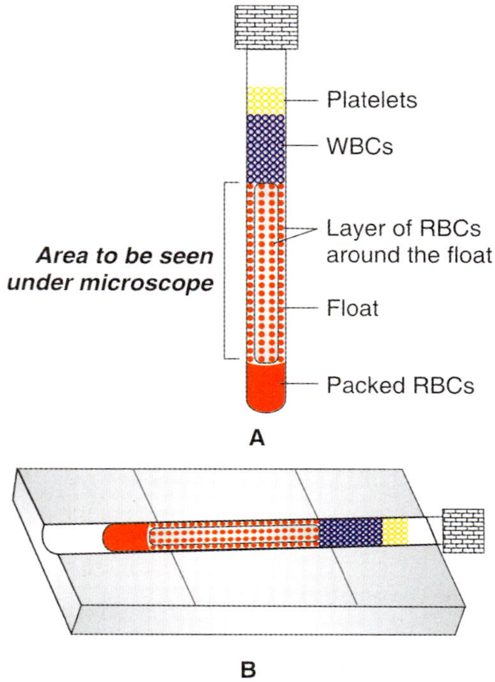

Fig. 5.12. Quantitative buffy coat (QBC) test.

The key feature of the method is centrifugation and thereby concentration of the red blood cells in a predictable area of the QBC tube, making detection easy and fast. Red cells containing plasmodia are less dense than normal ones and concentrate just below the leucocytes, at the top of the erythrocyte column. The float forces all the surrounding red cells into the 40 µm space between its outside circumference and the inside of the tube. Since the parasites contain DNA which takes up the acridine orange stain, they appear as bright specks of light among the non-fluorescing red cells. Virtually all of the parasites found in the 60 µl of blood can be visualized by rotating the tube under the microscope. A negative test can be reported within one minute and positive result within minutes. The comparison between peripheral blood smear and QBC test for the detection of malaria parasites is given in Table 5.2.

Table 5.2. Comparison between peripheral smear and QBC test for the detection of malaria parasites

	Peripheral smear	QBC
Method	Cumbersome	Easy
Time	Longer, 60–120 minutes	Faster, 15–30 minutes
Sensitivity	5 parasites/μl in thick film and 200/μl in thin film	Claimed to be more sensitive, at least as good as a thick film
Specificity	Gold standard	Artifacts may be reported as positive by not-so-well-trained technicians
Species identification	Accurate	Not possible
Cost	Inexpensive	Costly equipment and consumables
Acceptability	100%	Not so
Availability	Everywhere	Limited

The QBC method is reported to have a good sensitivity for the detection of malaria parasites, and has also been applied, to a lesser extent, to other parasites such as trypanosomes, microfilaria and *Babesia* spp.

OTHER TECHNIQUES

Other diagnostic methods include polymerase chain reaction and antibody detection by serology (indirect haemagglutination, indirect fluorescent antibody and enzyme-linked immunosorbent assay). However, serology only measures prior exposure and not specifically current infection.

Treatment

Chloroquine was the standard treatment for acute malaria for many years. **However, resistance to this drug in *P. falciparum* is widespread.** Less commonly *P. vivax* may also be chloroquine-resistant. **Quinine is the most reliable alternative to chloroquine** for the treatment of malaria caused by chloroquine-resistant strains. Tetracycline and clindamycin exhibit some anti-malarial activity and are used as an adjunct to quinine therapy. **Mefloquine** and **halofantrine** are also active against chloroquine-resistant strains, but resistance to these drugs has also been reported.

Chloroquine and quinine do not eliminate exo-erythrocytic parasites in the liver. For this primaquine (8-aminoquinoline drug) should be used. However, this drug may precipitate haemolysis in individuals who are deficient in the enzyme glucose-6-phosphate dehydrogenase.

Drug resistance in malaria parasites

Effective, affordable, and safe treatment of malaria, particularly falciparum malaria, is becoming increasingly difficult as resistance to chloroquine and other antimalarial drugs continues to spread throughout the tropics. Chloroquine-resistant *P. falciparum* was first reported in Columbia and Thailand in the late 1950s. It has now spread to more than 40 countries in Asia including India, South and Central America, East, West and Central Africa and the Pacific region. Resistance to multiple drugs is common in Southeast Asia. *P. vivax* resistance to chloroquine and to normal doses of primaquine is also spreading with reports of resistance from Thailand, Papua New Guinea, Indonesia, Myanmar, India, Somalia, Central and South America.

Most resistant strains of *P. falciparum* have developed due to:

1. Inadequate drug doses mainly as a result of unregulated drug distribution and prescribing.
2. Lack of adequate drugs.
3. Poor quality of drugs.
4. Incorrect taking of drugs by patients.
5. When insufficient drug is taken to kill the malaria parasites, the mutants survive and multiply. It is also thought that selective pressure favouring naturally occurring resistance mutations increase in areas of intense malaria transmission.

WHO definition and classification of drug resistance

Drug resistance has been defined by the World Health Organization as the ability of a parasite to multiply or to survive in the presence of concentrations of a drug that normally destroy parasites of the same species or prevent their multiplication. Three levels of resistance (R) are defined by the World Health Organization:

RI: Following treatment, parasitaemia clears but a recrudescence occurs.
RII: Following treatment, there is a reduction but not a clearance of parasitaemia.
RIII: Following treatment, there is no reduction of parasitaemia.

The above method of classifying resistance, based on counting trophozoites in blood films for up to 7 days after treatment and monitoring the patient for any subsequent recrudescence is referred to as *in vivo* testing.

Prophylaxis

Malaria control depends upon:

1. Spraying residual insecticides such as DDT or malathion.
2. Spraying the breeding sites with petroleum oils and Paris green (copper acetoarsenite) as larvicides.
3. Flooding and flushing of breeding places.
4. Eliminating breeding places such as lagoons and swamps.
5. Avoiding exposure to mosquito bites by:
   (a) Wearing long-sleeved clothing and trousers after sunset when the insects are most active.
   (b) Using bed nets impregnated with pyrethroids.
   (c) Using an electric mat to vaporize synthetic pyrethroids or burning mosquito coils.
   (d) Application of mosquito repellents containing diethyltoluamide to exposed skin.
6. Taking chemoprophylaxis. Chloroquine and the antifolate drugs pyrimethamine and proguanil have been widely used for antimalarial prophylaxis.
7. Early diagnosis and prompt treatment of patients.

In India, the National Malaria Control Programme operated very successfully for 5 years, bringing down the annual incidence of malaria from 75 million in 1953 to 2 million in 1958. Because of the spectacular success achieved in the control of malaria, the control programme was converted in 1958 into the National Malaria Eradication Programme with the objective of the eradication of the disease. By 1961, the incidence dropped to 50,000 cases and no deaths. However, there have been setbacks from 1970. By 1976, the incidence rose to 6.4 million cases and by 1995, it has covered virtually all parts of India. Particularly distressing is the spread of *P. falciparum* which has become increasingly drug-resistant.

Vaccine

Despite very intensive research since the mid 1970s, no effective malaria vaccine is yet available.

PLASMODIUM KNOWLESI

A fifth species, *P. knowlesi*, which normally infects long-tailed macaques (*Macaca fascicularis*) and pig-tailed macaques (*Macaca nemestrina*), is a significant cause of human malaria in Southeast Asia. It is transmitted by *Anopheles leucosphyrus* group of mosquitoes that reside in the upper canopy of the forests and has infrequent contact with humans. Similar to *P. falciparum*, the erythrocyte invasion by *P. knowlesi* is not restricted to young or old RBCs which allows the development of high levels of parasitemia. It has a short life cycle of 24 hours (quotidian), and the development of the parasite in RBCs is not synchronous. *P. knowlesi* infection is usually misidentified as *P. falciparum* or *P. malariae* because its early trophozoites resemble the ring forms of *P. falciparum* and the later stages mimic those of *P. malariae*. In contrast to *P. falciparum*, *P. knowlesi* does not appear to sequester in the microvasculature, and the neurologic complications seen with *P. falciparum* infection have not been described.

RBCs infected with *P. knowlesi* exhibit a normal morphology, and all developmental stages may be seen in peripheral blood.

P. knowlesi, similar to *P. falciparum* and *P. malariae*, does not appear to produce hypnozoites in the liver. Relapses from the liver are not known to occur.

Human *P. knowlesi* infections have been described in high numbers only in Malaysia; however, because of reports of infection in the neighbouring countries of Thailand, Singapore, Brunei, Indonesia, Myanmar, Vietnam and the Philippines, it appears that *P. knowlesi* is a natural parasite of macaques throughout the Southeast Asia region.

BABESIA

Babesia is named after Babes, who in 1888 described the intraerythrocytic parasite in the blood of cattle and sheep in Romania. It belongs to kingdom Protozoa, phylum Sporozoa, class Coccidia, order Piroplasmida (Table 1.5). In 1893, the parasite was shown to cause the tick-borne disease, **Texas cattle fever**, an acute haemolytic disease of cattle in southern United States. **This was the first arthropod-borne disease to have been identified.** *B. microti* has taken a prominent place among the 'emerging infections' of humans. More than 70 species of *Babesia* causing infections in numerous animal species such as deer, cattle, and rodents, and birds have been recognized. Human infection is caused by only three species – *B. microti*, *B. divergens* and *B. bovis*.

Geographical distribution

Human cases of babesiosis have been reported from Yugoslavia, Ireland, Scotland, France, and the United States.

Morphology and life cycle

Mature babesial sporozoites, which occur in the salivary glands of *Ixodes dammini* tick, are pear-shaped with the anterior end the broad end. Man and other vertebrate hosts acquire infection when the salivary babesial sporozoites are inoculated by the feeding vector tick. They enter the blood and invade erythrocytes, wherein they multiply asexually, and then lyse the erythrocytes, releasing the merozoites. These can reinfect other cells to maintain the infection. These parasites, though typically pear-shaped, may be spherical, ovoid, spindle-shaped, or amoeboid. They may be found singly, in pairs, or in multiples of two (Fig. 5.13). *Babesia* are divided informally between those with intra-erythrocytic forms that are 1.0–2.5 μm in diameter and those of 2.5– 5.0 μm. The appearance in Giemsa stained films may be mistaken for *Plasmodium falciparum* rings.

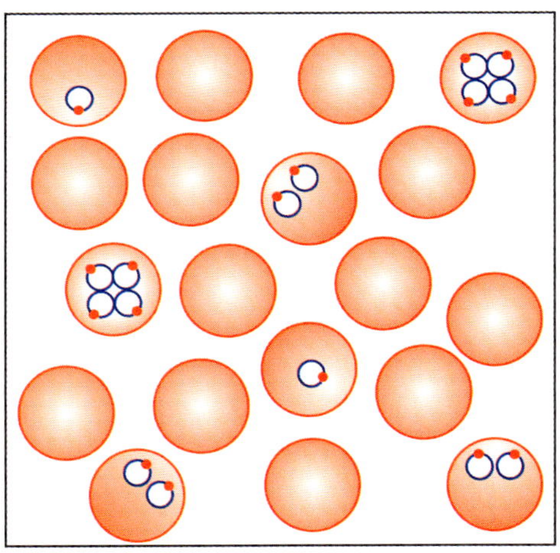

Fig. 5.13. Ring stages of *Babesia microti* in human blood smear.

The intra-erythrocytic parasites replicate when nucleus and other organelles migrate to a location under particular double membrane areas of the parent. These areas then develop and pinch off from the parental piroplasm in a process of budding. Asexually reproducing forms are known as **trophozoites** and their progeny is known as **merozoites**. In addition to these forms, there are also non-reproducing **gametocytes**. *Babesia* gametocytes, unlike those of *Plasmodium*, cannot be distinguished from asexual forms by light microscopy. **No pre- or exo-erythrocytic forms have been described for most *Babesia* spp., implying that the sporozoites directly invade erythrocytes. But in *B. equi*, an agent of equine babesiosis, and *B. microti* sporozoites appear to enter lymphocytes directly where they undergo a cycle of merogony before the resulting merozoites infect erythrocytes.**

Following the ingestion of parasitized erythrocytes by feeding *Ixodes dammini* tick larvae, the gametocytes emerge from erythrocytes within the gut of the tick and differentiate into **gametes**. Pairs of gametes fuse in a process of syngamy forming **zygotes** within the tick gut. These then develop into **ookinetes** 14–18 hours after the feeding larval tick becomes replete. Ookinetes enter salivary glands in 13 days after the larva becomes replete. In the salivary acini, ookinetes develop into **sporoblasts**. These remain dormant until the larval tick becomes a nymph and the nymphal tick attaches to a host. The state of dormancy, in case of *B. microti*, in its *I. dammini* vector, extends through the winter (9–10 months). After the attachment of infected nymphal tick, nuclear division occurs resulting in the formation of about 10,000 **sporozoites** from each sporoblast. Sporozoites are transmitted to man and other vertebrate host by the bite of feeding vector. Infection in the tick population can also be maintained by transovarian transmission. *Babesia* infection, in man, can also be acquired by blood transfusion.

Pathogenicity

Babesial infection (babesiosis) in humans is usually subclinical or very mild. Illness develops 1–4 weeks after the tick bite and is characterized by malaise, anorexia, headache, fatigue, nausea, vomiting, fever as high as 40°C without periodicity, shaking chill, drenching sweats, myalgia, arthralgia, anaemia, thrombocytopenia, haemoglobinuria and splenomegaly. Several factors determine the severity of infection:

- Human babesiosis is more severe in the elderly than in the young.
- HIV infection appears to promote the severe manifestations of babesial infection.
- In splenectomized individuals disease follows a severe course with rapid multiplication of parasites. They develop progressive haemolytic anaemia, jaundice and renal insufficiency.

Laboratory diagnosis

Examination of blood smear

Diagnosis of babesiosis can be made by demonstration of the parasite in Giemsa-stained thick and thin blood films. They may be found singly, in pairs or in multiples of two (Fig. 5.13). *Babesia* may be mistaken in humans for *P. falciparum* in its ring form in the red cells, though the presence of tetrad forms ('Maltese cross') in the red cells and the absence of parasite haemozoin (malarial pigment) are diagnostic. However, early ring stages of malaria parasites also lack pigment. *Babesia* trophozoites are quite variable in size (1–5 μm), and the smallest are smaller than *P. falciparum* rings. In case of *B. microti* infection parasitaemia ranges from 1%–20% in spleen intact patients, and reaches 85% in asplenic patients. Accolé form parasites and multiple infected parasites are more common in *Babesia*. At least 200–300 oil-immersion fields should be examined before the smears are considered negative.

Animal inoculation

Inoculation into hamster of blood from suspected cases facilitates diagnosis by amplifying the parasitaemia. The blood in stained smears, drawn from the tail of the animal should be examined microscopically at weekly intervals for at least 6 weeks before the test is declared negative. Demonstration of the characteristic organisms in the hamster blood proves infection.

Serological tests

Indirect fluorescent antibody test is useful for the diagnosis and distinguishing species of *Babesia* involved in individual cases. Infected hamster red cells are used as antigen.

Polymerase chain reaction

PCR detects *Babesia* DNA accurately and usually within a single working day. On the other hand, inoculation of hamster requires 1–6 weeks and blood sample for hamster inoculation must be taken prior to initiating treatment.

Treatment

Currently recommended therapy is with a combination of *clindamycin* and *quinine* for severe disease, and the combination of *azithromycin* and *atovaquone* for mild or moderate cases.

TOXOPLASMA GONDII

Toxoplasma gondii belongs to the kingdom Protozoa, phylum Sporozoa, class Coccidia and order Eimeriida (Table 1.5). It infects most species of warm-blooded animals, including humans. Members of the cat family, Felidae, are the only known definitive hosts for the sexual stage of *T. gondii* and thus are the main reservoirs of infection. Only one species exists. It was discovered by Nicolle and Manceaux in 1908 in Tunisia in a small rodent, *Ctenodactylus gundi*. The name *Toxoplasma* (from '*taxon*' meaning 'bow' and '*plasma*' meaning 'form') relates to the crescent shape of the tachyzoite stage of the parasite. It is worldwide in distribution and serologic data suggest that up to 70% of all individuals are exposed to *T. gondii* at some point during their lives, although most infections are benign or produce no symptoms.

Habitat

T. gondii is an obligate intracellular parasite, which is found inside the reticuloendothelial cells and many other nucleated cells.

Morphology

Tachyzoites (intracellular trophozoites or proliferative forms), tissue cysts and oocysts are important stages seen during the life cycle of the parasite (Figs. 5.14–5.16). All these stages are infectious to man.

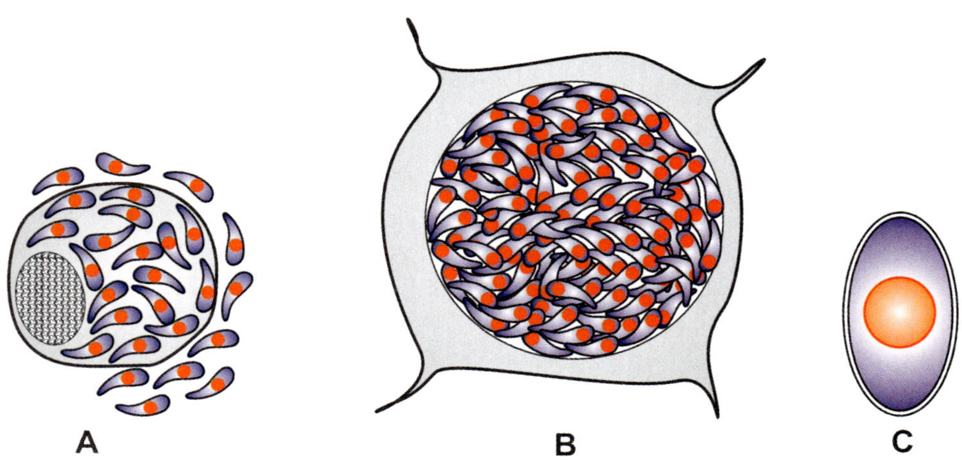

Fig. 5.14. Tachyzoites seen within and outside a cell (A), tissue cyst (B), and oocyst (C) of *Toxoplasma gondii*.

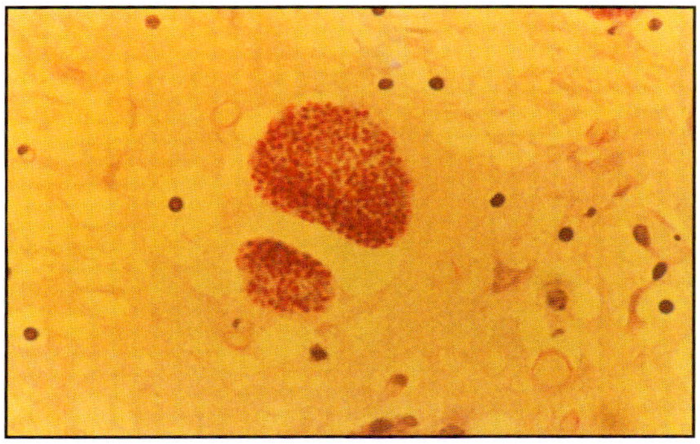

Fig. 5.15. Tissue cysts of *Toxoplasma gondii* in the brain (PAS stain, × 400).

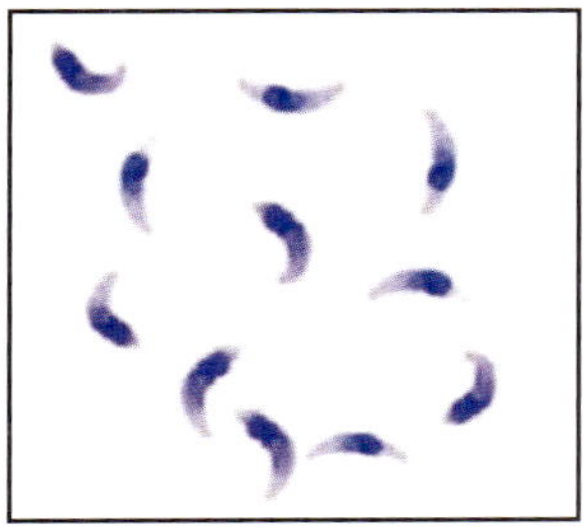

Fig. 5.16. *Toxoplasma gondii* tachyzoites, stained with Giemsa stain, from a smear of peritoneal fluid obtained from a mouse inoculated with *T. gondii* (PAS stain, × 400).

Tachyzoite

It is crescent-shaped with a pointed anterior and a rounded posterior end. It measures 6 µm in length and 2 µm in breadth. The nucleus is spherical or rounded and is usually situated towards the central area of the cell (Figs. 5.14 and 5.16).

Tachyzoite is the rapidly multiplying form seen during the acute stage of infection. It enters the host cell by active penetration of the host cell membrane. After entering the host cell the tachyzoite assumes an oval shape and becomes surrounded by a parasitophorous vacuole. It multiplies asexually within the host cell by repeated endodyogeny or internal budding, two daughter tachyzoites being formed within the parent cell. When the host cell becomes distended with the parasites it disintegrates releasing the trophozoites which infect other cells. Groups of proliferating tachyzoites within a host cell are known as **pseudocyst**.

Tissue cyst

Tissue cysts occur in chronic infection. These are formed when the parasites multiply and produce a wall within a host cell. The cyst wall is eosinophilic, argyrophilic and weakly PAS-positive. The organisms within the cyst are strongly PAS-positive and are known as **bradyzoites**. They are crescent-shaped, slender, measuring 7 µm in length and 1.5 µm in width, and have a nucleus situated towards the posterior end. Bradyzoites are the slowly multiplying forms of the trophozoites contained in tissue cyst, while tachyzoites are the rapidly dividing, proliferative forms of the trophozoite seen in acute infection.

Young tissue cysts may be as small as 5 µm in diameter and contain only 2 bradyzoites, while the older ones may contain hundreds of bradyzoites. In histological sections of brain, tissue cysts rarely reach a diameter of 60 µm (Fig. 5.15), whereas intramuscular cysts may reach a diameter of 100 µm.

Oocyst

This stage is present in cat and other felines and not in humans. It is oval or spherical, 10–12 µm in diameter and contains a sporoblast. The oocyst wall contains two colourless layers.

Tachyzoites and tissue cysts represent stages of asexual multiplication (schizogony), while the oocyst is formed by sexual reproduction (gametogony). All three forms occur in domestic cat and other felines which are the definitive hosts and which support both schizogony and gametogony. Only the asexual forms, tachyzoites and tissue cysts are present in other mammals, including man and birds, which are the intermediate hosts.

Cultivation

T. gondii can be cultured in laboratory animals, chick embryos and cell cultures. Mice, hamsters, guinea pigs and rabbits are all susceptible but mice are generally used as hosts because they are more susceptible. After intraperitoneal inoculation of any of the three infectious stages, i.e., tachyzoites, bradyzoites and oocysts of *T. gondii*, some strains grow in the peritoneal cavity producing ascites, and tissue cysts are prominent in the brain after eight weeks. Virulent strains usually produce illness in mice and sometimes kill them within 1–2 weeks. *T. gondii* tachyzoites multiply in many cell lines in cell culture. Virulent mouse strains rapidly destroy the cells whereas avirulent strains grow slowly causing minimal cell damage. The cysts can develop within three days of inoculation of tachyzoites in cell culture.

Life cycle

T. gondii has two types of life cycle (Fig. 5.17):

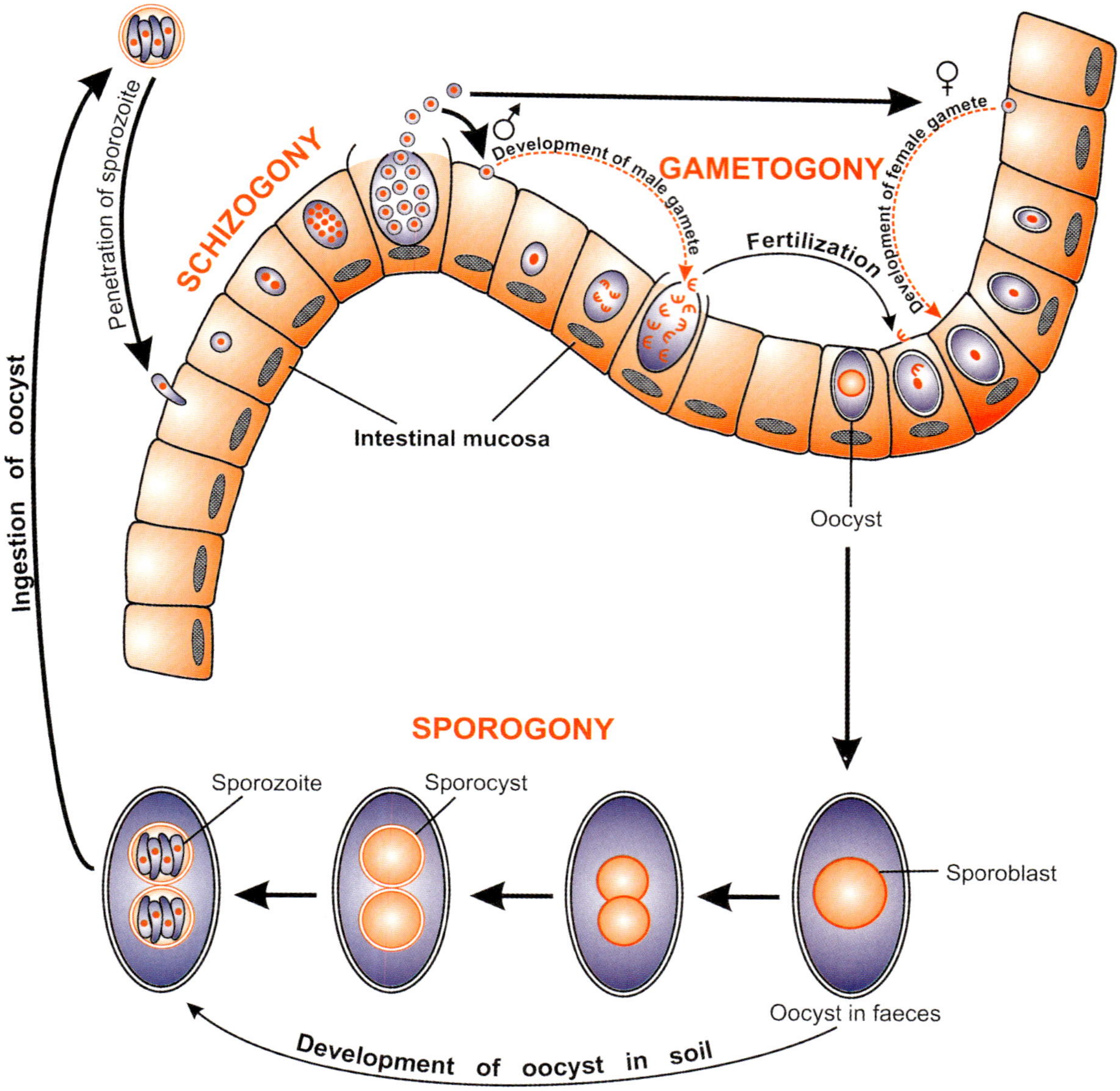

Fig. 5.17. Life cycle of *Toxoplasma gondii.*

1. Enteric cycle.
2. Exoenteric cycle.

Enteric cycle

Enteric cycle occurs in domestic cat and other felines which are definitive hosts. It includes both asexual multiplication (schizogony) and sexual reproduction (gametogony) within the mucosal epithelial cells of the small intestine. Cat acquires infection by ingestion of any of the three infectious stages of *T. gondii*, i.e., tachyzoites and bradyzoites from tissue cysts in the flesh of other animals (mostly rodents), and sporozoites from oocysts in cat faeces. These invade mucosal cells of cat's small intestine in which they undergo several cycles of asexual generation before the sexual cycle begins with the formation of male and female gametocytes which gives rise to male and female gametes respectively.

After sexual fusion (fertilization) of male and female gametes, oocysts develop, exit from host cell into the gut lumen, and pass out in the faeces. Freshly passed oocyst contains a sporoblast and is not infectious. It becomes infectious only after development in soil for 3–4 days. During this time, the sporoblast divides into two. These then become sporocysts by acquiring a cyst wall. Four sporozoites develop inside each sporocyst. The mature oocyst containing eight sporozoites is the infective form of the parasite. It can remain infective in the moist soil for about one year. When ingested, it can either repeat its cycle in a cat or if ingested by rodent or other mammal, including humans or certain birds, can establish an infection in which it reproduces asexually.

Exoenteric cycle

Exoenteric cycle occurs in humans, mice, rats, sheep, cattle, pigs, and certain birds, which are the intermediate hosts. Man acquires infection by:

- ingestion of food and drinks contaminated with cat's faeces containing sporulated oocysts, and
- by ingestion of undercooked meat (mutton, pork and rarely beef) containing tissue cysts. In the duodenum the oocysts release sporozoites, and tissue cysts release bradyzoites.

These pass through the gut wall, circulate in the body, and invade various cells, especially macrophages, where they form tachyzoites, multiply, break out and spread the infection to other organs. Subsequently, they enter into the neural and muscular tissues, such as the brain, eye, and skeletal and cardiac muscles where they multiply slowly (as bradyzoites) to form tissue cysts, initiating chronic stage of the disease. Tissue cysts may also develop in other organs such as lungs, liver and kidneys. Tissue cysts, when ingested by both definitive and intermediate hosts, are infective. Human infection may also be acquired by:

- organ transplantation or blood transfusion,
- transplacental transmission, and
- accidental inoculation of tachyzoites.

Maternal infection rate during the reproductive years is estimated to be between 3% and 5%.

Pathogenicity

T. gondii infection is widespread among humans and its prevalence varies from 16–80%. Most infections in humans are asymptomatic. However, fulminating fatal infections may develop in patients with congenital infections or in debilitated patients in whom underlying conditions may influence the final outcome of the infection.

Underlying conditions associated with toxoplasmosis in the compromised host include various types of malignancies (such as Hodgkin's disease, non-Hodgkin's lymphomas, leukaemias, or solid tumours), collagen vascular disease, organ transplantation, and AIDS. *T. gondii* is the most common cause of secondary CNS infection in patients with AIDS accounting for 38% of such patients. It is also the most common cause of intracerebral mass lesions in patients with HIV infection (accounting for 50–60% cases).

Congenital infection

Congenital infection develops when mothers are infected during pregnancy. Although the mother rarely has symptoms of infection, she does have a temporary parasitaemia. Focal lesions develop in the placenta and the foetus may become infected. In the foetus, there is generalized infection at first, but later it clears from visceral tissues and may localize in the central nervous system. Congenital infection leads to stillbirths, chorioretinitis, intracerebral calcification, psychomotor disturbances, and hydrocephaly or microcephaly. **Prenatal toxoplasmosis is a major cause of blindness and other congenital defects.**

The risk of congenital toxoplasmosis depends on the timing of the mother's acute infection. Transmission to the foetus increases with gestation age – 15–20% in the first trimester, 30–45% in the second, and 60–65% in the third. However, the severity of congenital disease decreases with gestation age. Infection during the first trimester generally results in stillbirth or major central nervous system anomalies. Second and third trimester infections induce less severe neurologic damage, though they are far more common. Clinical manifestations of these infections may be delayed long after birth. **Women who acquired their infection prior to pregnancy are essentially not at risk for delivering an infected infant, unless the woman is immunosuppressed.**

Postnatally acquired infection

Postnatally acquired toxoplasmosis is much less severe than congenitally acquired disease. The commonest manifestation is lymphadenopathy. Although any lymph node may be involved, the most frequently involved are the deep cervical lymph nodes. Lymphadenopathy may be associated with fever, malaise, headache, muscle pain, fatigue and sore throat. The illness is self-limited, though the lymphadenopathy may persist. Rarely there may be pneumonitis, myocarditis and meningoencephalitis, which may be fatal in some cases. Encephalitis is the most important manifestation of toxoplasmosis in immunosuppressed patients.

Acute infection with *T. gondii* can produce psychotic symptoms similar to those displayed by persons with schizophrenia. Exposure to cats in childhood is a risk factor for the development of schizophrenia.

Infections in immunocompromised patient

In immunocompromised patient, the CNS is primarily involved, with diffuse encephalopathy, meningoencephalitis, or cerebral mass lesions. More than 50% of these patients show altered mental state, motor impairment, seizures, abnormal reflexes, and other neurological sequelae.

Immune response

Infection with *T. gondii* stimulates the development of both humoral and cellular immune responses, with the cell-mediated response being the more predominant. These immune responses of the host can dramatically affect the course and severity of infection. In infected humans, IgM usually appears within 2 weeks after infection whereas IgG antibodies appear 2–3 weeks after infection and peak at approximately 6–8 weeks postinfection. The IgG titre then decreases gradually to a low level and remains at this level thereafter. IgA antibodies can be detected early in infection, and their level decreases between 3 and 9 months after infection. Therefore, **the detection of both IgA and IgM at the same time indicates the acute phase of toxoplasmosis, and the presence of IgG demonstrates proof of a prior infection with *T. gondii*.** IgE antibodies also appear early in infection, and then their level begins to decline. Therefore, the detection of IgE could also serve as an indicator for acute infection.

T lymphocytes mediate most immunity to *T. gondii*, largely via the mechanism of macrophage activation. Agents that interfere with either T-cell or monocyte function (steroids, antithymocyte globulin and lymphoma) predispose to toxoplasmosis. Among organ transplant recipients, toxoplasmosis is most common in heart recipients. Thus, the serological status of heart-donors and recipients should be assessed prior to transplantation.

Laboratory diagnosis

Specimens

Blood (buffy coat of heparinized sample), sputum, bone marrow, cerebrospinal fluid and biopsy material from lymph node, spleen and brain.

Microscopic examination

Smears and sections stained with Giemsa or other special stains, such as periodic acid-Schiff may show the organisms. Tachyzoites of *T. gondii* in the smear are crescent-shaped and in sections round to oval (Figs. 5.14A, 5.15 and 5.16). Tissue cysts (Figs. 5.14B and 5.15) are usually spherical and lack septa, and the cyst wall stains with silver stains. The bradyzoites are strongly PAS-positive. The densely packed cysts, chiefly in the brain or other parts of the central nervous system, suggest chronic infection. The immunohistochemical staining of parasites with fluorescent or other types of labelled *T. gondii* antiserum can aid in the diagnosis. Occasionally, *T. gondii* tachyzoites may be found in CSF in AIDS patients with *Toxoplasma* encephalitis.

Animal inoculation

T. gondii can be isolated by intraperitoneal inoculation of body fluids or ground tissues into young laboratory mice that are free from infection. Peritoneal fluid and spleen smears may show the tachyzoites after 7–10 days (Fig. 5.16). If no death occurs, the mice are observed for about six weeks, and tail or heart blood is then tested for specific antibody. The diagnosis is confirmed by demonstration of tissue cysts in the brain of inoculated mice.

Inoculation of tissue culture

T. gondii can also be isolated by inoculation of tissue culture.

Toxoplasma antigen detection

Toxoplasma antigen in blood or CSF may be demonstrated by ELISA.

Polymerase chain reaction (PCR)

Toxoplasma DNA can be detected in the blood and CSF by PCR.

Serology

Serodiagnosis of toxoplasmosis is based primarily on detection of *Toxoplasma*-specific antibodies in the serum. Commonly used methods are as under:

1. **Sabin-Feldman dye test:** This test depends upon the appearance in 2–3 weeks of antibodies that render the membrane of laboratory-cultured living *T. gondii* impermeable to alkaline methylene blue, so that organisms are unstained in the presence of positive serum. Equal amounts (0.1 ml) of diluted patient serum (1:16, 1:64, 1:128 and 1:256 dilutions), live trophozoites of *T. gondii* obtained from the peritoneal exudates of infected mice and accessory factor (normal guinea pig serum as source

of complement) are incubated for 1 hour at 37°C in a water bath. To each of the tubes is then added one drop of saturated alcoholic solution of methylene blue at pH 11. A drop of the mixture is then put on a slide, covered with a cover slip and examined under high power lens of microscope. The number of tachyzoites with stained and unstained cytoplasm is counted. The highest dilution of the serum in which 50% or more of the tachyzoites have unstained cytoplasm is taken as the titre. It is one of the first methods used to diagnose toxoplasmosis. This highly sensitive and specific test is a complement-mediated neutralizing antigen-antibody reaction. It becomes positive within 1–2 weeks after infection. It remains positive at lower titres for years.

2. **Latex agglutination test:** It is a simple test. It shows 94.4% agreement with the dye test. The latex particles are coated with inactivated *T. gondii* soluble antigen. This test does not require heat inactivation of serum samples.
3. **Other tests:** These include indirect haemagglutination assay, indirect fluorescent antibody assay and enzyme-linked immunosorbent assay.

Serologic screening

The finding of antibodies to *T. gondii* in a single serum sample merely establishes that the host has been infected at some time in the past, so it is best to collect two samples from the same individual, the second 2–4 weeks after the first. A 4–16-fold increase in antibody titre in the second sample indicates an active infection.

- If the IgG test is positive, no matter how much low the titre, and IgM test negative, the woman has been infected before pregnancy, there is no risk to her foetus and no treatment is needed.
- If both the IgG and IgM tests are positive, the tests should be repeated in 3 weeks time. If the titres have not risen, infection may be assumed to have occurred before pregnancy, and there is no risk to the foetus.
- If the IgG and IgM results are both negative, the woman is susceptible and the test should be repeated every 4–6 weeks to see if either or both become positive. If the woman is infected during pregnancy, the foetus is at high risk, and the woman should be given prophylactic treatment. When she delivers, her child should be examined, and if found to be infected, clinically or subclinically, should be treated.

Diagnosis of congenital infection

Diagnosis of congenital toxoplasmosis can be established by:

Polymerase chain reaction (PCR)

PCR of the amniotic fluid to detect the B_1 gene of the parasite.

Serology

The presence of IgM (which does not cross the placenta) in the infant's circulation is diagnostic but often this is not found. Specific IgG in the infant's circulation may be of maternal origin or due to infection. Testing of infant's blood at 2 monthly intervals will show whether the IgG antibody level is decreasing. At 6–10 months the infant's circulation should not contain maternal IgG and therefore persistence of IgG beyond this time is indicative of infection in the infant.

Diagnosis of toxoplasmosis in immunodeficient or immunosuppressed patient

1. An elevated serologic titre and the presence of clinical syndrome which includes neurologic symptoms. However, an immunosuppressed host may often fail to generate specific antibody response to acute infection, or this response may be delayed.
2. One of the most common diagnostic tests used for toxoplasmosis is the IFA procedure. Definitive diagnosis is usually accepted when there is a rising titre, an IgM-IFA titre of at least 1 : 64 or an IgM-ELISA titre of 1 : 256.
3. A finding that the Sabin-Feldman dye reaction is higher in the spinal fluid than in serum is also significant.
4. Demonstration of the actual trophozoites or isolation of the organisms from spinal fluid is very significant.

Treatment

Treatment of toxoplasmic encephalitis consists of the antifolates *pyrimethamine* and *sulphadiazine* along with *folinic acid*. Alternative drugs are azithromycin, clarithromycin, atovaquone or dapsone with either trimethoprim-sulphamethoxazole or pyrimethamine and folinic acid. These are less toxic but also less effective. *Spiramicin*, which concentrates in placental tissue, is used for treatment of acute acquired toxoplasmosis in pregnancy to prevent transmission to foetus. If foetal infection is detected, the combination of pyrimethamine, sulphadiazine and folinic acid is administered to the mother after the first 12–14 weeks of pregnancy and to newborn in the postnatal period.

Prevention

The measures recommended for prevention of toxoplasmosis include:

- Avoidance of human contact, particularly of pregnant women with negative serologic tests, with cat faeces and uncooked meat.
- Proper cooking of meat.
- Hands of the people handling meat, all cutting boards, sink tops, knives and other materials coming in contact with uncooked meat should be washed thoroughly with soap and water.

At present there is no effective subunit or killed vaccine for immunization against *T. gondii*.

SARCOCYSTIS

The *Sarcocystis* parasite was first described in the skeletal muscle of a house mouse (*Mus Musculus*) in Switzerland in 1843. Genus *Sarcocystis* belongs to the kingdom Protozoa, phylum Sporozoa, class Coccidea and order Eimeriida (Table 1.5). It has an obligatory prey-predator (two-host) life cycle. Asexual stages develop only in muscle and other cells of the intermediate (herbivorous) host, which in nature is often a prey animal, and sexual stages develop only in gut mucosal cells of the definitive (carnivorous) host. Humans serve as the definitive host for *S. hominis* and *S. suihominis*, and also serve as accidental intermediate hosts for several unidentified species of *Sarcocystis*. Cattle and pigs are the intermediate hosts of *S. hominis* and *S. suihominis* respectively.

Morphology

There are three morphological forms of *Sarcocystis* (Fig. 5.18):

1. Oocyst
2. Sporocyst
3. Sarcocyst

Oocyst

Oocyst is oval, colourless and thin-walled (< 1 μm). Within each oocyst develop two sporocysts each containing four sporozoites. It measures 13–19 μm in diameter in *S. hominis* and 10–13 μm in *S. suihominis*.

Sporocyst

Sporocyst is oval in shape. It measures 8–10 μm in diameter. Each sporocyst contains four banana-shaped **sporozoites**. Sporocysts found in human faeces are the infective form of the parasite.

Sarcocyst

Sarcocysts or muscular cysts of *S. hominis* and *S. suihominis* are found in cattle and pigs respectively. These are elongated, range from less than 0.1 mm to several centimeters long and are found along the length of the muscle fibre. The sarcocyst is always located within a parasitophorous vacuole in the host cell cytoplasm. It has a cyst wall and is divided into many compartments which contain many banana-shaped **bradyzoites**. The sarcocysts are most frequently found in the diaphragm, oesophagus and cardiac muscles of cattle and pigs.

Life cycle

Life cycle of *S. hominis* and *S. suihominis* is similar. It is passed in two hosts (Fig. 5.18). Definitive host is man and intermediate hosts are cattle and pigs in case of *S. hominis* and *S. suihominis* respectively. Man acquires infection by ingestion of raw or undercooked beef or pork containing sarcocysts. Bradyzoites liberated from the sarcocyst by digestion in the stomach and intestine, penetrate the cells of the intestinal mucosa and transform into male (micro) and female (macro) gametes. A macrogamete is fertilized by a microgamete and a zygote is formed. A wall develops around the zygote and an oocyst is formed. Within each oocyst develop two sporocysts each containing four sporozoites. The sporulated oocysts are shed into the lumen of the small intestine to release sporocysts in faeces of definitive host. These are infective to the intermediate host.

The intermediate host becomes infected by ingesting sporocysts in food or water. Sporozoites excyst from sporocysts in the small intestine. Without multiplication in the intestinal mucosa, sporozoites migrate to the blood stream and produce two generations of schizonts in the vascular endothelium. Merozoites liberated from schizonts enter the skeletal and cardiac muscle cells and develop into sarcocysts which contain numerous bradyzoites. The cycle is repeated by ingestion of raw or undercooked beef or pork, containing sarcocysts, by man.

Pathogenicity

S. hominis and *S. suihominis* cause intestinal **sarcocystosis**. It is usually asymptomatic but patient may develop nausea, pain abdomen and diarrhoea 3–6 hours after ingesting uncooked beef and within 24 hours of ingestion of uncooked pork. Sporocysts are excreted in the faeces of the patient 14–18 days and 11–13 days after ingestion of uncooked beef and pork respectively. The disease is self-limiting.

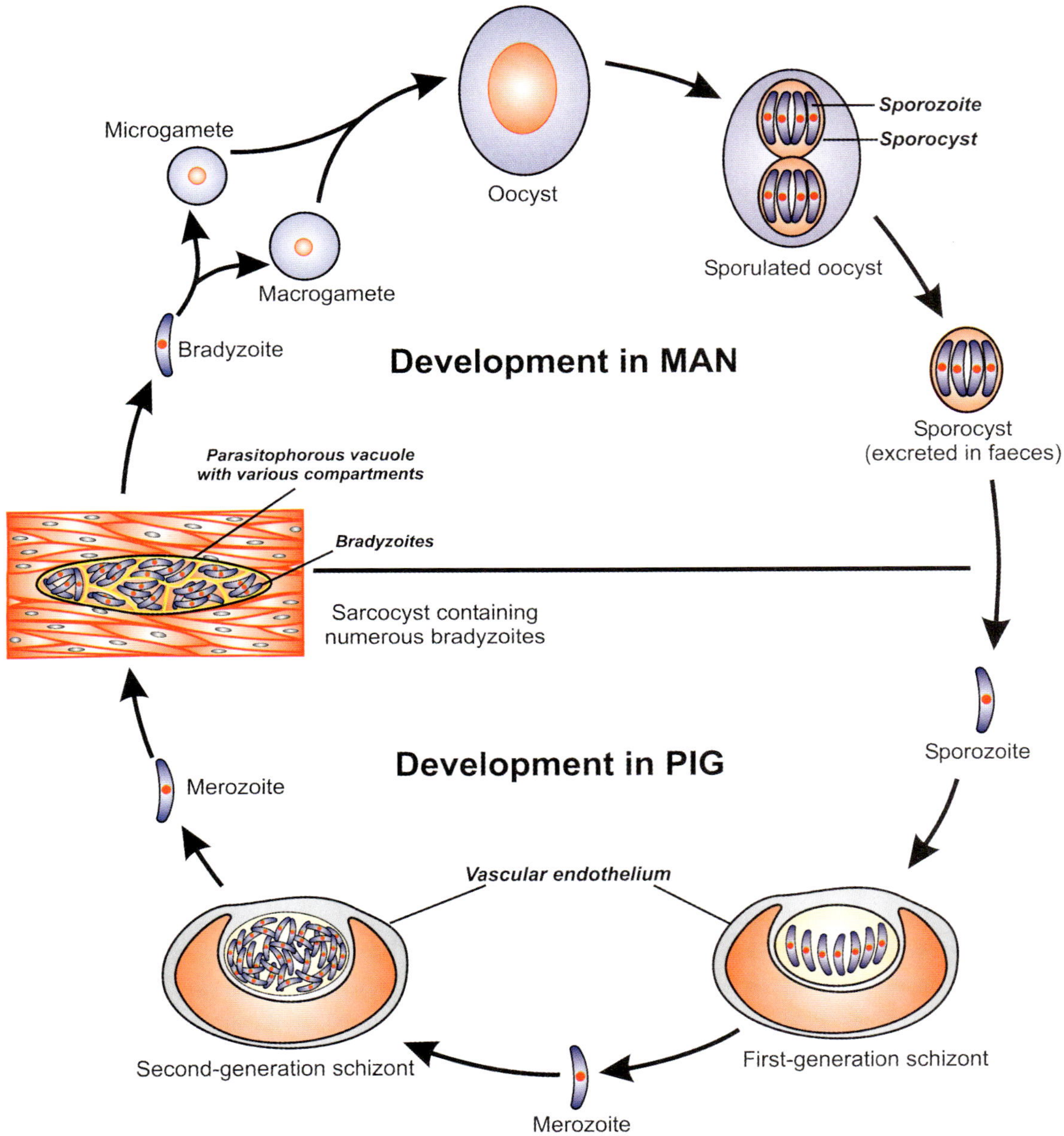

Fig. 5.18. Life cycle of *Sarcocystis suihominis*.

Laboratory diagnosis

The diagnosis of intestinal sarcocystosis is easily made by demonstration of characteristic **sporocysts in faeces**. It is not possible to distinguish one species of *Sarcocystis* from another by the examination of sporocysts.

Prevention

Intestinal sarcocystosis can be prevented by not eating uncooked beef or pork.

MUSCULAR SARCOCYSTOSIS

As mentioned earlier, man may also serve as accidental intermediate host for several unidentified species referred to collectively as ***S. lindemanni***. Man acquires infection by ingestion of food and drinks contaminated with sporocysts excreted in the faeces of cats, dogs or other carnivorous animals which are believed to be the definitive hosts of the parasite. The life cycle of *S. lindemanni* is similar to that of *S. hominis* and *S. suihominis* with the exception that **in case of *S. linde-***

***manni* man is intermediate host and cats and dogs are definitive hosts**.

S. lindemanni may cause muscular sarcocystosis. It is generally asymptomatic. In some cases muscular pain, muscular weakness, focal myositis and pericarditis have been observed.

Diagnosis of human muscular sarcocystosis can be made by demonstration of sarcocysts in the skeletal and cardiac muscle at biopsy or autopsy. Intact sarcocysts in skeletal or cardiac muscle of humans measure up to 100 × 325 µm and are usually not accompanied by an inflammatory reaction. Each sarcocyst contains many bradyzoites, approximately 7–16 µm long. Inflammation follows disintegration of the cysts and death of intracystic bradyzoites.

Muscular sarcocystosis can be prevented by avoidance of contamination of food and drink with faeces of cat, dog or other carnivorous animals.

ISOSPORA BELLI

Isospora belli was first described by Virchow in 1860 and was named by Wenyon in 1923. It belongs to the kingdom Protozoa, phylum Sporozoa, class Coccidia and order Eimeriida (Table 1.5). It is a coccidian parasite of the intestinal epithelium. Both sexual and asexual reproduction in the intestinal epithelium can occur, resulting in tissue damage. The end product of gametogenesis is the oocyst, which is the diagnostic stage present in faecal specimens. *I. belli* is distributed worldwide.

Morphology

Unsporulated oocysts of *I. belli* are ellipsoidal, measuring 20–33 × 10–19 µm (Fig. 5.19 and Table 5.3). Inside each oocyst develop two sporoblasts which later on convert into sporocysts. Each sporocyst is 9–14 × 7–12 µm and contains four crescent-shaped sporozoites. The oocyst is surrounded by a thin, smooth, two-layered cyst wall.

Life cycle

Man acquires infection by ingestion of food or water contaminated with sporulated oocysts from contaminated soil (Fig. 5.19). Eight sporozoites are released from two sporocysts in the upper small intestine and invade the epithelial cells of the distal duodenum and proximal jejunum and initiate schizogony. Upon rupture of the schizont, the merozoites are released, invade new epithelial cells, and continue the cycle of asexual multiplication. After a minimum of one week, the sexual stage (gametogony) begins with the development of micro- and macrogametes. Fertilization results in the development of oocysts that are excreted in the stool. Usually the oocyst contains only one immature sporont, but two may be present. Continued development occurs in 3–4 days outside the body with the development of two mature sporocysts each containing four sporozoites. **The sporulated oocyst is the infective stage of the parasite.**

Pathogenicity

I. belli infects both immunocompetent and immunocompromised adults and children. Infection may be asymptomatic in immunocompetent individuals or it may lead to a mild, self-limiting diarrhoea lasting for 6 weeks to 6 months. Persistent non-bloody diarrhoea indistinguishable from that caused by microsporidia and *Cryptosporidium parvum*, is the major manifestation in immunocompromised individuals. Vomiting, headache, fever and malaise may also be present and dehydration follows when diarrhoea is severe. In AIDS patients, extra-intestinal infections can occur, though they are rare. Necropsy occasionally reveals infection of mesenteric lymph nodes, liver, and spleen. Biliary disease has also been reported.

Laboratory diagnosis

Stool examination

Diagnosis can be established by:

- The demonstration of characteristic *I. belli* oocysts in the faeces by examination of unstained or iodine-stained direct smear preparations and by zinc sulphate centrifugal flotation as well as formalin-ether sedimentation methods.
- Oocysts can also be detected in faecal smears following acid-fast staining or staining with auramine-rhodamine. Oocysts tentatively identified by using auramine-rhodamine stains should be confirmed by wet smear examination or acid-fast stain, particularly if the stool contains other cells or excess artifact material. With acid-fast stain oocysts appear red in colour.

Unstained oocysts are autofluorescent, appearing violet under ultraviolet light and green under green or blue-violet light (Table 5.3).

Biopsy

- Various life cycle stages can be detected within the epithelial cells of intestinal mucosa obtained by biopsy

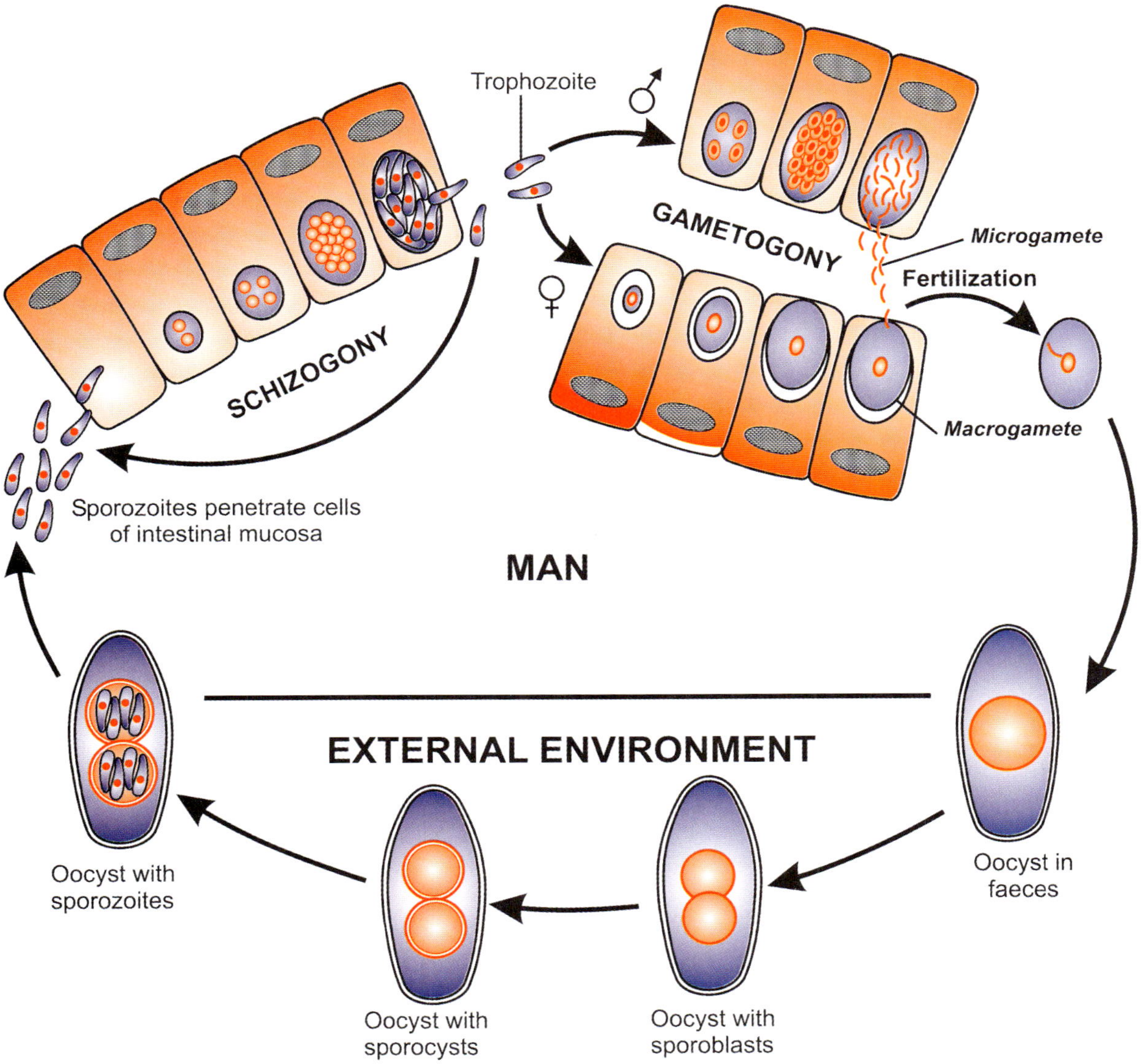

Fig. 5.19. Life cycle of *Isospora belli*.

(Table 5.4). It is quite possible to have a positive biopsy specimen but not recover the oocysts in the stool because of the small number of organisms present. These organisms are acid-fast and can also be demonstrated by using auramine-rhodamine stains.

- Trophozoites of *I. belli* have also been reported to occur in tracheobronchial, mediastinal and mesenteric lymph nodes, gallbladder, liver and spleen in the AIDS patients.

Polymerase chain reaction (PCR)

A highly sensitive and specific method for diagnosis has employed PCR with primers for small-subunit rRNA sequences of *I. belli*.

Treatment

Co-trimoxazole is usually effective if antimicrobial treatment is necessary.

CYCLOSPORA CAYETANENSIS

Cyclospora cayetanensis was first identified by Ortega, Gilman and Sterling in 1994. It belongs to the kingdom Protozoa, phylum Sporozoa, class Coccidia and order Eimeriida (Table 1.5). In recent years, human cyclosporiasis has emerged as an important infection. The distribution is worldwide (United States, Caribbean, Southeast Asia, eastern Europe, Australia, Nepal).

Table 5.3. Differential characters of oocysts of *Cryptosporidium* spp., *Cyclospora cayetanensis* and *Isospora belli*

Cryptosporidium species	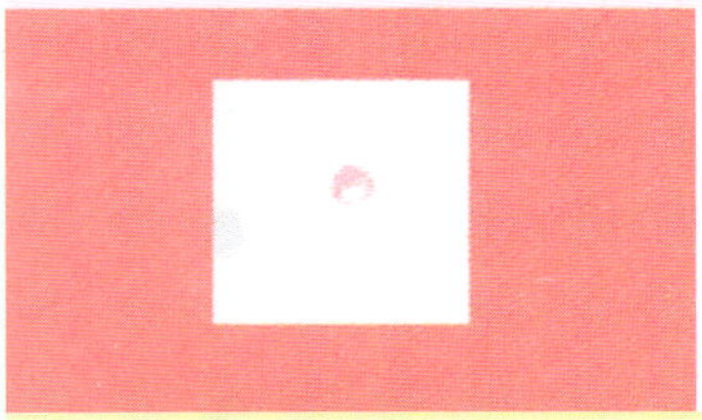	• Spherical or oval. • 4–5 µm in diameter. • 4 sporozoites. • Acid-fast. • Infective when passed in the faeces. • Under ultraviolet illumination, unstained oocysts are autoflourescent.
Cyclospora cayetanensis	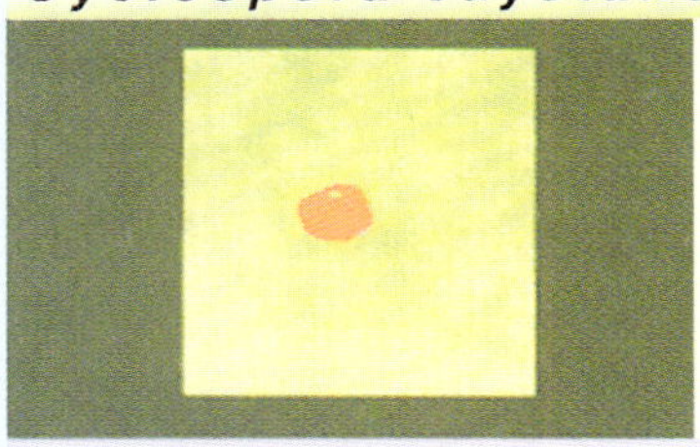	• Spherical or oval. • 8–10 µm. • 2 sporocysts (4–6 µm), each sporocyst has 2 sporozoites. • Acid-fast • Not infective when passed in the faeces. • Under ultraviolet illumination, unstained oocysts are autofluorescent.
Isospora belli		• Ellipsoidal. • 20–33 × 10–19 µm. • 2 sporocysts (9–14 × 7–12 µm), each sporocyst has 4 sporozoites. • Acid-fast • Not infective when passed in the faeces. • Under ultraviolet illumination, unstained oocysts are autofluorescent.

Table 5.4. Biopsy findings in the small intestine in patients infected with *Cryptosporidium* spp., *Cyclospora cayetanensis* and *Isospora belli.*

Cryptosporidium spp.	• In H&E stained sections, the parasites appear as small spherical, basophilic bodies 1–3 µm in diameter. • They are intracellular but extracytoplasmic and are found in parasitophorous vacuoles in the microvillous region of small intestine, with jejunum being most heavily infected site.
Cyclospora cayetanensis	• Developmental stages may be seen in the jejunal enterocytes. • These resemble developmental stages of *Isospora belli*
Isospora belli	• Various life cycle stages can be detected within the epithelial cells of intestinal mucosa obtained by biopsy. • These can be demonstrated by modified acid-fast and auramine rhodamine staining.

Morphology

Oocysts of *C. cayetanensis* are nonrefractile, spherical to oval, slightly wrinkled bodies (mulberry appearance) measuring 8–10 µm in diameter (almost twice the size of the oocysts of *Cryptosporidium* spp.). They contain two ovoid sporocysts, 4–6 µm in size. Each sporocyst contains two sporozoites (Table 5.3). Thus each sporulated oocyst contains four sporozoites.

Life cycle

Life cycle of *C. cayetanensis* is similar to that of *I. belli* in that oocysts are excreted unsporulated and require a period of time outside the host for maturation to occur. Man acquires infection by ingestion of food or water contaminated with sporulated oocysts from contaminated soil. In the intestine the oocyst releases sporozoites, which invade the enterocytes to form type I merozoites, and these form type II merozoites. The type II merozoites differentiate within the mucosal cells into sexual stages – the microgametes and macrogametes. The macrogamete is fertilized by the microgamete and produces a zygote. Unsporulated oocysts are then formed which are excreted in faeces. Sporulation occurs outside the body within approximately 7–13 days. The cycle is thus repeated.

Pathogenicity

It causes self-limiting diarrhoea, fever, fatigue, abdominal cramps lasting for 3–4 days and is associated with poor sanitation. As with other coccidian parasites, infection is more severe in immunocompromised patients, particularly with AIDS. In patients with AIDS, symptoms may persist for as long as 12 weeks. Biliary infection with accompanying symptoms has been observed in AIDS patients.

Laboratory diagnosis

Stool examination

Diagnosis can be made by microscopic detection of oocysts in stool:

- Oocysts may be detected by light microscopic examination of unstained faecal material (wet mount), where they appear as refractile, spherical to oval, slightly wrinkled bodies measuring 8–10 µm in diameter.
- Under ultraviolet illumination unstained oocysts of *C. cayetanensis* are autofluorescent, giving a rapid and inexpensive diagnostic method.
- Oocysts of *C. cayetanensis* are acid-fast and stain light pink to deep red in colour. Older cells may fail to stain.
- Oocysts stain orange red with safranin.
- They do not stain with iron-haematoxylin, Grocott-Gomori methenamine silver, iodine, or periodic acid-Schiff.
- *Cyclospora* oocysts may be excreted intermittently and in small numbers. Thus a single negative specimen does not rule out the diagnosis. Three or more specimens at 2- or 3-day intervals may be required.
- Concentration procedures should be used to maximize recovery of oocysts. The method most familiar to laboratories is the formalin-ether sedimentation technique.

Jejunal biopsy

It reveals blunting of jejunal villi, villous atrophy, and crypt hyperplasia of varying degrees. Developmental stages resembling those of *I. belli* may be seen in jejunal enterocytes (Table 5.4).

Treatment

Co-trimoxazole appears to be effective in management of serious infection.

CRYPTOSPORIDIUM PARVUM

Cryptosporidium belongs to the kingdom Protozoa, phylum Sporozoa, class Coccidia and order Eimeriida (Table 1.5). In 1907, Tyzzer first described this parasite in the gastric crypts of a laboratory mouse. Subsequently, it has been found in chickens, turkeys, rats, guinea pigs, horses, pigs, calves, sheep, rhesus monkeys, dogs, cats, and humans. Cryptosporidiosis is a zoonosis and is transmitted via the faecal-oral route. This infection is now well recognized as causing disease in humans, particularly in those who are in some way immunosuppressed or immunodeficient.

Cryptosporidiosis has been implicated as one of the more important opportunistic infections in patients with AIDS. Calves and perhaps other animals serve as potential sources of human infections. There are at least 16 different species of *Cryptosporidium*, however, *C. parvum* and *C. hominis* are the species most commonly infecting humans. Other species of *Cryptosporidium* which have also been reported to cause human disease are *C. felis*, *C. meleagridis*, *C. canis* and *C. muris*. *Cryptosporidium* spp. are distributed worldwide. Direct person-to-person transmission is also likely and may occur through direct or indirect contact with stool material. Direct transmission may occur during sexual practices involving anal-oral contact. The first cases of human cryptosporidiosis were reported in 1976.

Habitat

C. parvum differs from other coccidia that infect warm-blooded vertebrates in that the developmental stages do not occur deep within host cells but are confined to an intracellular, extracytoplasmic location. Each stage is within a parasitophorous vacuole in the microvillous region of epithelial cells of the small intestine. The organisms have also been found, but less frequently, in the stomach, large intestine and lungs.

Morphology

The parasite released in the faeces is known as oocyst. It is colourless, spherical or oval and measures 4–5 µm in diameter. It contains four crescent-shaped naked or nonencysted sporozoites (sporocysts not present) (Table 5.3). The anterior end of the sporozoite is pointed and the posterior end which contains a prominent nucleus is rounded. The oocyst wall of *C. parvum* is composed of an electron-lucent middle zone surrounded by two electron-dense layers. Oocyst does not stain with iodine and is acid-fast (Fig. 5.20).

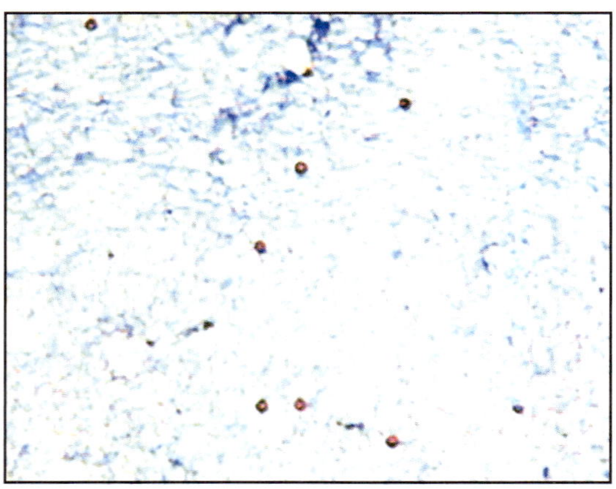

Fig. 5.20. Oocyst of *Cryptosporidium parvum* in faecal smear stained with modified acid-fast stain, × 400.

Life cycle

C. parvum undergoes both asexual (schizogony) and sexual (gametogony) multiplication (Fig. 5.21) in a single host (man, cattle, cat or dog). Man acquires infection by direct contact with infected animal or by ingestion of food or water contaminated with faeces containing oocysts of the parasite. After excysting from oocysts in the lumen of the intestine, sporozoites invade the epithelial cells, and develop into trophozoites (uninucleate meronts) within parasitophorous vacuoles in the microvillous region of the mucosal epithelium. These trophozoites multiply asexually (schizogony) by nuclear division to produce type I meronts. Eight merozoites are released from each type I meront. These enter adjacent host cells to form additional type I meronts or to form type II meronts.

Four merozoites are released from each type II meront. They enter host cells to form the sexual stages (gametogony), microgamonts and macrogamonts. A microgamont produces 12–16 microgametes and a macrogamont transforms into only one macrogamete. After fertilization of a macrogamete by a microgamete an environmentally resistant, thick-walled oocyst is formed that undergoes sporogony to form sporulated oocyst containing four sporozoites. Sporulated oocyst released in faeces transmits the infection from one host to another.

About 20% zygotes do not form a thick oocyst wall, but have only a unit membrane surrounding four sporozoites. These thin-walled oocysts represent **auto-infective life cycle** forms that can maintain the parasite in the host without repeated oral exposure to thick-walled oocysts present in the environment.

Intracellular stages of *C. parvum* are intracellular but extracytoplasmic and are found within parasitophorous vacuoles in the microvillous region of the host cell (Table 5.4). On the other hand, *Isospora* spp. occupy parasitophorous vacuoles deep (perinuclear) within the host cells. Oocysts of *C. parvum* undergo sporogony within the host cell and are infective when released in the faeces, whereas oocysts of *Isospora belli* sporulate only after they are released from the host and exposed to oxygen and temperature below 37°C for 1–14 days.

Pathogenicity

Humans become infected either from direct contact with infected animals or from ingestion of faecally contaminated food or water. Calves and other animals serve as a major source for human infections, and human-to-human transmission can occur. Oocysts of *C. parvum* are not eliminated by chlorination and may persist in posttreatment water supplies. Symptomatic intestinal and respiratory cryptosporidiosis has been seen in both immunocompetent and immunodeficient patients of all ages. However, once the primary infection has been established, the immune system of

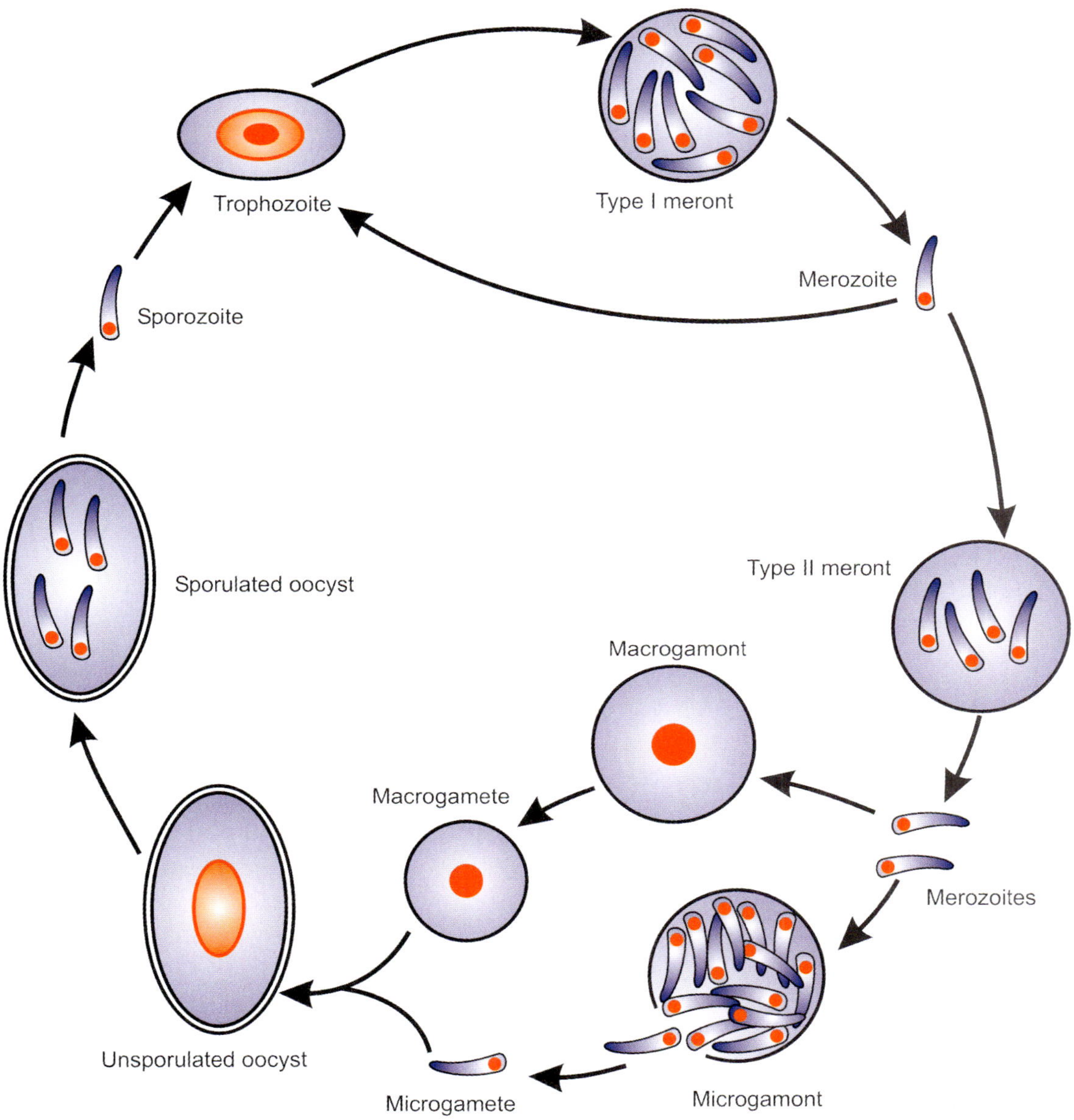

Fig. 5.21. Life cycle of *Cryptosporidium* spp.

the host plays a very important role in determining the length and severity of the illness.

People who are immunocompetent usually develop a short-term, self-limited diarrhoea lasting approximately 2 weeks. In contrast, those who are immunocompromised initially develop the same type of illness; however, it becomes more severe with time and results in a prolonged, life-threatening, cholera-like illness. These severe infections have been seen in patients undergoing immunosuppressive chemotherapy with drugs that affect both T- and B-lymphocyte function, in patients with hypogammaglobulinemia and in those with AIDS. Individuals whose immunosuppressive therapy has been discontinued rapidly clear the body of *C. parvum* once their immune system function is restored.

Immune response to cryptosporidiosis is probably an antibody-dependent cell-mediated cytotoxic effect of unknown mechanism. About 2–5% of AIDS patients develop cryptosporidiosis.

Most severely immunocompromised patients cannot overcome the infection and the illness becomes progressively worse with time. In these patients, *C. parvum* infections are not always confined to the gastrointestinal tract; additional symptoms (respiratory cryptosporidiosis, cholecystitis, hepatitis, and pancreatitis) have been associated with extraintestinal infections. In infection of the gall bladder oocysts are passed in the stool. Biological factors which impact the epidemiology of *Cryptosporidium* are given in Table 5.5.

Table 5.5. Biological factors which impact the epidemiology of *Cryptosporidium*

- Small (4–5 μm), environmentally resistant, and fully sporulated/infectious oocysts when passed
- Large livestock animal and human reservoir host populations
- Ubiquitous
- Able to cross-infect multiple host species
- Low infective dose (≤ 10–100 oocysts)
- Resistance to disinfectants
- Lack of effective therapy; resistance to available drugs

Laboratory diagnosis

Stool examination

For diagnosis, three consecutive specimens of stool should be examined.

Wet mount

A direct wet mount of stool shows highly refractile, spherical or oval oocysts measuring 4–5 μm in diameter. If the specimen represents the typically watery diarrhoea, numerous organisms are found caught up in mucus. Therefore, wet mount should be prepared from the mucus.

Concentration methods

Stool concentration techniques that can be used for identification of *C. parvum* oocysts include floatation of oocysts in Sheather's sugar solution, in zinc sulphate solution (specific gravity 1.18–1.2) or in saturated sodium chloride solution (specific gravity 1.27). Stool concentration techniques using sedimentation include formalin-ether sedimentation and formalin-ethyl acetate sedimentation. Because of the small size of oocysts of *C. parvum,* stool sample should be centrifuged at 500 *g* for at least 10 minutes.

Staining procedures

A large number of staining procedures have been employed for demonstration of oocysts of *C. parvum* in the faecal smear but modified acid-fast staining is the method of choice. By this method, oocysts appear bright red and yeasts take up blue colour. The 4–5 μm in diameter oocysts of *C. parvum* can be readily differentiated microscopically from those of *C. cayetanensis* and *I. belli*, as they are half the size of the former and 4–6 times smaller than the latter (Table 5.3). Red stained oocysts can also be demonstrated in the sputum, bronchial washings and duodenal or jejunal aspirations by modified acid-fast staining methods.

Fluorescence microscopy

Less common staining methods, such as auramine-rhodamine and acridine orange have also been described. Immunofluorescent antibody (IFA) procedure employing *Cryptosporidium*-specific polyclonal or monoclonal antibodies is a specific and most sensitive method for accurate identification of *C. parvum* in the faeces.

Sputum examination

Respiratory cryptosporidiosis has been reported in AIDS patients. Sputum specimens from immunodeficient patients with undiagnosed respiratory illness should be collected in 10% formalin and examined for *Cryptosporidium* oocysts by the same techniques as used for stool samples.

Histopathological examination

Various life cycle stages of *C. parvum* can be detected in the microvillous region of intestinal mucosa obtained by biopsy. In haematoxylin and eosin-stained sections the parasites appear as small, spherical, basophilic bodies 1–3 μm in diameter. They are intracellular but extracytoplasmic and are found in parasitophorous vacuole in the microvillous region of epithelial cells of small intestine with jejunum being most heavily infected site (Fig. 5.22 and Table 5.4).

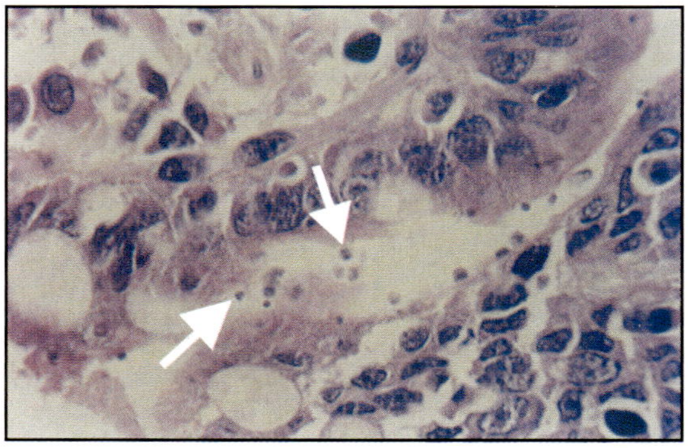

Fig. 5.22. *Cryptosporidium parvum* on the intestinal mucosal surface (haematoxylin and eosin stain, × 400).

Serodiagnosis

Antibodies specific to *C. parvum* can be detected by:

- IFA assays using endogenous stages of the parasite in tissue sections as antigens or intact oocysts as antigens.
- Specific anti-*Crytosporidium* IgG or IgM or both may be detected by enzyme-linked immunosorbent assay using crude oocyst preparations as antigens.
- Cryptosporidial antigen in the faecal samples can be detected by ELISA.

Polymerase chain reaction (PCR)

PCR technology offers alternative to conventional diagnosis of *Cryptosporidium* in both clinical and environmental samples. Compared with microscopic examination by conventional acid-fast staining procedures, PCR is more sensitive and easier to interpret but requires more "hands on" time and expertise, as well as being more expensive. PCR has been used to detect *Cryptosporidium* DNA in fixed, paraffin-embedded tissue.

Treatment

Cryptosporidium infection in the immunocompetent host is self-limiting and requires only supportive treatment to prevent dehydration. The most effective therapy for cryptosporidiosis in AIDS patients is restoration of their immune function through highly active antiretroviral therapy (HAART). *Nitazoxanide* has shown activity in treating cryptosporidiosis in immunocompetent children and is possibly effective in immunocompetent adults. Its efficacy in children and adults with HIV infection and AIDS is not clearly established.

BLASTOCYSTIS SPECIES

Geographical distribution

Worldwide.

Classification

Blastocystis hominis is strict anaerobic protozoan found in human intestine. Over the years, it was considered to be related to fungus *Blastomyces* spp. *Blastocystis* has recently been placed in the kingdom Stramenopila (Table 1.5), based on analysis of 18S ribosomal ribonucleic acid and other molecular evidence.

Morphology

It shows great morphological diversity. Four main morphological types have been described – vacuolar, granular, amoeboid and cyst form. *B. hominis* morphology also differs between fresh faecal specimens and cultures. Whether these different morphological types are all involved in the life cycle or whether some are merely artifactual or degenerative forms is not clear.

Vacuolar form

The vacuolar form is seen in faecal specimens and is predominant form in culture. This form is usually spherical with a large size variation from 2 μm to more than 200 μm (average size between 4 and 15 μm). It has a thin band of cytoplasm around a large vacuole that occupies at least 90% of the cell volume. The nucleus shows a typical crescent-shaped band of condensed chromatin on one side. It often has a surface slime layer or capsule surrounding the cell membrane.

Granular form

This form can be regarded simply as a vacuolar form with granules in the central vacuole. The size range is similar and the granules are visible in unstained preparations. In older cultures, the granular form is often the most frequently found morphotype.

Amoeboid form

It is only rarely encountered. Extended pseudopodia are often seen in amoeboid forms of *B. hominis*. The amoeboid form has been reported to feed on bacteria and cellular debris from dead cells.

Cyst form

The classic form found in human stool is the cyst, which varies tremendously in size from 6 to 40 μm. It shows a thick wall and a bilayered membrane between the wall and the cytoplasm. It may have one or more nuclei. Some cysts possess external capsular layer. Cysts are occasionally found in long-term cultures.

Life cycle

The thick-walled cyst present in the stools is believed to be responsible for external transmission, possibly by the faecal-oral route through ingestion of contaminated water or food. The cysts infect epithelial cells of the digestive tract and multiply asexually. Vacuolar forms of the parasite give origin to multi-vacuolar and amoeboid forms. The multivacuolar form develops into a precyst that gives origin to a thin-walled cyst, thought to be responsible for autoinfection. The amoeboid form gives origin to a precyst, which develops into thick-walled cyst by schizogony. The thick-walled cyst is excreted in faeces.

Pathogenicity

It is usually non-pathogenic but may cause diarrhoea, nausea, abdominal pain, cramps and discomfort, and flatulence in persons with immunodeficiency. It is being increasingly reported from persons with HIV infection.

Laboratory diagnosis

Diagnosis is based on finding the parasite in faeces. The vacuolar form of *B. hominis* is usually easily recognized in either saline or iodine wet preparations. Permanently stained smears (trichrome and iron haematoxylin staining) are preferred over wet mount preparations because faecal debris may be mistaken for the organisms in the latter.

Further Reading

1. Beare, N.A.V., Lewis, D.K., et al. 2003. Retinal changes in adults with cerebral malaria. *Ann. Trop. Med. Parasitol.*, **97**, 313–15.
2. Beg, M.A., Khan, R., et al. 2002. Cerebral involvement in benign tertian malaria. *Am. J. Trop. Med. Hyg.*, **67**, 230–2.
3. Clark, I.A., Alleva, L.M., et al. 2004. Pathogenesis of malaria and clinically similar conditions. *Clin. Microbiol. Rev.*, **17**, 509–39.
4. Dubey, J.P., Saville, W.J.A., et al. 2000. Completion of the life cycle of *Sarcocystis neurona*. *J. Parasitol.*, **86**, 1276–80.
5. Eberhard, M.L., Ortega, Y.R., et al. 2000. Attempts to establish experimental *Cyclospora cayetanensis* infection in laboratory animals. *J. Parasitol.*, **86**, 577–82.
6. Franzen, C., Muller, A., et al. 2000. Taxonomic position of the human intestinal protozoan parasite *Isospora belli* as based on ribosomal RNA sequence. *Parasitol. Rev.*, **86**, 669–76.
7. Gray, J.S., Von Stedingk, L.V., et al. 2002. Transmission studies of *Babesia microti* in *Ixodes ricinus* ticks and gerbils. *J. Clin. Microbiol.*, **40**, 1259–63.
8. Hänscheid, T. and Grobusch, M.P. 2002. How useful is PCR in the diagnosis of malaria? *Trends Parasitol.*, **18**, 395–400.
9. Hunter, P.R. and Nichols, G. 2002. Epidemiology and clinical features of *Cryptosporidium* infection in immunocompromised patients. *Clin. Microbiol. Rev.*, **15**, 145–54.
10. Midha, N., Ichhpujani, R.L., Singh, P., Arora, D.R., Arora, B. and Chugh, T.D. 1981. Evaluation of fluorescent microscopy for the identification of malarial parasites. *J. Com. Dis.*, **13**, 241–43.
11. Montoya, J.G. 2002. Laboratory diagnosis of *Toxoplasma gondii* infection and toxoplasmosis. *J. Infect. Dis.*, **185**, Suppl. 573–82.
12. Muller, A., Bialek, R., et al. 2000. Detection of *Isospora belli* by polymerase chain reaction using primers based on small-subunit ribosomal RNA sequences. *Eur. J. Clin. Microbiol.*, **19**, 631–4.
13. Tenter, A.M., Heckeroth, A.R. and Weiss, L.M. 2000. *Toxoplasma gondii*: from animals to humans. *Int. J. Parasitol.*, **30**, 695–9.

Important Questions

1. Discuss morphology, life cycle, pathogenicity and laboratory diagnosis of:
   (a) Malaria parasites
   (b) *Babesia* spp.
   (c) *Toxoplasma gondii*
   (d) *Cryptosporidium parvum*
   (e) *Isospora belli*
2. Tabulate differences between:
   (a) Human malaria parasites
   (b) *Plasmodium falciparum* and *Babesia* spp.
3. Write short notes on:
   (a) Blackwater fever
   (b) Pernicious malaria
   (c) Relapse and recrudescence of malaria
   (d) Host immunity to malaria
   (e) Prophylaxis of malaria
   (f) Muscular sarcocystosis
   (g) *Cyclospora cayetanensis*
   (h) *Sarcocystis*
   (i) *Blastocystis hominis*
   (j) *Plasmodium knowlesi*

Multiple Choice Questions

1. Which is the infective form of the malaria parasite?
   (a) Oocyst.
   (b) Sporozoite.
   (c) Bradyzoite.
   (d) Tachyzoite.
2. Resting stage of the malaria parasite is known as:
   (a) sporozoite.
   (b) trophozoite.
   (c) merozoite.
   (d) hypnozoite.

3. Relapse of malaria is **not** seen in infection with:
   (a) *Plasmodium vivax*.
   (b) *Plasmodium ovale*.
   (c) *Plasmodium falciparum*.
   (d) All of the above.
4. For infection of mosquito, the blood of human carrier must contain atleast:
   (a) 6 gametocytes/ml.
   (b) 8 gametocytes/ml.
   (c) 10 gametocytes/ml.
   (d) 12 gametocytes/ml.
5. Malaria infection can be transmitted by:
   (a) bite of infected female *Anopheles* mosquito.
   (b) blood transfusion.
   (c) vertical transmission through placental defect.
   (d) All of the above.
6. *Plasmodium falciparum* is the most pathogenic of the human *Plasmodium* spp. because:
   (a) it causes a high level of parasitaemia.
   (b) it invades erythrocytes of all ages.
   (c) its erythrocytic schizogony takes place in the capillaries of internal organs.
   (d) All of the above.
7. Which forms of *Plasmodium falciparum* are generally absent in peripheral blood film of the patient?
   (a) Early trophozoite or ring stage.
   (b) Schizonts.
   (c) Crescents.
   (d) None of the above.
8. Crescent-shaped or banana-shaped gametocytes are seen in infection with:
   (a) *Plasmodium vivax*.
   (b) *Plasmodium falciparum*.
   (c) *Plasmodium ovale*.
   (d) *Plasmodium malariae*.
9. Maurer's dots in red blood cells are seen in infection with:
   (a) *Plasmodium vivax*.
   (b) *Plasmodium falciparum*.
   (c) *Plasmodium malariae*.
   (d) *Plasmodium ovale*.
10. Quartan periodicity of malaria is seen in infection with:
   (a) *Plasmodium vivax*.
   (b) *Plasmodium falciparum*.
   (c) *Plasmodium malariae*.
   (d) *Plasmodium ovale*.
11. Which drug is used to eliminate exo-erythrocytic parasites in the liver?
   (a) Chloroquine.
   (b) Quinine.
   (c) Primaquine.
   (d) Mefloquine.
12. Which was the first arthropod-borne disease to be identified?
   (a) Leishmaniasis.
   (b) Trypanosomiasis.
   (c) Malaria.
   (d) Babesiosis.
13. Babesiosis is transmitted by bite of:
   (a) female *Anopheles* mosquito.
   (b) sandfly.
   (c) reduviid bug.
   (d) tick.
14. Which is the infective stage of parasite in babesiosis?
   (a) Sporozoite.
   (b) Merozoite.
   (c) Tachyzoite.
   (d) Bradyzoite.
15. Which animal is used for diagnosis of babesiosis?
   (a) Hamster.
   (b) Guinea pig.
   (c) Mouse.
   (d) Rabbit.
16. In the intermediate host *Toxoplasma gondii* lives inside the:
   (a) lumen of small intestine.
   (b) lumen of large intestine.
   (c) reticuloendothelial cells and many other nucleated cells.
   (d) red blood cells.
17. Oocysts of *Toxoplasma gondii* are seen in:
   (a) domestic cat and other felines.
   (b) humans.
   (c) sheep.
   (d) cattle.
18. During which trimester/s of pregnancy infection with *Toxoplasma gondii* is more severe?
   (a) First.
   (b) Second.
   (c) Third.
   (d) Second and third.

19. Commonest manifestation of postnatally acquired infection with *Toxoplasma gondii* is:
    (a) lymphadenopathy.
    (b) pneumonitis.
    (c) myocarditis.
    (d) meningoencephalitis.

20. Intermediate host for *Sarcocystis hominis* is:
    (a) man.
    (b) cattle.
    (c) pig.
    (d) cat.

21. Man acts as accidental intermediate host in infection with:
    (a) *Sarcocystis hominis*.
    (b) *Sarcocystis suihominis*.
    (c) *Sarcocystis lindemanni*.
    (d) All of the above.

22. How many sporozoites are seen in mature oocyst of *Sarcocystis suihominis*?
    (a) Two.
    (b) Four.
    (c) Six.
    (d) Eight.

23. Muscular sarcocystosis is caused by:
    (a) *Sarcocystis hominis*.
    (b) *Sarcocystis suihominis*.
    (c) *Sarcocystis lindemanni*.
    (d) All of the above.

24. Sporulated oocysts of *Isospora belli* contain:
    (a) one sporocyst.
    (b) two sporocysts.
    (c) three sporocysts.
    (d) four sporocysts.

25. Each sporulated oocyst of *Cyclospora cayetanensis* contains:
    (a) two sporozoites.
    (b) four sporozoites.
    (c) six sporozoites.
    (d) eight sporozoites.

26. Which statement is **true** about *Cryptosporidium parvum*?
    (a) Developmental stages of the parasite are extracellular.
    (b) Both asexual and sexual multiplication of the parasite occurs in a single host.
    (c) Each oocyst contains eight naked sporozoites.
    (d) It causes meningoencephalitis in AIDS patients.

27. Which of the following stains is used for demonstration of *Cryptosporidium* oocysts in stool?
    (a) Modified Ziehl-Neelsen stain.
    (b) Haematoxylin and eosin
    (c) Iron haematoxylin.
    (d) Gram's.

28. A 40-year-old patient developed high fever of sudden onset. Peripheral blood film showed all stages of malaria parasite. The mature schizonts were 9–10 μm in diameter and contained 12–24 merozoites each. The malaria pigment was yellowish-brown in colour. Which of the following malaria parasites is the causative agent?
    (a) *Plasmodium falciparum*
    (b) *Plasmodium vivax*
    (c) *Plasmodium ovale*
    (d) *Plasmodium malariae*

29. Schuffner's dots in red blood cells are seen in infection with:
    (a) *Plasmodium vivax*
    (b) *Plasmodium falciparum*
    (c) *Plasmodium malariae*
    (d) *Plasmodium ovale*

30. Ziemann's dots in red blood cells are seen in infection with:
    (a) *Plasmodium vivax*
    (b) *Plasmodium falciparum*
    (c) *Plasmodium malariae*
    (d) *Plasmodium ovale*

31. James's dots in red blood cells are seen in infection with:
    (a) *Plasmodium vivax*
    (b) *Plasmodium falciparum*
    (c) *Plasmodium malariae*
    (d) *Plasmodium ovale*

32. Cerebral malaria is caused by:
    (a) *Plasmodium vivax*
    (b) *Plasmodium falciparum*
    (c) *Plasmodium malariae*
    (d) *Plasmodium ovale*

33. The situation in which the RBC infection with *Plasmodium* spp. is not eliminated by immune system or by therapy and their numbers in the RBCs begin to increase again with subsequent clinical symptoms is called:
    (a) gametogony.
    (b) secondary exo-erythrocytic schizogony.
    (c) relapse.
    (d) recrudescence.

34. Which of the following parasites can be transmitted vertically?
   (a) *Echinococcus granulosus.*
   (b) *Toxoplasma gondii.*
   (c) *Giardia lamblia.*
   (d) *Entamoeba histolytica.*
35. In which of the following parasites domestic cat is the definitive host?
   (a) *Plasmodium falciparum.*
   (b) *Leishmania donovani.*
   (c) *Toxoplasma gondii.*
   (d) *Trichomonas vaginalis.*
36. Sabin-Feldman dye test is used for the diagnosis of:
   (a) toxoplasmosis.
   (b) histoplasmosis.
   (c) leishmaniasis.
   (d) Chagas' disease.
37. All of the following are common causes of diarrhoeal disease in persons with HIV infection **except**:
   (a) *Isospora belli.*
   (b) *Cyclospora cayetanensis.*
   (c) *Cryptosporidium parvum.*
   (d) *Toxoplasma gondii.*
38. Which of the following parasites is **not** a sporozoan?
   (a) *Balantidium coli.*
   (b) *Plasmodium falciparum.*
   (c) *Isospora belli.*
   (d) *Cryptosporidium parvum.*
39. Malaria parasites can be detected in the peripheral blood when the parasite density is at least:
   (a) 1 parasite/μl.
   (b) 5 parasites/μl.
   (c) 10 parasites/μl.
   (d) 100 parasites/μl.
40. More than one ring stage of *Plasmodium* in an infected RBC is common in:
   (a) *Plasmodium falciparum.*
   (b) *Plasmodium vivax.*
   (c) *Plasmodium ovale.*
   (d) *Plasmodium malariae.*
41. Definitive host of *Toxoplasma gondii* is:
   (a) Dog.
   (b) Cat.
   (c) Cattle.
   (d) Man.
42. *Toxoplasma gondii* can be cultured on:
   (a) NNN medium.
   (b) Boeck and Drbohlav's diphasic medium.
   (c) Diamond's medium.
   (d) Intraperitoneal inoculation of mice.
43. Schizonts of *Plasmodium falciparum* are generally **not** seen in peripheral blood because:
   (a) these are ingested by monocytes.
   (b) these are killed by antibodies.
   (c) these are absent in its life cycle.
   (d) erythrocytic schizogony of *Plasmodium falciparum* takes place in the capillaries of internal organs.
44. *Plasmodium vivax* can cause:
   (a) cerebral malaria.
   (b) algid malaria.
   (c) blackwater fever.
   (d) None of the above.
45. Malaria parasites can be cultured in:
   (a) human red blood cells.
   (b) *Anopheles* mosquito cell lines.
   (c) human amnion cells.
   (d) Vero cell lines.
46. Who first found and described malaria parasite?
   (a) Charles Laveran.
   (b) Ronald Ross.
   (c) Robert Koch.
   (d) Carlos Chagas.
47. Which form of malaria parasite is present in the saliva of infected mosquito?
   (a) Merozoite.
   (b) Sporozoite.
   (c) Tachyzoite.
   (d) Bradyzoite.
48. Which form of malaria parasite present in peripheral blood of the patient is capable of further development in female *Anopheles* mosquito?
   (a) Gametocytes.
   (b) Merozoites.
   (c) Schizonts.
   (d) Ring forms.
49. Primary exoerythrocytic schizogony or pre-erythrocytic schizogony of *Plasmodium* spp. occurs in:
   (a) brain.
   (b) liver.
   (c) spleen.
   (d) kidney.

50. Relapse of malaria due to *Plasmodium vivax* and *P. ovale* is due to:
   (a) antigenic variation.
   (b) drug resistance.
   (c) hypnozoites.
   (d) All of the above.

51. Oocysts of which of the following parasites are infective when passed in stools?
   (a) *Isospora belli.*
   (b) *Cyclospora cayetanensis.*
   (c) *Cryptosporidium parvum.*
   (d) All of the above.

52. Which of the following parasites preferably infect young red blood cells?
   (a) *Plasmodium falciparum.*
   (b) *Plasmodium vivax.*
   (c) *Plasmodium ovale.*
   (d) *Plasmodium malariae.*

53. In which of the following parasites band forms are seen in red blood cells?
   (a) *Plasmodium falciparum.*
   (b) *Plasmodium vivax.*
   (c) *Plasmodium malariae.*
   (d) *Plasmodium ovale.*

54. Malignant tertian malaria is caused by:
   (a) *Plasmodium falciparum.*
   (b) *Plasmodium vivax.*
   (c) *Plasmodium malariae.*
   (d) *Plasmodium ovale.*

55. Quartan malaria is caused by:
   (a) *Plasmodium falciparum.*
   (b) *Plasmodium vivax.*
   (c) *Plasmodium malariae.*
   (d) *Plasmodium ovale.*

56. Benign tertian malaria is caused by:
   (a) *Plasmodium falciparum.*
   (b) *Plasmodium vivax.*
   (c) *Plasmodium malariae.*
   (d) *Plasmodium ovale.*

57. Which of the following parasites causes cerebral malaria, pernicious malaria and blackwater fever?
   (a) *Plasmodium falciparum.*
   (b) *Plasmodium vivax.*
   (c) *Plasmodium malariae.*
   (d) *Plasmodium ovale.*

58. A genetic deficiency known as glucose-6-phosphate dehydrogenase trait confers some protection against:
   (a) *Plasmodium falciparum.*
   (b) *Plasmodium vivax.*
   (c) *Plasmodium malariae.*
   (d) *Plasmodium ovale.*

59. Presence of abnormal haemoglobin like thalassemia haemoglobin and foetal haemoglobin confers resistance against:
   (a) *Plasmodium falciparum.*
   (b) *Plasmodium vivax.*
   (c) *Plasmodium malariae.*
   (d) all of the above.

60. Modified Ziehl-Neelsen staining is used for staining oocysts of:
   (a) *Isospora belli.*
   (b) *Cyclospora cayetanensis.*
   (c) *Cryptosporidium parvum.*
   (d) All of the above.

61. Which of the following parasites **does not** occur in human intestine?
   (a) *Giardia lamblia.*
   (b) *Entamoeba histolytica.*
   (c) *Cyclospora cayetanensis.*
   (d) *Toxoplasma gondii.*

62. Which of the following statements about malaria is correct?
   (a) Infection is transmitted by *Culex* mosquito.
   (b) The parasites develop first in liver.
   (c) Once infected, immunity is lifelong.
   (d) The most dangerous species is *Plasmodium vivax.*

63. Which of the following malaria parasites has the shortest incubation period?
   (a) *Plasmodium vivax.*
   (b) *Plasmodium falciparum.*
   (c) *Plasmodium malariae.*
   (d) *Plasmodium ovale.*

64. Recrudescence of malaria is caused by:
   (a) *Plasmodium vivax.*
   (b) *Plasmodium falciparum.*
   (c) *Plasmodium malariae.*
   (d) All of the above.

65. Which of the following statements is correct for the protozoan parasite *Toxoplasma gondii*?
   (a) It is obligate intracellular parasite producing tachyzoites 6 μm in length and 2 μm in breadth.
   (b) It produces infective oocysts.

(c) It infects cat, pigs, sheep and man.
(d) All of the above.

66. Which of the following tests would be most useful for examination of *Cryptosporidium parvum* oocysts in stool?
(a) Trichrome stain.
(b) Modified acid-fast stain.
(c) Gram stain.
(d) Methylene blue stain.

67. One of the major features that can be used to differentiate *Cyclospora cayetanensis* and *Cryptosporidium parvum* is:
(a) shape.
(b) colour.
(c) size.
(d) refractility.

68. Which of the following parasites should be of special interest to pregnant women?
(a) *Isospora belli.*
(b) *Toxoplasma gondii.*
(c) *Ascaris lumbricoides.*
(d) *Endolimax nana.*

69. An AIDS patient complained of watery diarrhoea (15–20 motions/day). Modified acid-fast staining of the stools revealed oocysts 4–5 μm in diameter. What is the probable organism?
(a) Microsporidia.
(b) *Isospora belli.*
(c) *Cyclospora cayetanensis.*
(d) *Cryptosporidium parvum.*

70. Following statement is true about which of the following parasites?
It infects most species of warm-blooded animals, including humans. Members of cat family, Felidae, are the only definitive hosts for the sexual stage of this parasite and thus are main reservoir of infection.
(a) *Cyclospora cayetanensis.*
(b) *Isospora belli.*
(c) *Toxoplasma gondii.*
(d) *Cryptosporidium parvum.*

ANSWERS TO MCQs

1 (b), 2 (d), 3 (c), 4 (d), 5 (d), 6 (d), 7 (b), 8 (b), 9 (b), 10 (c), 11 (c), 12 (d), 13 (d), 14 (a), 15 (a), 16 (c), 17 (a) 18 (a), 19 (a), 20 (b), 21 (c), 22 (d), 23 (c), 24 (b), 25 (b), 26 (b), 27 (a), 28 (b), 29 (a), 30 (c), 31 (d), 32 (b), 33 (d), 34 (b), 35 (c), 36 (a), 37 (d), 38 (a), 39 (b), 40 (a), 41 (b), 42 (d), 43 (d), 44 (d), 45 (a), 46 (a), 47 (b), 48 (a), 49 (b), 50 (c), 51 (c), 52 (b), 53 (c), 54 (a), 55 (c), 56 (b), 57 (a), 58 (a), 59 (d), 60 (d), 61 (d), 62 (b), 63 (b), 64 (d), 65 (d), 66 (b), 67 (c), 68 (b), 69 (d), 70 (c).

6

Balantidium coli

Balantidium coli

- *Geographical distribution*
- *Habitat*
- *Morphology*
- *Culture*
- *Life cycle*
- *Pathogenicity*
- *Laboratory diagnosis*
- *Treatment*
- *Prophylaxis*

BALANTIDIUM COLI

Balantidium coli belongs to the kingdom Protozoa, phylum Ciliophora, class Litosmomatea and order Vestibuliferida (Table 1.5). This was first discovered by Malmsten in 1857 in the faeces of two patients with acute dysentery.

Geographical distribution

B. coli is worldwide in distribution. Because pigs are an animal reservoir, human infections occur more frequently in areas where pigs are raised.

Habitat

B. coli inhabits the large intestine of man, monkeys and pigs. It is generally believed that pigs act as the main reservoir for human infections.

Morphology

B. coli is the only pathogenic ciliate and is the largest protozoal parasite inhabiting the large intestine of man. It has a trophozoite and a cyst stage (Fig. 6.1). The trophozoite is found in dysenteric stool. It is actively motile and is the invasive stage. On the other hand, the cyst is found in chronic cases and carriers. It is the resistant form and the infective stage.

Trophozoite

It is an oval organism, measuring 60×45 µm or more. The anterior end is somewhat pointed and has a groove (*peristome*) leading to a mouth (*cytostome*) terminating in a short funnel-shaped gullet (*cytopharynx*) extending up to anterior one-third of the body. There is no intestine. The posterior end is broadly rounded and has an excretory opening known as *cytopyge* (Fig. 6.1) through which the residual contents of food vacuoles empty periodically. The body is covered with a delicate pellicle showing longitudinal striations. Embedded in the pellicle are short cilia of relatively uniform length that, in the living organism, maintain a constant

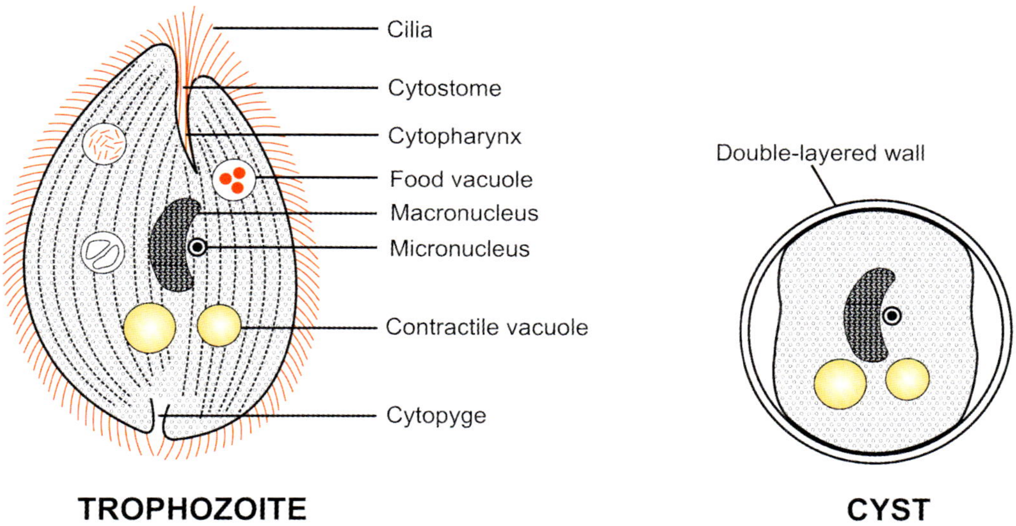

Fig. 6.1. Morphological forms of *Balantidium coli.*

synchronized motion that vigorously propels the protozoan forward. The cilia that line the mouth part are longer and are called adoral cilia. These are used for propelling food into the cytopharynx. The cytoplasm of the trophozoite has:

1. ***Two nuclei:*** A macronucleus which is large and situated near the middle of the body. It may be kidney-shaped, spherical, curved or elongate. The micronucleus is small, round and lies in close proximity to the macronucleus.
2. ***Two contractile vacuoles:*** Which may lie side by side or one above the other. These vacuoles are responsible for maintaining the proper osmotic pressure in the cell by drawing excess water from the cytoplasm and ejecting it to the exterior.
3. ***Numerous food vacuoles:*** The food particles on being ingested become surrounded by a vacuolar membrane and digestion takes place inside the vacuoles. The parasite is capable of ingesting a variety of food particles, such as bacteria, starch grains, fat droplets, cell debris of the intestinal wall, red blood cells, etc.

Cyst

The cyst of *B. coli* is spherical or oval measuring 40–60 μm in diameter. It is surrounded by a thick and transparent double-layered wall. Newly formed cyst shows movement, but as the cyst matures the cilia are absorbed and the movement ceases. The macronucleus, micronucleus and vacuoles are present in the cyst also. Unlike encystation in amoebae, in *B. coli* this is not preceded by complete discharge of undigested foods.

Culture

B. coli can be cultured in all the media that support the growth of *E. histolytica*.

Life cycle

B. coli passes its life cycle in two stages, but in one host only. Pig is the natural host and man is incidental host. Transmission occurs from pig-to-pig, pig-to-man, man-to-man and man-to-pig. Pig-to-pig transmission is very common. The cyst is the infective form of the parasite. Man acquires infection by ingestion of food or water contaminated with the faeces containing the cysts of *B. coli* (faecal-oral route). **Excystation** occurs in the small intestine and multiplication occurs in the large intestine. From each cyst, a single trophozoite is formed (Fig. 6.2). The trophozoites feed on bacteria and faecal debris which may remain either in the lumen or invade submucosa of the large intestine.

B. coli reproduces by transverse binary fission. First the micronucleus divides into two, then the macronucleus and finally the cytoplasm separates into two daughter organisms by a transverse partition in the middle of the body. The daughter organism formed from the anterior half retains the cytostome of the original parasite but develops a new excretory pore, whereas the one formed from the posterior end develops a new mouth. Successive divisions produce a large number of trophozoites.

Sexual union (**syngamy**) is an important aspect of this parasite's life cycle. It occurs by a process of conjugation, in which two cells come in contact with each other at their anterior ends and exchange nuclear

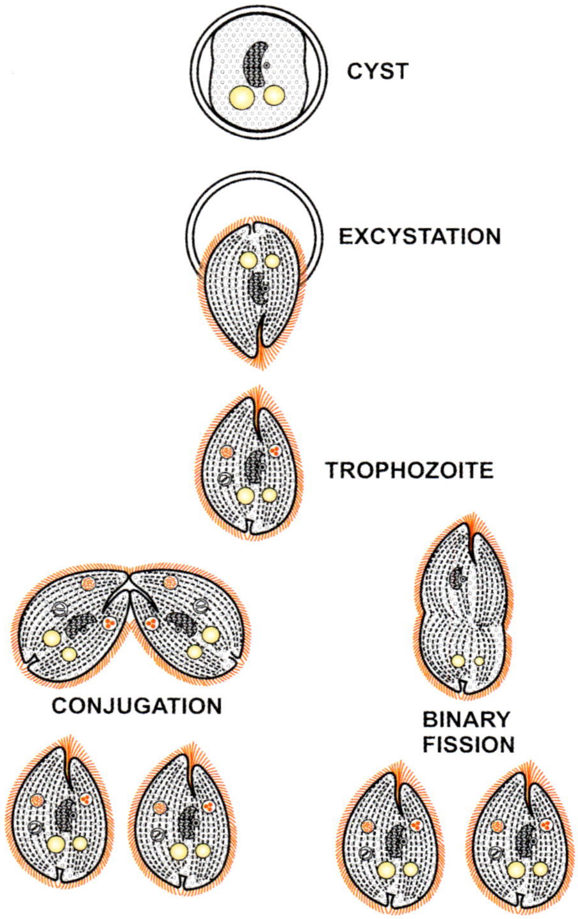

Fig. 6.2. Life cycle of *Balantidium coli*.

material. Conjugation lasts for a few moments, after which the cells detach. There is no increase in numbers as a result of conjugation.

Encystation of the trophozoite occurs as it is being transported down the intestine. In this process, the organism partially rounds up, then, without completely retracting the cilia, it secretes a tough cyst wall. In the infected person the parasite may be passed in the faeces as a trophozoite or a cyst. The trophozoite does not encyst outside the body and disintegrates. The passed cyst survives and may contaminate food and water and, as a result, may then be passed to other humans or animals.

Pathogenicity

Most infections with *B. coli* are apparently harmless. However, rarely, the trophozoites invade the mucosa and submucosa of the large intestine and terminal ileum and produce ulcers or subsurface abscesses in the mucous or submucous coats that sometimes extend to the muscular layer. The ulcers are round, ovoid, or irregular in shape with undermined edges. The floor of the ulcer is covered with pus and necrotic material. The abscesses are usually small and, when incised, are found to be filled with a mucoid material containing numerous balantidia. The intervening mucosa may or may not be inflamed.

On microscopic examination, parasites are frequently seen in clusters in the submucosa or at the bases of the crypts. They can easily be recognized because of the presence of the macronucleus which stains deeply with haematoxylin and eosin. The cellular response is mainly lymphocytic with some plasma cells being present. Neutrophils are few unless there is a superimposed bacterial infection. Sometimes the parasites may invade the regional lymph nodes and then they may be detected inside the lymphatic tissues. *B. coli* can produce **hyaluronidase**, which probably helps it in its invasion of the host tissues by dissolution of the intercellular ground substance.

Chronic recurrent diarrhoea, alternating with constipation, is the most common clinical manifestation, but there may be bloody mucoid stools, tenesmus, anorexia, nausea, epigastric pain, vomiting and intestinal colic. In a majority of patients, recovery occurs in 3–4 days even without treatment but extreme cases may mimic severe intestinal amoebiasis. In patients with acute infection, extraintestinal involvement such as liver abscess formation, peritonitis, pleuritis and pneumonia may occur.

Laboratory diagnosis

Stool examination

Diagnosis is based on faecal examination, which reveals mainly trophozoites in acutely infected patients and cysts in chronic cases and carriers. It is, generally, easy to recognize *B. coli* in stool specimens because of its large size (60 × 45 μm or more), an outer membrane covered with short cilia, and its large kidney-shaped macronucleus. When observed in wet mounts, the trophozoite has a rotatory, boring motility. In iodine mounts, the trophozoite stains yellowish-brown in colour, and the macronucleus is easily visible. The cyst (40–60 μm in diameter) can also be recognized by the large macronucleus.

Biopsy

Diagnosis can also be made by the examination of biopsy specimens taken with the help of a sigmoidoscope or by examination of scrapings of an ulcer.

Culture

Balantidium can be cultured in all the media that support the growth of *Entamoeba histolytica*. However, culture is rarely attempted for diagnosis as the parasites are more easily detected in faeces by microscopy and in tissues on histological examination.

Treatment

Tetracycline 500 mg four times a day for 10 days or metronidazole 750 mg three times a day may be used for the treatment of *B. coli* infection.

Prophylaxis

Preventive measures include:

- Hygienic rearing of pigs and preventing the human-pig contact which can lead to human infection.
- Prevention of contamination of food and water with pig and human faeces.
- Treatment of humans shedding cysts. This will prevent human-to-human transmission.

Further Reading

1. Gutierrez, Y. 2000. *Diagnostic Pathology of Parasitic Infections*, 2nd edn., Oxford University Press, New York, 263–70.
2. Zaman, V. 1993. *Balantidium coli*, *Parasitic Protozoa*, 2nd edn., Vol.3, eds. Kreier, J.P. and Baker, J.R., Academic Press, New York, 43–60.

Important Questions

Discuss morphology, life cycle, pathogenicity and laboratory diagnosis of *Balantidium coli*.

Multiple Choice Questions

1. Which of the following acts as the main reservoir of *Balantidium coli* infection in human beings?
   (a) Man.
   (b) Monkey.
   (c) Pig.
   (d) Cow.
2. Which of the following is the largest protozoal parasite inhabiting the large intestine of man?
   (a) *Entamoeba histolytica*.
   (b) *Entamoeba coli*.
   (c) *Balantidium coli*.
   (d) *Giardia lamblia*.
3. Which is the natural host of *Balantidium coli*?
   (a) Pig.
   (b) Man.
   (c) Cow.
   (d) Dog.
4. Which of the following parasites may cause dysentery?
   (a) *Cryptosporidium parvum*.
   (b) *Balantidium coli*.
   (c) *Cyclospora cayetanensis*.
   (d) *Isospora belli*.

ANSWERS TO MCQs

1 (c), 2 (c), 3 (a), 4 (b).

7

Microsporidia

MICROSPORIDIA

Microsporidia belong to the kingdom Fungi, phylum Microspora and class Microsporea (Table 1.5). They are obligate intracellular parasites. To date, more than 1200 species belonging to 143 genera have been described infecting a wide range of vertebrate and invertebrate hosts. Eight genera have been reported to cause disease in man (Table 7.1).

Microsporidia are being increasingly recognized as opportunistic infectious agents worldwide. Cases of microsporidiosis have been reported in developed as well as in developing countries, including Argentina, Australia, Botswana, Brazil, Canada, Czech Republic, France, Germany, India, Italy, Japan, The Netherlands, New Zealand, Spain, Sri Lanka, Sweden, Switzerland, Thailand, Uganda, United Kingdom, United States of America, and Zambia.

Morphology and Life cycle

Microsporidia are unicellular obligate intracellular parasites. In host cells the parasites develop and multiply producing a large number of infective spores. Spores are highly resistant and are the only life cycle stage able to survive outside the host cell and is the infective stage.

They are small, ranging from 1.5–2.5 μm × 2.5–4.0 μm. They are oval to cylindrical and possess a thick double-layered spore wall that renders it environmentally resistant. The outer layer, or exospore, is proteinaceous and electron-dense and, the inner layer, or endospore, is chitinous and electron-lucent. The plasma membrane lines the inside of the spore wall. Within the cytoplasm the spore possesses a coiled polar tube. It has a spring-like tubular extrusion mechanism by which the infective material, 'sporoplasm', is injected into host cell (Fig. 7.1). The coiled tube is everted and penetrates the host cell.

Inside the host cell, the invading parasite grows into a spherical or oblong schizont, with two to eight or

Table 7.1. Microsporidia causing human disease

Genus	Species	Main sites of infection
1. *Enterocytozoon*	*bieneusi*	Small intestinal epithelium, bile duct epithelium and rarely nasal polyps and bronchial epithelium
2. *Encephalitozoon*	*hellem*	Corneal and conjunctival epithelia, nasal polyps, kidney, tracheobronchial tree
	intestinalis	Epithelia of the gut from small intestine to colon, macrophages in the lamina propria, kidney, eyes and gall bladder
	cuniculi	Liver, peritoneum, kidney, intestine, eyes
3. *Trachipleistophora*	*hominis*	Skeletal muscle, heart muscle, corneal epithelium, kidney, nasopharynx
	anthropophthera	Brain, kidney, heart, pancreas, thyroid, parathyroid, liver, spleen, bone marrow
4. *Pleistophora*	*ronneafiei*	Skeletal muscle
5. *Brachiola*	*vesicularum*	Skeletal muscle
	conori (synonym *Nosema conori*)	Smooth and cardiac muscle, kidney, liver, lungs, adrenal cortex
	algerae	
6. *Vittaforma*	*corneae* (synonym *Nosema corneum*)	Corneal stroma of the eye
7. *Nosema*	*ocularum*	Corneal stroma of the eye
8. *Microsporidium*	*ceylonensis*	Corneal stroma of the eye
	africanum	Corneal stroma of the eye

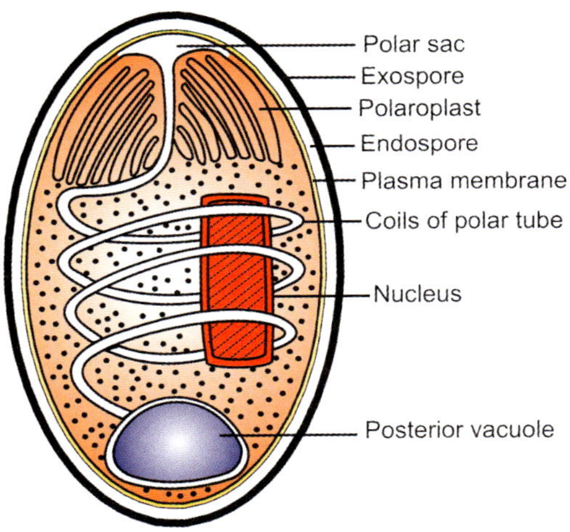

Fig. 7.1. Microsporidian spore.

more nuclei which become separate merozoites, followed by a complex series of asexual and sexual divisions leading to more spore production.

The spores stain poorly with haematoxylin and eosin but can be better visualized with Gram, acid-fast, periodic acid-Schiff, Giemsa, or modified trichrome stains. They are Gram-positive and acid-fast. Identification of species and genera is based upon electron microscopic morphology of spores, nuclei, and coiled polar filament.

Pathogenicity

Microsporidia have been recognized as causing disease in animals as early as the 1920s but were not recognized as agents of human disease until the AIDS pandemic began in the mid-1980s. Approximately 30% of AIDS patients and those with cryptosporidiosis may also have infections with microsporidia. In this group of patients with **chronic diarrhoea**, microsporidian infection must be considered. Currently 14 microsporidian species (Table 7.1) have been identified in man, most, but not all, are associated with HIV infection.

The first case of microsporidiosis from India was a patient with diarrhoea and was reported by Sehgal et al in 2001. Main sites of infection by microsporidia are given in Table 7.1. Infection is probably by spores being ingested, inhaled, or inoculated (eyes). The spores are highly resistant in the environment. Transplacental transmission also occurs. Microsporidian species most frequently reported in association with AIDS are *E. bieneusi*, *E. hellem* and *E. intestinalis*.

Intestinal microsporidiosis is the commonest infection caused mainly by *E. bieneusi*. It produces persistent diarrhoea with wasting. *E. bieneusi* is normally restricted to the small intestinal enterocytes, whereas *E. intestinalis* spreads into the lamina propria. Both these species have been found to spread from the intestine along the epithelium to the gall bladder, and the pancreatic and bile ducts. Although rarer, spread to the respiratory system has been documented with both species.

In AIDS patients, ocular involvement is often the presenting sign of microsporidiosis. Infection of corneal and conjunctival epithelia is commonly caused by *E. hellem*, but *E. intestinalis*, *E. cuniculi* and *Trachipleistophora hominis* may also cause it. These infections cause a bilateral **keratoconjunctivitis**. However, Sridhar and Sharma (2003) reported a case of microsporidial keratoconjunctivitis of left eye in an HIV-seronegative, 40-year-old female (Figs. 7.2 and 7.3). *E. hellem* has also been reported from lungs.

Another presentation can be **myositis**. *Pleistophora* spp., *T. hominis*, *B. vesicularum* and *B. conori* infections produce symptoms of severe muscle pain and weakness.

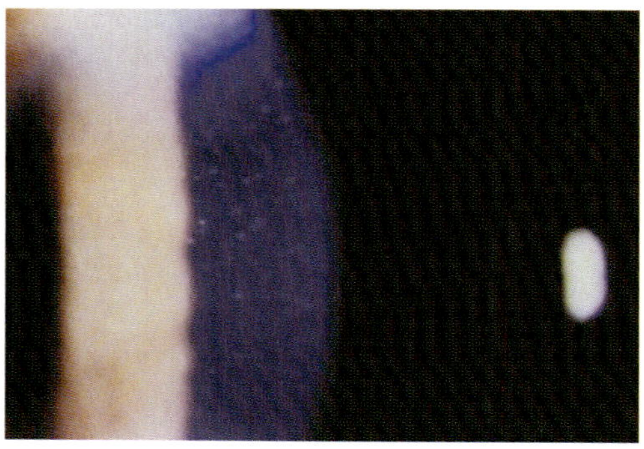

Fig. 7.2. Slit-lamp view of the left eye showing coarse epithelial lesions of the cornea. (*Courtesy:* Dr. S. Sharma)

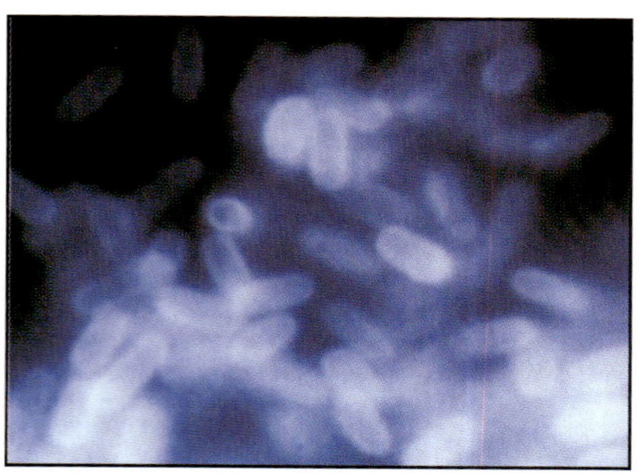

Fig. 7.3. Corneal scrapings showing microsporidial spores in potassium hydroxide and calcoflour white stain, × 1000. (*Courtesy:* Dr. S. Sharma)

Antibodies appear to be significantly less protective than the cell-mediated immune response in controlling microsporidial infections.

Laboratory diagnosis

Small-intestinal biopsy

Enteric infection is the most common type of microsporidial infection. It can be diagnosed by light microscopic and electron microscopic examination of small-intestinal biopsy sections or touch preparations of biopsy. Tiny intracytoplasmic spores are best demonstrated using Brown-Brenn or Brown-Hopps tissue Gram stains, Gomori methanamine silver, acid-fast, periodic acid-Schiff or Giemsa-stained touch preparations. They stain poorly with haematoxylin and eosin.

Electron microscopy (EM) continues to serve as the "gold standard" for confirming infection and for attempting to classify the organisms seen in tissues. The identification of spores with a polar tube is characteristic of all genera. However, this option is not available to all laboratories and the sensitivity of EM may not be equal to that of other methods when examining stool or urine.

Corneal scrapings

Microsporidian spores can be detected in the corneal scrapings stained with potassium hydroxide and calcofluor white (Fig. 7.3), and Gram staining.

Stool and duodenal-jejunal content examination

Microsporidial spores in the stool samples and the contents of the duodenum-jejunum using Enterotest method (which is often used to obtain luminal contents for detection of *Giardia*) can be detected by staining with modified trichrome stain, Giemsa or fluorescent dyes. These can also be detected by indirect immunofluorescence antibody stains using polyclonal antisera.

Microsporidial spores can also be detected in urine and nasopharyngeal swabs by above staining techniques.

Culture of microsporidia

Microsporidial spores from clinical specimens such as urine, nasal polyps, nasopharyngeal aspirates, faeces and muscle biopsies can be cultured in various cell lines.

Polymerase chain reaction

Microsporidial DNA can be amplified by PCR.

Serological testing

A variety of serological tests (carbon immunoassay, indirect immunofluorescent-antibody test (IFA), enzyme-linked immunosorbent assay (ELISA), counterimmunoelectrophoresis (CIE), and Western blotting) have been used to detect IgG and IgM antibodies to microsporidia, particularly to *E. cuniculi*. IFA and ELISA have been the most useful because of the simplicity of the test methods.

Treatment

Infection with microsporidia has been treated successfully with albendazole, an inhibitor of β-tubulin polymerization. Immunocompromised individuals with intestinal microsporidiosis due to *E. bieneusi* (which does not respond as well to albendazole) have been treated successfully with the antimicrobial fumagillin.

Further Reading

1. Dengjel, B., Zehler, M. et al. 2001. Zoonotic potential of *Enterocytozoon bieneusi*. *J. Clin. Microbiol.*, **39**, 4495–9.
2. Frazen, C. and Muller, A. 1999. Molecular techniques for detection, species differentiation and phylogenetic analysis of microsporidia. *Clin. Microbiol. Rev.*, **12**, 243–85.
3. Gumbo, T., Gangaidzo, I.T. et al. 2000. *Enterocytozoon bieneusi* infection in patients without evidence of immunosuppression: two cases from Zimbabwe found to have positive stools by PCR. *Ann. Trop. Med.* Parasitol., **94**, 699–702.
4. Lores, B., Lopez-Miragaya, I., 2002. Intestinal microsporidiosis due to *Enterocytozoon bieneusi* in elderly human immunodeficiency virus-negative patients from Vigo, Spain. *Clin. Infect. Dis.*, **34**, 918–21.
5. Muller, A., Bialek, R., et al. 2001. Detection of microsporidia in travelers with diarrhoea. *J. Clin. Microbiol.*, **39**, 1630–32.
6. Sadler, F., Peake, N. et al. 2002. Genotyping of *Enterocytozoon bieneusi* in AIDS patients from northwest of England. *J. Infect.*, **44**, 39–42.
7. Sehgal, R., Yadav, C. et al. 2001. Prevalence of "newer coccidia" and microsporidia in patients with diarrhoea in northern India. J. *Parasitic Diseases*, **25**, 21–5.
8. Sianongo, S., McDonald, V. and Kelly, P. 2001. A method for diagnosis of microsporidiosis adapted for use in developing countries. *Trans. R. Soc. Trop. Med. Hyg.*, **95**, 605–7.
9. Sridhar, M.S., Sharma, S. 2003. Microsporidial keratoconjunctivitis in an HIV-seronegative patient treated with debridement and oral itraconazole. *Am. J. Ophthalmol.*, **136**, 745–6.
10. Visvesvara, G.S. 2002. *In vitro* cultivation of microsporidia of clinical importance. *Clin. Microbiol.* Rev., **15**, 401–13.

Important Questions

Name various microsporidian genera causing human disease. Discuss morphology, life cycle, pathogenicity and laboratory diagnosis of these.

Multiple Choice Questions

1. How many genera of microsporidia have been reported to cause disease in man?
   (a) Two.
   (b) Four.
   (c) Seven.
   (d) Eight.
2. *Enterocytozoon bieneusi* tends to preferentially infect:
   (a) enterocytes.
   (b) brain.
   (c) kidneys.
   (d) conjunctiva.
3. What is the infective stage of microsporidia in the stool?
   (a) Cyst.
   (b) Oocyst.
   (c) Spore.
   (d) Trophozoite.
4. Which of the following parasites is **not** seen in faecal specimens:
   (a) *Entamoeba histolytica.*
   (b) *Cyclospora cayetanensis.*
   (c) *Toxoplasma gondii.*
   (d) *Enterocytozoon bieneusi.*

ANSWERS TO MCQs

1 (d), 2 (a), 3 (c), 4 (c).

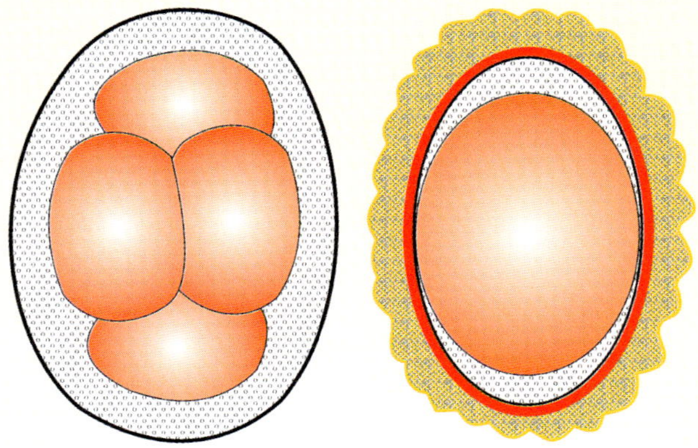

SECTION 3
Helminthology

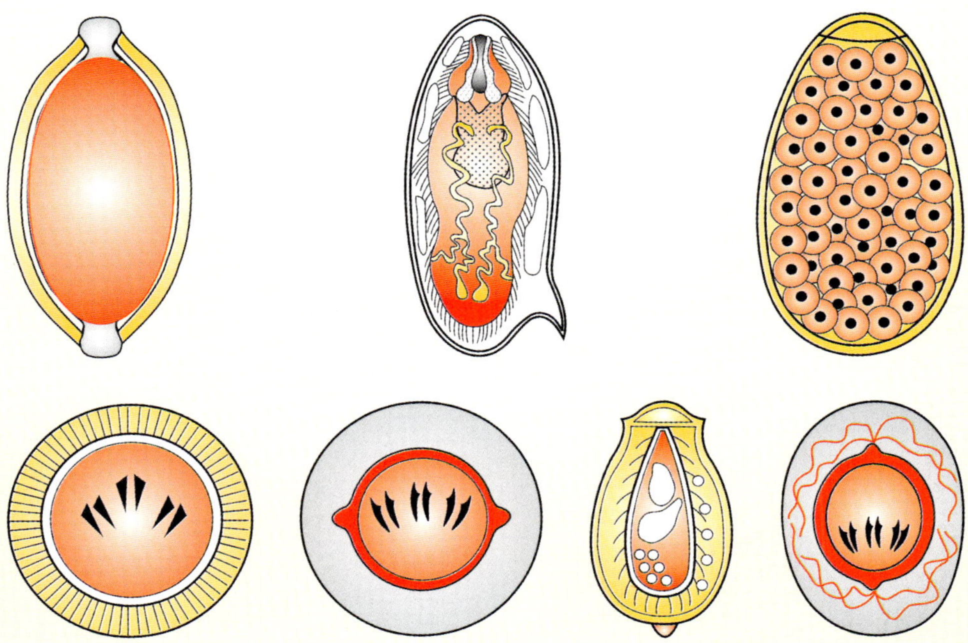

8

Introduction to Helminths

Helminths or parasitic worms belong to the kingdom Animalia. They are multicellular, bilaterally symmetrical, elongated, flat or round animals. Helminths which occur as parasites in humans belong to two phyla (Table 1.6):

1. Phylum Platyhelminthes
2. Phylum Nemathelminthes

PHYLUM PLATYHELMINTHES

The platyhelminthes or flatworms are dorsoventrally flattened, leaf-like or tape-like. Their alimentary canal is incomplete or entirely lacking and body cavity is absent. They are mostly hermaphrodites (monoecious). Human pathogenic helminths of this phylum belong to two classes – the Cestoidea and the Digenea.

PHYLUM NEMATHELMINTHES

Nematodes are unsegmented, dioecious worms which are usually filiform. They have a body cavity with a high hydrostatic pressure, complete alimentary canal with an anteriorly terminal mouth and posteriorly sub-terminal anus, no circulatory system, a simple excretory system and a body wall consisting of an outer layer of longitudinal muscles. Phylum Nemathelminthes is divided into 2 classes – the Adenophorea and the Secernentea (Tables 1.6 and 8.1). Both these classes have parasitic members though the majority of animal parasites belong to the latter.

Tabel 8.1. Differences between nematodes of class Adenophorea and class Secernentea

	Adenophorea	**Secernentea**
Eggs	With plug at either end	Without plug at either end
Excretory system	Without lateral canals	With lateral canals
Caudal papillae	Absent or few	Numerous
Stage of larva infective to final host	First larval stage	Third larval stage

Differences between cestodes, trematodes and nematodes are given in Table 8.2.

GENERAL CHARACTERISTICS OF HELMINTHS

Most helminthic worms are macroscopic ranging in size from less than 1 mm to 1 m or larger. The external surface of some helminths is covered with a protective cuticle, which is acellular and may be smooth or possess ridges, spines, or tubercles. The protective covering of flat helminths is known as **tegument**. Often helminths possess elaborate attachment structures, such as hooks, suckers, teeth, or plates. These structures are usually located anteriorly and may be useful in classifying and identifying the helminths. They have primitive nervous and excretory systems. Some have alimentary tracts; however, none have a circulatory system. Larval forms of these worms include:

- Rhabditiform, filariform and microfilaria in nematodes;
- Cysticercus, cysticercoid, coenurus, coracidium, procercoid, plerocercoid and hydatid cyst in cestodes; and
- Miracidium, sporocyst, redia, cercaria and metacercaria in trematodes.

All helminths with a few exceptions produce eggs. These are excreted in different secretions or excretions of the body.

Life cycle of helminths may be completed in one or more than one hosts. Cestodes with the exception of *Hymenolepis nana* complete their life cycle in two different hosts. For most of the cestodes man is the definitive host but for *Echinococcus granulosus* man acts as intermediate host. For *Taenia solium* man is the definitive host but may act as intermediate host also.

Trematodes complete their life cycle in one definitive host (man) and two intermediate hosts – freshwater snail or mollusc as first intermediate host and fish or crab as second intermediate host.

Nematodes complete their life cycle in one host except in filarial nematodes and *Dracunculus medinensis*, which complete their life cycle in man and insect vector as second host for the former and cyclops as second host for the latter.

The pathological lesions in helminthic diseases are due to direct damage caused by helminths and indirect damage from host response, for example hypersensitivity reaction to the helminths. The role of malnutrition in helminthic infections may be great, both with respect to the parasite and its host. Alteration of diet or dietary deficiencies are important factors governing susceptibility to certain helminths, in spontaneous loss of the worms or in partial or complete refractoriness to infection.

Malnutrition interferes with antibody production, may decrease inflammatory reaction and, in this way, lowers resistance. The clinical manifestations of helminthic diseases are variable. These may be acute or chronic. In many helminthic infections, allergic manifestations are important. The specific diagnosis of helminthic diseases is usually based on the morphological recognition of helminths in relevant specimens and on the immunological test.

Chemotherapy is the method of choice for the treatment of helminthic diseases. Surgery is indicated in a few helminthic infections such as hydatid disease and cysticercosis.

Table 8.2. Differences between cestodes, trematodes and nematodes

	Cestodes	Trematodes	Nematodes
Shape	Tape-like, segmented	Leaf-like, unsegmented	Elongated, cylindrical, unsegmented
Sexes	Monoecious (not separate)	Monoecious except schistosomes which are dioecious	Dioecious (separate)
Head	Suckers, often with hooks	Suckers, no hooks	No suckers, no hooks. Some species have well-developed buccal capsule.
Alimentary canal	Absent	Present but incomplete; no anus	Present and complete with an anteriorly terminal mouth and posteriorly subterminal anus.
Body cavity	Absent	Absent	Present
Mode of infection	Infection generally by encysted larvae	Infection mainly by larval stages, entering intestinal tract, sometimes through skin	Infection by ingestion of eggs, or penetration of larvae through surfaces, or arthropod vector, or ingestion of encysted larvae

Further Reading

1. Coombs, I. and Crompton, D.W.T. 1991. *A guide to human helminths*, Taylor and Francis, London.
2. Miller, R.1975. Worms and Diseases. *A manual of Medical Helminthology*, Heinemann Medical, London.

Important Questions

Write short notes on:

(a) General characters of helminths.
(b) Phylum Platyhelminthes.
(c) Phylum Nemathelminthes.

Multiple Choice Questions

1. Miracidium larval form is seen in :
   (a) cestodes.
   (b) nematodes.
   (c) trematodes.
   (d) sporozoa.
2. Two intermediate hosts are essential to complete the life cycle in:
   (a) cestodes, except *Diphyllobothrium latum*.
   (b) nematodes.
   (c) trematodes.
   (d) sporozoa.
3. Two different hosts are essential to complete the life cycle in the following helminths **except**:
   (a) *Hymenolepis nana*.
   (b) *Echinococcus granulosus*.
   (c) *Taenia saginata*.
   (d) *Dracunculus medinensis*.

ANSWERS TO MCQs

1 (c), 2 (c), 3 (a).

9

Cestodes or Tapeworms

General characteristics of cestodes
- *Life cycle*
- *Pathogenicity*
- *Laboratory diagnosis*
- *Prophylaxis*

Classification of cestodes
Diphyllobothrium latum
Spirometra
Taenia saginata and *Taenia solium*
Taenia asiatica
Taenia multiceps
Hymenolepis nana
Hymenolepis diminuta
Dipylidium caninum
Echinococcus granulosus
Echinococcus multilocularis
Echinococcus vogeli

GENERAL CHARACTERISTICS OF CESTODES

Cestodes belong to the kingdom Animalia and phylum Platyhelminthes. They are segmented, dorsoventrally compressed and tape-like, hence called tapeworms. They vary from a few millimetres to several metres in length. The most conspicuous features of tapeworms are the lack of a mouth or digestive cavity. Adult cestodes, or tapeworms, live attached to the mucosa in the small intestine and absorb food from the intestine of the host. They belong to the class Cestoidea and orders Pseudophyllidea and Cyclophyllidea (Tables 1.6 and 9.1).

Adult worm

Adult worm consists of three parts:

1. Scolex (head)
2. Neck
3. Strobila (body or trunk)

Scolex (Head)

It is a more or less distended muscular organ. It serves as an organ of attachment. In the parasites of the order Pseudophyllidea, the scolex does not possess suckers. On the other hand, it normally possesses a pair of longitudinal grooves (bothria) which help in the attachment of the parasite to the small intestine of the host. Scolex of the parasites of the order Cyclophyllidea normally possesses four suckers. Rostellum (apical protrusion on scolex) is usually present, but may be absent. The rostellum may be armed with hooks or not.

Neck

It is the portion of the worm which lies immediately behind the scolex and from which proglottids of the body are continuously generated. The scolex and neck are important structures, since infection persists as long as these portions of the worm remain attached to the host's intestinal wall, even though the greater portion of the strobila may have become free and been evacuated.

Strobila

Strobila (body or trunk) is composed of a chain of proglottids or segments. Three types of proglottids are recognized – immature, mature and gravid. Those near the neck are young immature segments where male and female organs are not differentiated. Behind them are mature segments. These are larger units, each of which contains one and in some species two full sets of male and female genital organs. Therefore, each individual worm is hermaphrodite (monoecious). The gravid proglottids are those farthest away from the scolex. In them the primary genitalia have atrophied and are completely occupied by the uterus filled with eggs. There is no specialized alimentary or digestive system. Nutrients are absorbed through the worm's integument. The scolex is strictly an organ for attachment, and it does not serve for procurement of food. Body cavity is absent. Rudimentary excretory and nervous systems are present.

Egg

In pseudophyllidean cestodes the egg is ovoid, operculated and does not contain any embryo when first laid. The membrane covering the embryo, which is formed outside, has a ciliated epithelium. In cyclophyllidean cestodes the egg is not operculated and has two coverings – the inner which surrounds the embryo is known as embryophore and the outer is thin and is known as egg-shell. The egg, when first laid, contains a six-hooked (hexacanth) embryo known as oncosphere. It does not have ciliated epithelium. In some cases the egg-shell is so thin that it is lost before the egg reaches the exterior with the faeces. In such cases the embryophore becomes thick and radially striated for the protection of the embryo.

Life cycle

Cestodes complete their life cycle in two different hosts. However, *Hymenolepis nana* is an exception which is capable of completing its life cycle in a single host. Man is definitive host for most tapeworms which cause human infection. An important exception is *Echinococcus granulosus* (dog tapeworm) for which dog is the definitive host and man is the intermediate host. For *Taenia solium* (pork tapeworm) man is ordinarily the definitive host, but sometimes man acts as the intermediate host and harbours the larval form of this parasite.

The intermediate hosts are mammals, fish or arthropods. They harbour larval stages of the parasite. In majority of the cestode infections, only one intermediate host is needed. However, in *Diphyllobothrium latum*, two intermediate hosts are required.

Pathogenicity

Tapeworm infections are acquired either by ingestion of the eggs or of larval stages present in meat, fish, etc. Adult tapeworms are intestinal parasites. They tend to do little physical damage to their host. Large infections can, however, lead to obstruction of the bowel. They may cause diarrhoea and loss of appetite. In some cases, absorption of certain nutrients, e.g., vitamin B_{12} in case of *D. latum* infection results in pernicious anaemia. The presence of encysted larval tapeworms in tissues is much more serious, particularly in certain organs such as the brain, liver and lungs, since the cysts can, in some cases, reach a large size.

Laboratory diagnosis

Intestinal infection with adult worms can be diagnosed by demonstration of eggs and sometimes proglottids in the faeces. Extraintestinal infections caused by the larvae can be diagnosed by biopsy, serology and radio-imaging.

Prophylaxis

Avoidance of eating raw or inadequately cooked food, meat, fish or drinking of contaminated water will prevent transmission of infection to man. Thorough cooking prevents infection. Sanitary disposal of human faeces containing the viable eggs of these tapeworms protects communities. Avoidance of contact with the faeces of man and dog prevents infection with *T. solium* and *E. granulosus* respectively.

CLASSIFICATION OF CESTODES

Cestodes can be classified in two ways:

1. Systematic classification
2. According to habitat

Systematic classification

Tapeworms that infect man, belong to two orders – Pseudophyllidea and Cyclophyllidea, the former bearing a pair of longitudinal grooves called bothria and the latter cup-like suckers on their scolices. Simplified systematic classification is given in Table 9.1.

According to habitat

Tapeworms may be classified on the basis of the habitat of the adult worms and larval stages in man (Table 9.2).

DIPHYLLOBOTHRIUM LATUM

Common names: The fish tapeworm; the broad tapeworm. The name fish tapeworm relates to the fact that fish is the source of infection to humans, and the broad (*latum*) tapeworm to the fact that the proglottids are much wider than they are long, unlike the *Taenia* species.

The head of the worm was found by Bonnet as early as 1777 but its life cycle was described by Janicke and Rosen in 1917. Several other *Diphyllobothrium* species have been reported to infect humans, but less frequently; they include *D. pacificum*, *D. cordatum*, *D. ursi*, *D. dendriticum*, *D. lanceolatum* and *D. yonagoensis*.

Geographical distribution

Diphyllobothrium latum is endemic in Europe, Russia, Japan, Tropical Africa, and North and South America.

Habitat

Adult worm lives in the small intestine (ileum or jejunum) of man; also in dog, cat, fox and other fish-eating animals.

Table 9.1. Systematic classification of cestodes

Order	Family	Genus	Species
Cyclophyllidea	Taeniidae	*Taenia*	*T. solium* *T. saginata* *T. asiatica* *T. multiceps*
		Echinococcus	*E. granulosus* *E.multilocularis* *E. vogeli*
	Hymenolepididae	*Hymenolepis*	*H. nana* *H. diminuta*
	Dipylidiidae	*Dipylidium*	*D. caninum*
Pseudophyllidea	Diphyllobothriidae	*Diphyllobothrium*	*D. latum*
		Spirometra	*S. mansoni* *S. theileri* *S. erinace*

Table 9.2. Classification of tapeworms on the basis of the habitat of the adult worms and larval stages in man

Order	Adult worms in the intestine of man	Larval stages in man
Pseudophyllidea	*Diphyllobothrium latum*	*Spirometra mansoni* *S. theileri* *S. erinace*
Cyclophyllidea	*Taenia solium* *T. saginata* *T. asiatica* *Hymenolepis nana* *H. diminuta* *Dipylidium caninum*	*Echinococcus granulosus* *E. multilocularis* *E. vogeli* *T. solium* *T. multiceps*

Morphology

Adult worm

D. latum is the **longest tapeworm found in man**. It measures up to 10 metres or more in length. It can live for 5–13 years in its host. When freshly expelled from the human intestine, the worm is ivory coloured. It consists of scolex, neck and strobila.

Scolex: The scolex is almond-shaped or spoon-shaped and measures 2–3 mm in length and 1 mm in breadth. It bears two slit-like grooves (bothria) demarcated by lateral lip-like folds, one dorsal and the other ventral. There are no rostellum and hooklets (Fig. 9.1).

Neck: It is situated immediately behind the scolex. It is thin, unsegmented and several times the length of the head.

Strobila: It has 3,000 or more proglottids (segments), consisting of immature, mature and gravid segments in that order from the front to backwards. The typical mature proglottid is broader (10–20 mm) than long (2–4 mm) and is practically filled with male and female reproductive organs. A coiled uterus in the form of a compact-rosette is seen centrally within each segment. Eggs are discharged periodically through the uterine pore of each functional proglottid. A single worm may discharge as many as one million eggs daily. The terminal segments are shrunken and empty owing to the constant discharge of eggs through the uterine pore. Later the dried-up segments break off from the body, in chains, and are passed in the faeces.

Egg

Egg of *D. latum* is yellowish-brown in colour (bile-stained), oval or elliptical in shape, measures 70 μm in length and 45 μm in breadth and has thin and smooth shell. It contains an immature embryo. There is an inconspicuous operculum at one end (operculated egg) with a small knob at the other end (Figs. 9.1 and 9.2). **It does not float in saturated solution of common salt.** The freshly passed egg is not infective to man.

Larval stages

The egg develops into first-, second-, and third-stage larva. The first-stage larva is known as **coracidium**. It develops from the egg in water. The second-stage larva is known as **procercoid**. It develops from coracidium inside small copepods, mainly of the genera *Diaptomus* and *Cyclops* (first intermediate host). The third-stage larva is known as **plerocercoid** or **sparganum**. It develops from procercoid in freshwater fish, the second intermediate host. It is the infective form of the parasite.

Life cycle

The worm passes its life cycle in one definitive host and two intermediate hosts (Fig. 9.1).

Definitive hosts

Man is the main definitive host and contributes most to the spread of infection, but freshwater fish-eating animals such as dogs, cats, foxes, bears and pigs may also act as definitive hosts of *D. latum*.

Intermediate hosts

D. latum is unique among human tapeworms for its freshwater aquatic life cycle involving two intermediate hosts.

- ***First intermediate host:*** Small copepods, mainly of the genera *Diaptomus* and *Cyclops*.
- ***Second intermediate host:*** Freshwater fishes (pike, perch, salmon, lawyer, trout, etc.).

Adult worm resides in the small intestine (ileum or jejunum) of man and other definitive hosts. It lays operculated eggs which are passed alongwith the faeces in water. A spherical ciliated embryo containing three pairs of hooklets (hexacanth embryo or oncosphere) develops within each egg-shell in 1–2 weeks. It is known as coracidium. Eggs also develop and survive well in environments such as those provided by damp soil and ooze at the water margin of lakes, ponds and streams.

The fully developed coracidium leaves the egg via operculum, swims about in the water and is ingested by small copepods. In order to continue its development it must be ingested by an appropriate copepod within about 12 hours. In the intestine of copepod, the ciliated embryophore is shed and oncosphere penetrates the intestine and enters the body cavity (haemocoel). Here, in the course of 2–3 weeks, it is transformed into procercoid larva measuring 0.5 mm in length.

When copepods with infective procercoid larvae are eaten by a suitable second intermediate host (a freshwater fish), the procercoid penetrates the intestine of the fish and comes to lie free between the muscle fibres, where it grows into infectious plerocercoid larva measuring 10–20 mm × 2–3 mm. It is not encysted or encapsulated, has a well developed and normally contracted, partly invaginated scolex. If a small infected fish is eaten by a larger suitable fish, the plerocercoids are, to some degree, able to penetrate the intestine of this second host and survive without further development i.e. this host is **paratenic host** (a host in

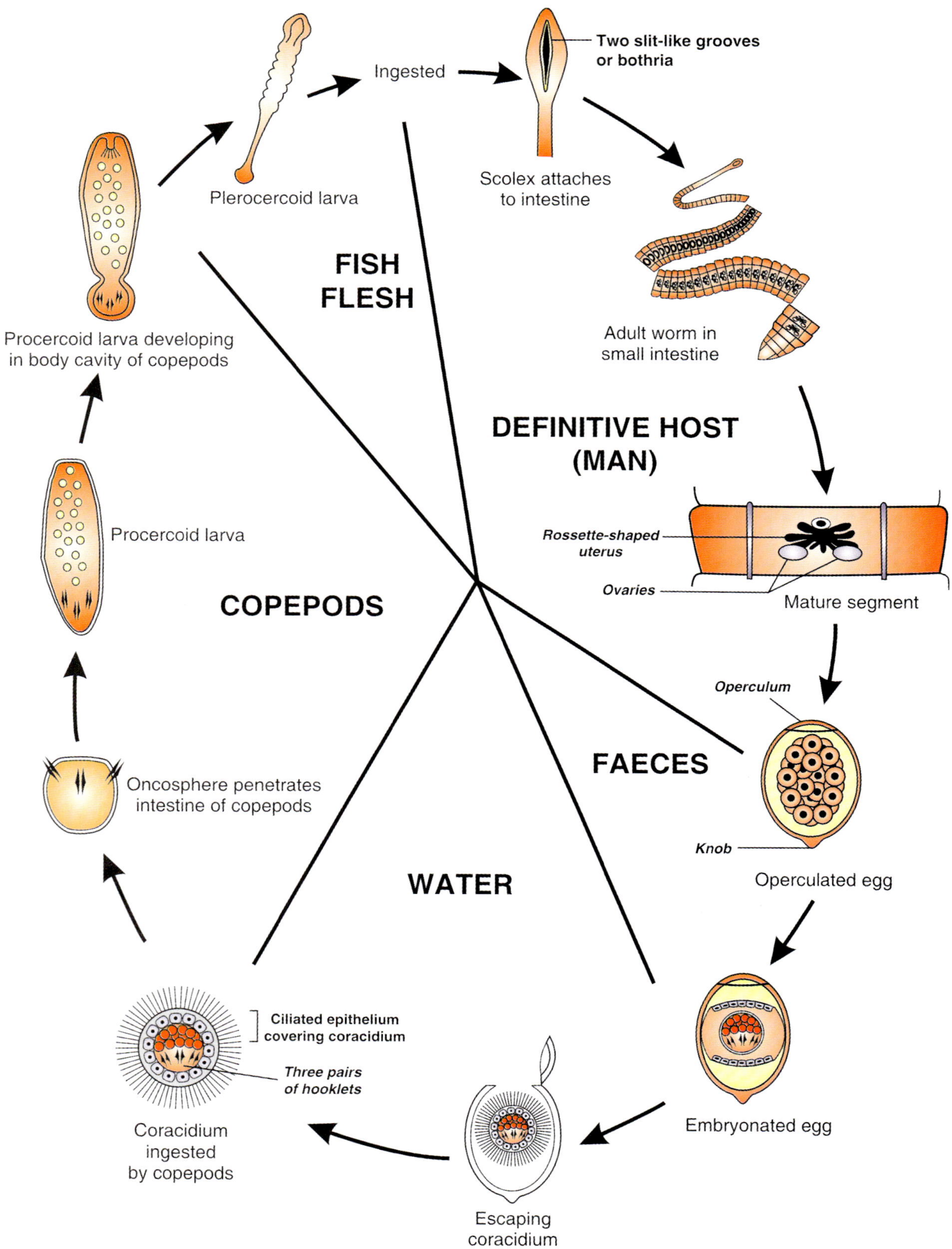

Fig. 9.1. Life cycle of *Diphyllobothrium latum*.

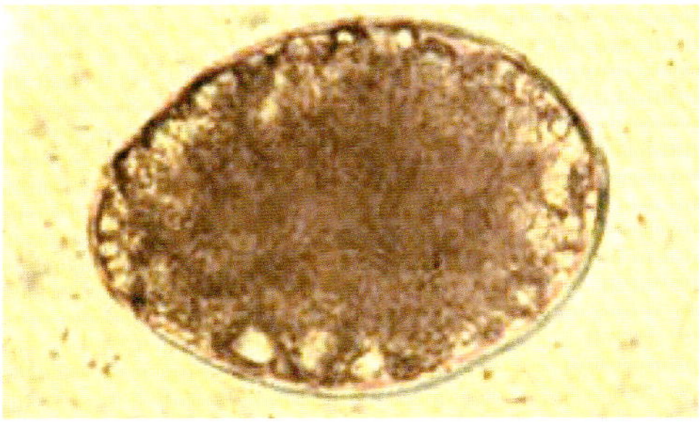

Fig. 9.2. Egg of *Diphyllobothrium latum* (saline wet mount, ×400).

which the parasite does not mature or is not essential for its life cycle).

Humans become infected when they eat undercooked, raw or lightly salted meat or roe from infected freshwater fishes. Inside the intestine of man the plerocercoid larva develops into an adult worm and after having attained sexual maturity in about 5–6 weeks, begins to lay eggs which are passed alongwith the faeces. The cycle is thus repeated.

Pathogenicity

Infection caused by *D. latum* in man is known as diphyllobothriasis. Patient may develop fatigue, weakness, diarrhoea and numbness of the extremities. Some patients develop mechanical obstruction of the bowel by a large number of the worms that become tangled together. The worms may remain active for many years or may be discharged spontaneously.

In a few cases pernicious anaemia may develop due to manifest vitamin B_{12} deficiency. *D. latum* has been shown to absorb as much as 80–100% of a single oral dose of vitamin B_{12}, thereby competing with the host for this important vitamin. The size of the tapeworm and its proximity to the stomach influences the amount of B_{12} absorption by the parasite. Large tapeworms in close proximity to the stomach reduce B_{12} availability to the host leading to parasite-induced **pernicious anaemia**. Infection at the jejunal level causes impairment of the interaction between the extrinsic and intrinsic factors of Castle, hence the pernicious type of anaemia. Inadequate supply of vitamin B_{12} in the diet may contribute to the development of tapeworm-induced pernicious anaemia.

Laboratory diagnosis

The laboratory diagnosis of diphyllobothriasis in humans can be made by identification of the characteristic operculated eggs (Figs. 9.1 and 9.2) or proglottids in the faeces. Eggs are usually numerous and readily demonstrated in a direct faecal smear. If egg operculum is difficult to see, the coverslip of the wet preparation can be tapped and the pressure may cause the operculum to pop open, thus making it more visible. Occasionally, portions of the worm up to several metres long may be vomited.

Treatment

Therapy with praziquantel readily eliminates the worm and ensures haematological remission.

Prophylaxis

Preventive measures include:

1. Thorough cooking of freshwater fish.
2. Freezing of fish or roe intended to be eaten raw or semi-raw at –18°C for 24–48 hours kills any plerocercoids that may be present.
3. Preventing the contamination of lakes, ponds and river water by human faeces.
4. Effective sanitary disposal of faeces.
5. Protection of water supplies from faecal pollution.
6. Chemotherapy of infected humans.

SPIROMETRA

Genus *Spirometra* occurs in humans as a **plerocercoid larva** known as **sparganum**. Species of medical importance are *S. mansoni*, *S. theileri* and *S. erinacei*.

Geographical distribution

Sparganosis has been reported mostly from Japan and Southeast Asia and less often from America and Australia. A few cases have also been reported from India.

Life cycle

Adult worms live in the intestinal tract of cats and dogs, producing large number of eggs which pass out with the faeces and hatch in water to release a ciliated larva known as **coracidium** (Fig. 9.3). If the coracidium is eaten by a suitable copepod, they develop in the body cavity as a **procercoid larva**. When the infected copepod is ingested by the second intermediate host (frog, fish, snake) the larva migrates to various organs of the body where it develops into plerocercoid larva. When a cat or dog eats the second intermediate host the plerocercoid larva develops into **adult worm**.

Pathogenicity

Man acquires infection by:

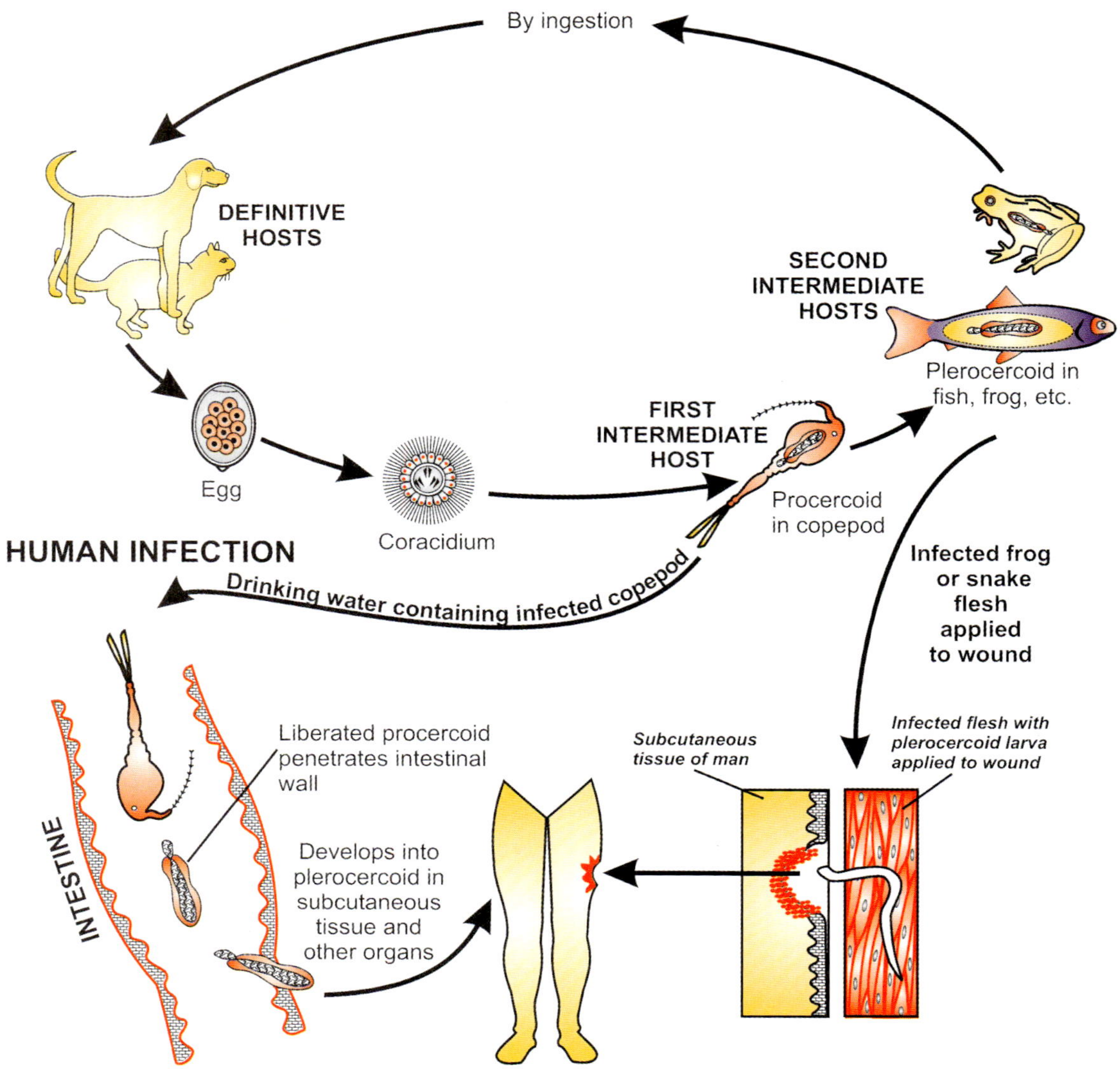

Fig. 9.3. Life cycle of *Spirometra* spp.

- Drinking water containing infected copepods.
- Eating raw or poorly cooked flesh of second intermediate host.
- Using frog or snake flesh as a poultice on a wound or injured eye.

The disease caused by plerocercoid larvae (spargana) of *Spirometra* is known as **sparganosis**. Humans act as the end-stage host for the larval stage, sparganum. In the human intestine, the procercoid larvae are liberated from the copepods. They penetrate the intestinal wall and usually migrate to the subcutaneous tissue and other organs, and develop into spargana. These become encysted in fibrous nodules reaching 2 cm in diameter. These may be painful. The condition is much more serious if the larvae end up in the eye, lymphatic system, brain, etc. When frog or snake flesh is used as a poultice on a wound or injured eye, the spargana migrate from vertebrate host tissues into human tissues. Inflammation and secondary infection are the usual outcome.

Laboratory diagnosis

The definitive diagnosis is made only after surgical removal of a sparganum and identifying white, ribbon-like worm that measures up to 30 cm in length by 3 mm in breadth. **The absence of suckers and hooklets differentiates spargana from cysticercus and coenrus.** Species diagnosis can be made by feeding living spargana to a cat or dog and subsequently examining the adult worm.

Prophylaxis

Sparganosis can be prevented by filtering water, and avoiding the consumption or contact with raw flesh which might harbour plerocercoid larvae.

Treatment

Surgical removal of the nodule containing larvae is the method of choice for treatment of the infection.

TAENIA

Genus *Taenia* has 32 recognized species, of which *T. saginata*, *T. solium*, *T. asiatica* and *T. multiceps* cause human infection.

TAENIA SAGINATA AND TAENIA SOLIUM

Common names: *Taenia saginata* – The beef tapeworm; the unarmed tapeworm of man. *Taenia solium* – The pork tapeworm; the armed tapeworm of man.

Geographical distribution

T. saginata has a worldwide distribution in countries where cattle are raised and inadequately cooked beef is eaten. The name 'beef tapeworm' comes from the fact that beef is the main source of infection. *T. solium* is not as widely distributed as *T. saginata*. It occurs mainly in southern Africa, China, India, Central America, Chile, Brazil, Papua New Guinea, and non-Islamic Southeast Asia where human faeces reach pigs and pork is eaten raw or undercooked. *T. solium* is known as 'pork tapeworm' because pork is the main source of infection. It does not occur in Muslims and Jews, who do not eat pork. It is estimated that as many as 100 million people are infected with *T. saginata* and *T. solium*.

Habitat

Adult worms of both *T. saginata* and *T. solium* live in small intestine (upper jejunum) of man (Fig. 9.4). They remain attached to the intestinal mucosa with their suckers.

Morphology

Adult worm

The adult worms consist of scolex (head), neck and strobila which is made up of a large number of proglottids (segments). The differentiating features of *T. saginata* and *T. solium* are given in Figs. 9.5 and 9.6, and Table 9.3.

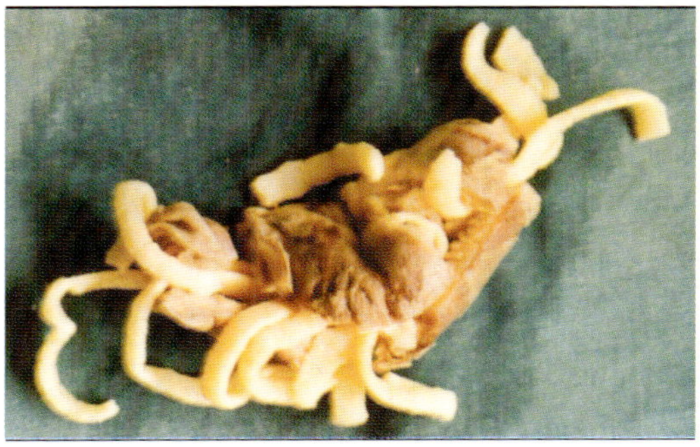

Fig. 9.4. *Taenia solium* causing obstruction of small intestine.

Eggs

Eggs (Figs. 9.5–9.7) of both species are indistinguishable. They are spherical, **brown in colour (bile-stained)** and measure 31–43 μm in diameter. They are surrounded by embryophore which is brown, thick-walled and radially striated. Outside this may be present thin transparent shell which represents the remnant of yolk mass. Inside the embryophore is present hexacanth embryo (oncosphere) with three pairs of hooklets. **It does not float in saturated solution of common salt.** The eggs of *T. solium* are infective to pig and also to man, while those of *T. saginata* are infective only to cattle.

Life cycle of *T. saginata*

T. saginata passes its life cycle in two hosts. The definitive host is man who harbours the adult worm. The intermediate host is cattle. Eggs or gravid segments are passed out with the faeces on the ground (Fig. 9.5). These are ingested by cows or buffaloes while grazing in the field. When they reach the duodenum, the embryophore of the eggs ruptures and liberates **oncospheres**. With the help of their hooklets they penetrate the wall of the intestine and enter into portal vessels or mesenteric lymphatics. Then they reach general circulation via liver, right side of the heart, lungs and left side of the heart. From general circulation, they are filtered out in striated muscles where, in 10–12 weeks, they develop into bladder worm known as **Cysticercus bovis**.

The mature cysticerci are ovoid in shape, milky-white, opalescent and measure 7.5–10 mm in breadth and 4–6 mm in length. They have unarmed scolices (scolices without hooklets) invaginated in them. These cysticerci are frequently found in the muscles of mastication, the cardiac muscle, diaphragm and tongue. The cysticerci can live in flesh of cattle for about 8

Table 9.3. Differentiating features of *T. saginata* and *T. solium*

	T. saginata	*T. solium*
Length	4–6 metres or more	2–4 metres or more
Scolex	Large, quadrate without rostellum and hooklets. Possesses four suckers which may be pigmented.	Small, globular, with rostellum armed with a double row of 25–30 alternating large and small hooklets. Possesses four suckers which are not pigmented.
Neck	3–7 mm in length	5–10 mm in length
Proglottids:		
• Measurement of gravid segment	20 mm in length and 5 mm in breadth	12 mm in length and 6 mm in breadth
• Number	1,000–2,000	800–1,000
• Expulsion	Expelled singly	Expelled in chains of 5 or 6
• Number of lateral branches of uterus	15–30	5–10
• Vaginal sphincter	Present	Absent
• Ovaries	Two, without any accessory lobe	Two, with an accessory lobe
• Testes	300–400 follicles	150–200 follicles
Larva	Cysticercus bovis, present in cow and not in man	Cysticercus cellulosae, present in pig and may also develop in man.

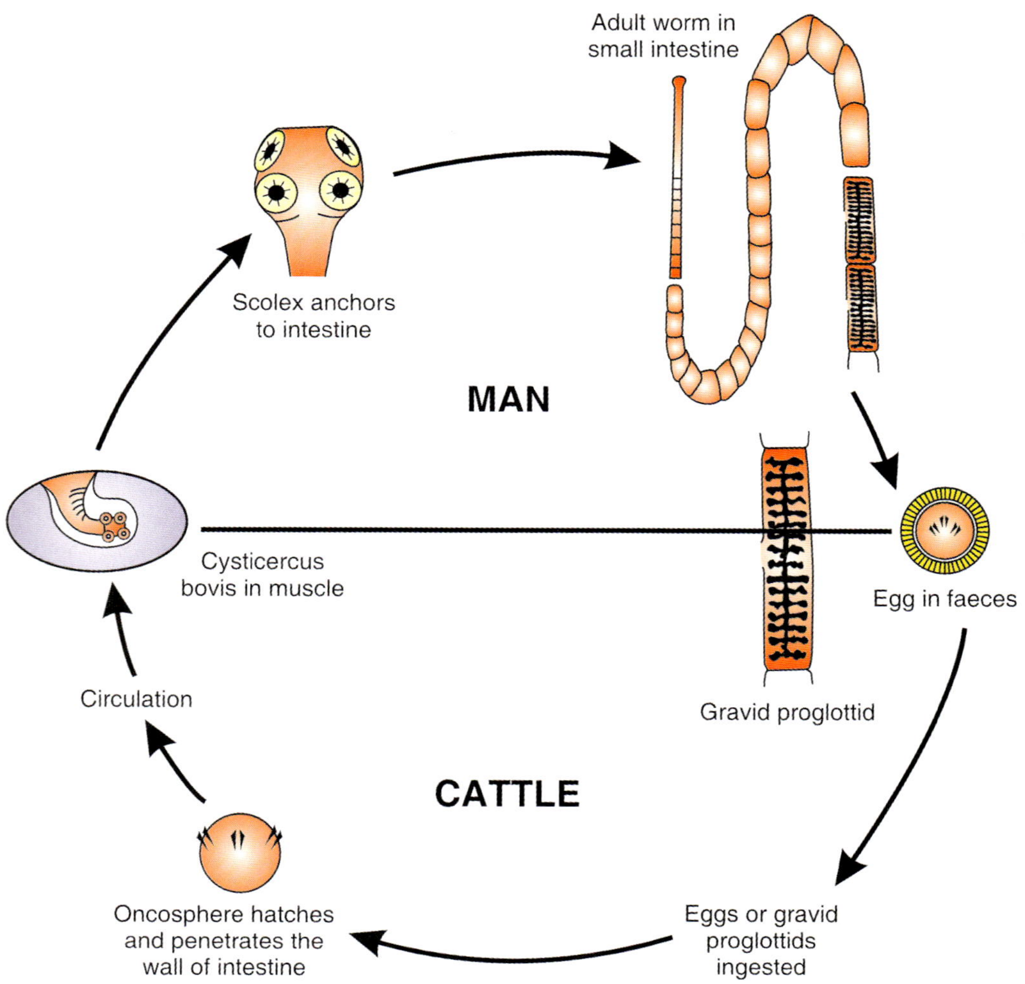

Fig. 9.5. Life cycle of *Taenia saginata*.

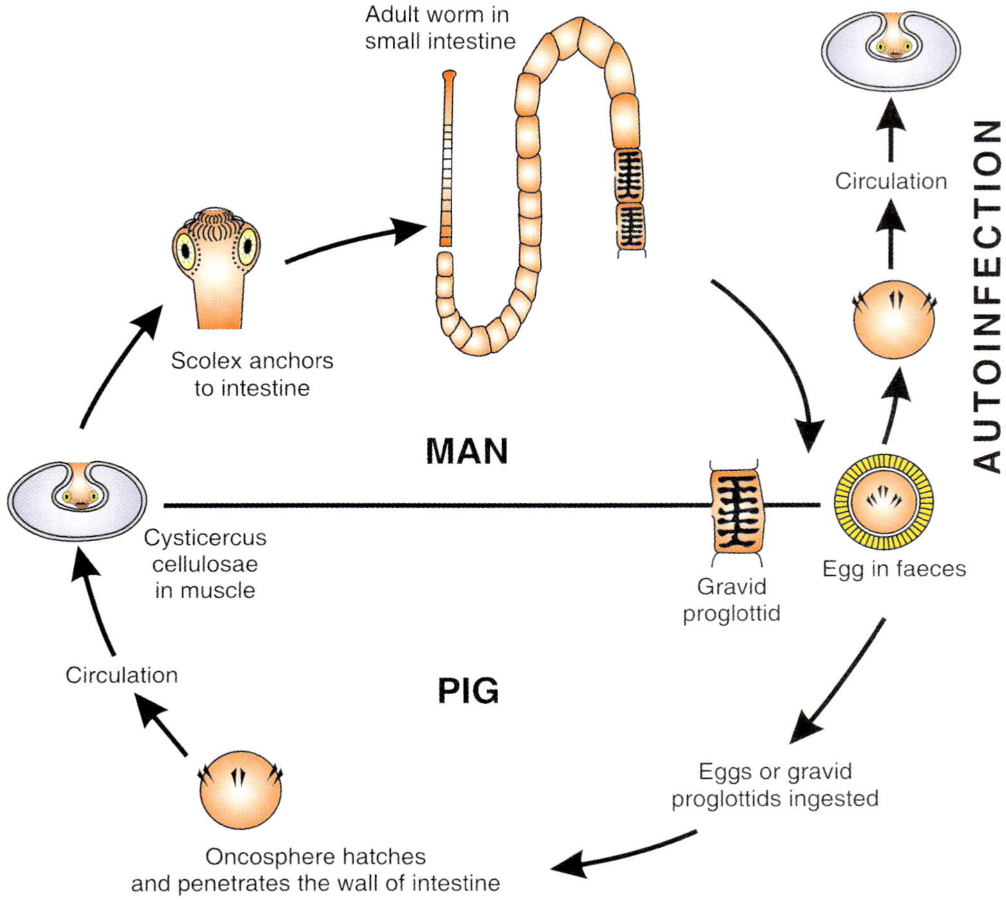

Fig. 9.6. Life cycle of *Taenia solium*.

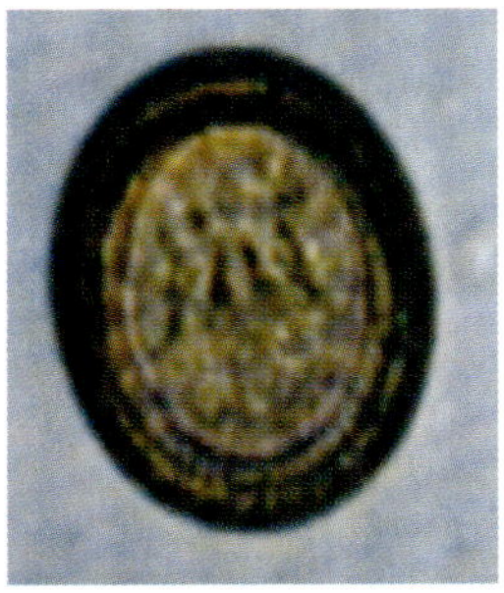

Fig. 9.7. Egg of *Taenia* (saline wet mount, × 400).

months, but can develop further only when ingested by man, its definitive host. **Cysticercus bovis is unknown in humans.**

Man acquires infection by eating raw or undercooked beef containing encysted larval stage (cysticercus bovis). The larvae hatch out in the small intestine, the scolices exvaginate and anchor to the mucosal surface by means of their suckers and develop into adult worms. They grow to sexual maturity in 2–3 months, lay eggs which are passed out in faeces along with the gravid segments and the cycle is repeated.

Life cycle of *T. solium*

The parasite passes its life cycle in two hosts (Fig. 9.6). The definitive host is man and the intermediate host is usually the pig but man may occasionally serve as the intermediate host also.

The adult worm lives in the small intestine of man and the gravid segments come out with the faeces in chains of 5 or 6. Whole segment or eggs from disintegrated segment are eaten up by pig, a highly coprophagus animal. When they reach duodenum, the embryophore of the eggs ruptures and liberates oncospheres. With the help of their hooklets they penetrate the wall of the intestine and enter into portal vessels or mesenteric lymphatics. Then they reach general circulation via liver, right side of the heart, lungs and left side of the heart. From general circulation, they are filtered out in striated muscles where, in 7–9 weeks, they develop into bladder worm known as **cysticercus cellulosae**. The muscles which are most commonly selected are those of the tongue, neck, shoulder and ham. The cardiac muscle is also involved.

Mature cysticercus cellulosae (Figs. 9.8–9.10) is an opalescent, ellipsoidal body and measures 8–10 mm in breadth and 5 mm in length. Its long axis lies parallel to the muscle fibres. It has an invaginated scolex with its four suckers and a rostellum with a double row of alternating large and small hooklets.

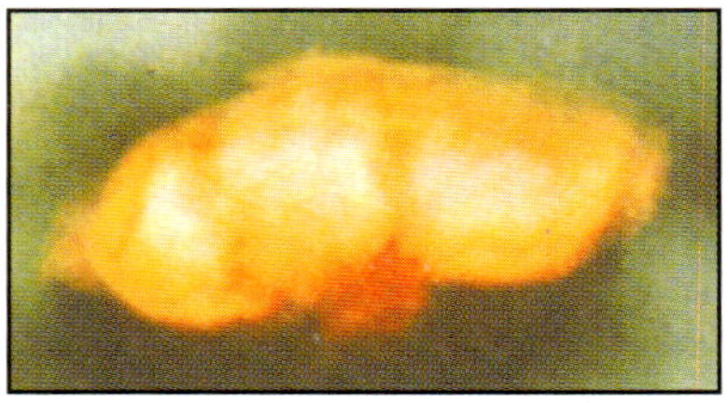

Fig. 9.8. Cysticerci (three in number) in the abdominal muscle.

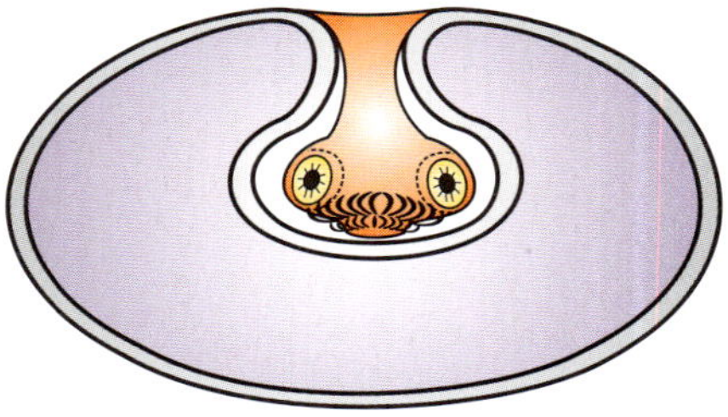

Fig. 9.9. Cysticercus cellulosae.

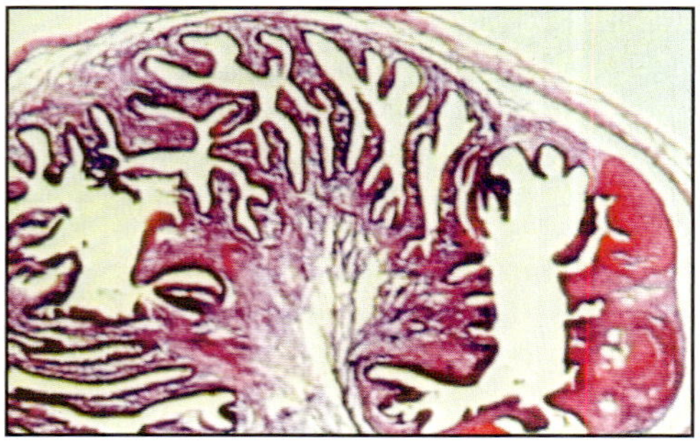

Fig. 9.10. Microscopic appearance of cysticercus cellulosae (haematoxylin and eosin stain, × 100).

Man acquires infection by eating raw or undercooked pork containing encysted larval stage (cysticercus cellulosae). The larvae hatch out in the small intestine, the scolices exvaginate and anchor to the mucosal surface by means of their suckers and hooklets, and develop into adult worms. They grow to sexual maturity in 2–3 months. Gravid segments pass out with the faeces in chains of 5 or 6 and the cycle is repeated.

Cysticercus cellulosae can also develop in man as follows:

- By ingesting the eggs with contaminated water or food.
- A man harbouring adult worms may autoinfect oneself either by unhygienic personal habits or by reverse peristaltic movements of the intestine whereby the gravid segments are thrown into the stomach, equivalent to the swallowing of thousands of eggs. Further development to cysticercus cellulosae in man is similar to that in pig.

Pathogenicity

Adult worms in the small intestine usually produce no symptoms. But at times, they may cause vague abdominal discomfort, indigestion, persistent diarrhoea or diarrhoea alternating with constipation and loss of appetite. Large infections may lead to obstruction of the bowel (Fig. 9.4).

Cysticercosis is a disease caused by larval stage of *T. solium*, an important public health problem of the tropical countries including India. Cysticercus cellulosae may develop in any organ and the effects produced depend on the location of cysticerci. They usually occur in large numbers, sometimes they may occur singly. They usually develop in the subcutaneous tissues and muscles forming visible nodules (Fig. 9.8). It may also develop in brain (Fig. 9.11) leading to epileptic attacks and in anterior and vitreous chambers of the eye. *In India, it is regarded as the second most important cause of intracranial space-occupying lesions following tuberculosis and the most common cause of epilepsy. It is estimated that 5–20% of all cases with epilepsy in India have neurocysticercosis.*

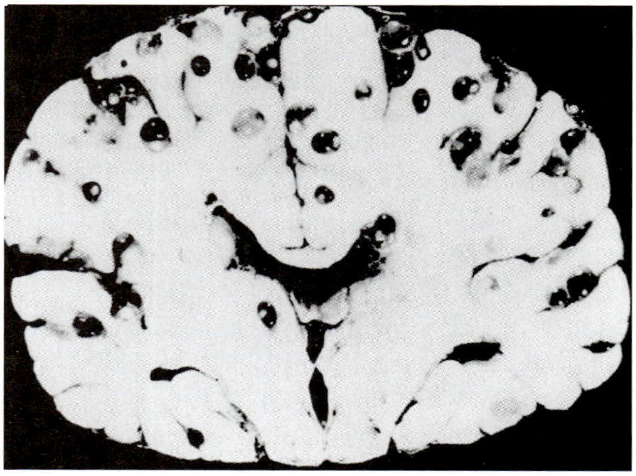

Fig. 9.11. Multiple cysticercus cellulosae in brain.

Laboratory diagnosis

1. The diagnosis of *T. saginata* and *T. solium* infections can be carried out by:
   - **Demonstration of characteristic eggs** (Figs. 9.5–9.7) in the stool by direct smear and concentration method by sedimentation technique (formalin-ether sedimentation). **They do not float in saturated solution of common salt.** However, for detecting eggs, anal swabs are superior to the methods using faeces.
   - Since eggs of both *T. saginata* and *T. solium* are similar, therefore, for the species diagnosis, the **demonstration of gravid proglottids and scolices** is essential (Figs. 9.5 and 9.6, and Table 9.3).
2. **The diagnosis of cysticercosis** can be carried out by:
   - **Biopsy of subcutaneous nodule:** It may reveal cysticerci (Figs. 9.8–9.10).
   - **X-ray of skull and soft tissue:** It may reveal calcified cysticerci.
   - **CT scan of the brain:** It can accurately locate the lesion in the brain.
   - **Differential leucocyte count:** It reveals eosinophilia.
   - **Serological tests:** Serological tests such as indirect haemagglutination (IHA), indirect fluorescent antibody (IFA) and enzyme-linked immunosorbent assay (ELISA) can be used for demonstration of specific antibodies in the serum.

TAENIA ASIATICA

T. asiatica (Asian tapeworm) was first discovered by Eon and Rim in 1993. Since it showed similarity to *T. saginata*, it was believed to be a different strain of *T. saginata*, but, subsequently, it was demonstrated to be a separate species. It is found in Taiwan, Korea, Indonesia, Thailand, China, Malaysia and the Philippines. Adult *T. asiatica* resembles *T. saginata* except that the scolex of the former is larger and possesses rostellum with no hooklets, and the cysticercus – named **Cysticercus viscerotropica** is different in morphology and development. *T. asiatica* shows two unique characters:

1. Humans, like for other *Taenia* spp., are the definitive hosts; however, in contrast, both cattle and pigs serve as intermediate hosts.
2. The preferred locations of cysticerci are liver, serosa and lungs in pigs, and liver in cattle.

Laboratory diagnosis

Stool examination

It shows eggs resembling those of *T. saginata* and *T. solium*. The definitive identification of *T. asiatica* can be made by demonstration of:

- rostellum with no hooklets on the scolex;
- a large number of uterine branches (more than 57); and
- a prominent posterior protuberance in gravid proglottids of the parasite.

Examination of cysticercus viscerotropica

It shows wart-like formation on the surface.

Polymerase chain reaction (PCR)

It can be used for detection of ribosomal 5.8S gene.

Treatment

Praziquantel is the drug of choice for treatment of infection by *T. saginata*, although niclosamide can also be used. Niclosamide is preferred for treatment of intestinal infections with *T. solium*. Albendazole is the drug of choice for treating cysticercosis.

Prophylaxis of *T. saginata* infection

1. All beef to be eaten by man should be inspected for cysticerci. However, inspection procedures for bovine cysticercosis do not always detect infection.
2. Thorough cooking of beef ensures complete protection.
3. Proper sanitary disposal of faeces. Cattle should not be allowed to feed or graze on ground polluted by human faeces or sewage. This will control cattle infection.
4. In order to break the parasitic life cycle, infected people should be treated.

Prophylaxis of *T. solium* infection

1. Personal hygiene.
2. General sanitary measures.
3. Avoid food and water contamination with *T. solium* eggs.
4. Strict veterinary inspection of pork in all slaughter houses with condemnation of "measly pork" (infected pig).
5. Thorough cooking of pork ensures complete protection.
6. Pickled or salted pork is not necessarily safe.
7. Pigs should not have access to human faeces.

8. Avoid eating raw vegetables grown on soil irrigated by sewage water.
9. In order to break the parasitic life cycle, infected people should be treated.

TAENIA MULTICEPS

Synonym

Multiceps multiceps

Morphology

The adult *T. multiceps* measures 40–60 cm in length. The scolex of the parasite is pyriform in shape, has four suckers and a rostellum armed with double row of 22–30 hooklets. Gravid proglottids are 8–10 mm in length and 3–4 mm in width. The eggs are 31–36 μm in diameter.

Definitive hosts are the dog, wolf and fox and intermediate hosts are sheep, cattle, horses and other herbivorous animals. Humans become infected by ingesting food or water contaminated with dog's faeces containing *T. multiceps* eggs. Oncospheres hatch in the intestine, penetrate the intestinal wall, and eventually lodge in various organs of the body but usually in CNS where the migrating larvae develop into a coenurus (Fig. 9.12), which is a bladder worm with multiple scolices, but no brood capsules or daughter cyst. Each scolex is capable of developing into an adult worm if eaten by definitive host.

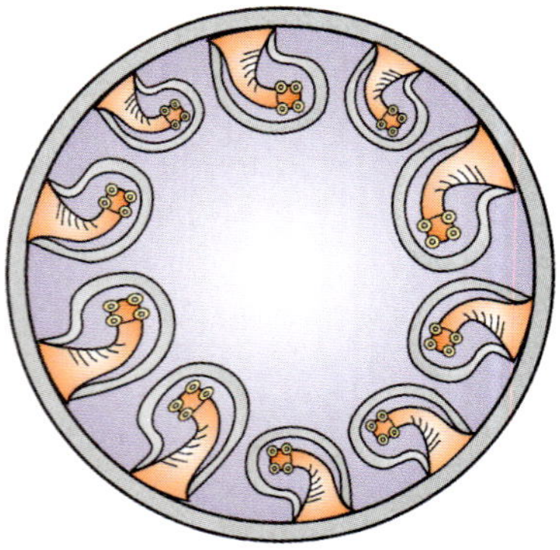

Fig. 9.12. Coenurus.

Infection caused by *T. multiceps* has been reported from France, Africa, England, Brazil and the United States. Symptoms are often those of space-occupying lesion, including headache, vomiting, and localizing neurologic symptoms, such as hemiplegia, paraplegia, aphasia, and seizures. The diagnosis is usually made following surgical removal of the cyst and histologic recognition of the coenurus.

HYMENOLEPIS NANA

Common name

The dwarf tapeworm.

Morphology

H. nana is the **smallest tapeworm** infecting humans. The name *Hymenolepis* refers to thin membrane covering the egg (*hymen*, membrane, *lepis*, covering) and *nana* to small size (*nanus*, dwarf or small). It was first discovered by Bilharz (1851) in the small intestine. It infects not only humans but also rodents such as mice and rats. In rodents the tapeworm is regarded by some as a special strain (*H. nana* var. *fraterna*), but cross-infections in both directions are possible.

Geographical distribution

H. nana has a worldwide distribution and is one of the more common causes of cestode infections in humans, particularly in children.

Habitat

In humans the adult tapeworms are found in the small intestine (distal portion of ileum). It is also found in rodents, especially in mice and rats.

Morphology

Adult worm

The adult tapeworm is small reaching only 4–5 cm in length and 1 mm in diameter. Like other tapeworms, it is made up of scolex, neck and strobila (Fig. 9.13).

Scolex

It is globular, has four cup-shaped suckers and a retractile rostellum armed with a single row of 20–30 hooklets.

Neck

It is long and slender and is situated posterior to the scolex.

Strobila

It consists of about 200 proglottids. A mature proglottid measures 0.15–0.3 mm in length and 0.8–1 mm in breadth. Genital pores are marginal and are situated on the same side. The uterus is a transverse sac with lobulated walls and the testes are round and three in number.

Life span of the adult worm is about two weeks. In an infected person 1,000–8,000 worms may be present.

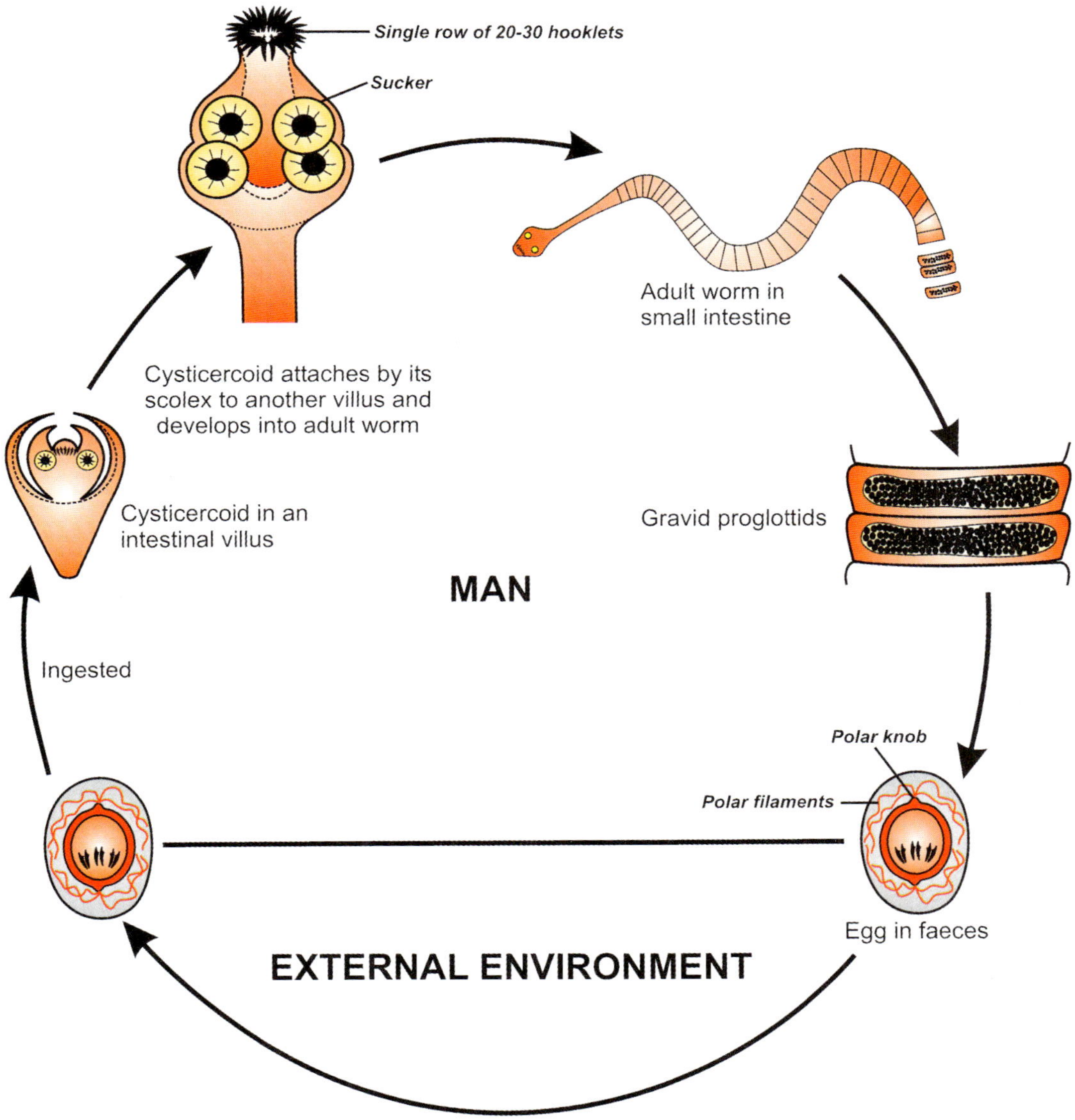

Fig. 9.13. Life cycle of *Hymenolepis nana*.

Egg

It is spherical or oval, hyaline, 35–40 µm in diameter. It has a smooth, thin and **colourless outer shell** and an inner membrane (embryophore), containing a hexacanth embryo (oncosphere). The space between two membranes is filled with yolk granules and 4–8 polar filaments emanating from polar thickenings at either end of embryophore. It is **non-bile-stained and floats in saturated solution of common salt** (Figs. 9.13 and 9.14).

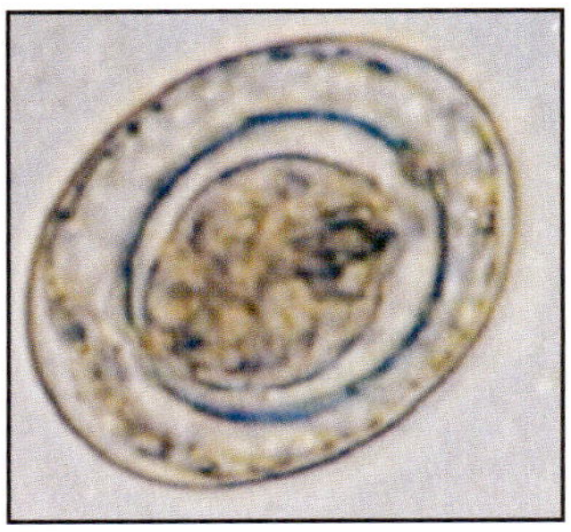

Fig. 9.14. Egg of *Hymenolepis nana* (saline wet mount, ×400).

Life cycle

H. nana **is the only cestode which is capable of completing its life cycle in a single host** (Fig. 9.13).

Adult worm resides in small intestine (distal portion of ileum) of man and rodents, especially mice and rats.

H. nana has two types of life cycle:

- Direct cycle
- Indirect cycle

Direct cycle

Eggs, and proglottids with eggs are passed in the faeces of infected humans and rodents. Man acquires infection by ingestion of food or water contaminated with these (faecal-oral route). In the lumen of small intestine, a free oncosphere (hexacanth embryo) is liberated from the egg. It penetrates into a villus of the small intestine and develops into **cysticercoid larva** in about four days. Thereafter, the villus ruptures and the cysticercoid becomes free in the lumen of the small intestine.

Later, it attaches by its scolex to another villus further down, and in the course of two weeks or more develops into an adult tapeworm. Strobilization is rapid and in about 30 days after the infection, the eggs, and proglottids with eggs begin to appear in faeces and the cycle is repeated.

H. nana also can cause autoinfection, with a subsequent increased worm burden. Eggs are able to hatch in the intestine, develop into a cysticercoid larva, and then grow into adult worms without leaving the host. This can lead to **hyperinfection** with very heavy worm burdens and severe clinical symptoms.

Indirect cycle

H. nana has an indirect life cycle with an insect as the intermediate host. Insects include grain- and flour-eating beetles such as species of *Tribolium* and *Tenebrio*, fleas such as *Xenopsylla cheopis*, *Pulex irritans* and *Ctenocephalides canis*, and moths. These insects or their larvae eat eggs of *H. nana*. They crush the egg shell, and enzymes in the gut stimulate the oncosphere to free itself from the enclosing membrane. In the gut lumen, the oncosphere penetrates the gut wall by means of its six hooklets and glandular secretions. In the body cavity of the insect, the oncosphere transforms into **cysticercoid larva**, which is infective to final host. Man is infected by accidental ingestion of these infected beetles, fleas and moths. In the intestine the cysticercoid larva is released and develops into adult worm.

Pathogenicity

H. nana, even in large numbers, is well tolerated. The mechanism by which symptoms are produced is an allergic reaction, and in heavy infections enteritis may be produced. The infection is more common in children. Patient develops headache, dizziness, anorexia, pruritus of nose and anus, abdominal pain, diarrhoea, restlessness, epileptiform convulsions and eosinophilia in excess of 5%.

Laboratory diagnosis

The diagnosis is made by demonstration of characteristic eggs in faeces by direct microscopy, salt floatation and formalin-ether sedimentation methods. *Eggs are infectious, therefore, unpreserved stools should be handled with care.*

Treatment

Praziquantel is effective against *H. nana* infections, but higher doses than used for other tapeworm infections usually are required. Albendazole is partially efficacious against *H. nana*.

Prophylaxis

Personal hygiene, sanitary improvements, uncontaminated food and water and rodent control are the measures for prevention of *H. nana* infection.

HYMENOLEPIS DIMINUTA

Common name: The rat tapeworm.

H. diminuta is a cosmopolitan parasite of rat and mouse. It has been reported occasionally from man.

Habitat

The adult worm resides in the distal portion of the ileum with the scolex embedded in the mucosa.

Morphology

Adult worm

H. diminuta is larger than *H. nana*. It measures 20–60 cm in length. Like *H. nana*, the scolex of *H. diminuta* has four suckers and a retractile rostellum (Fig. 9.15), but unlike *H. nana*, the scolex of *H. diminuta* has no hooklets on its rostellum (unarmed rostellum). The number of proglottids varies from 800–1,000. The terminal proglottids measure 0.75 mm in length and 3.5 mm in width and have internal structure similar to that of *H. nana*.

Egg

The eggs are larger than those of *H. nana*. These are subspherical, have a **slightly yellowish (bile-stained) transparent outer membrane** (shell), measuring 60–80 µm in diameter and have an inner membrane around

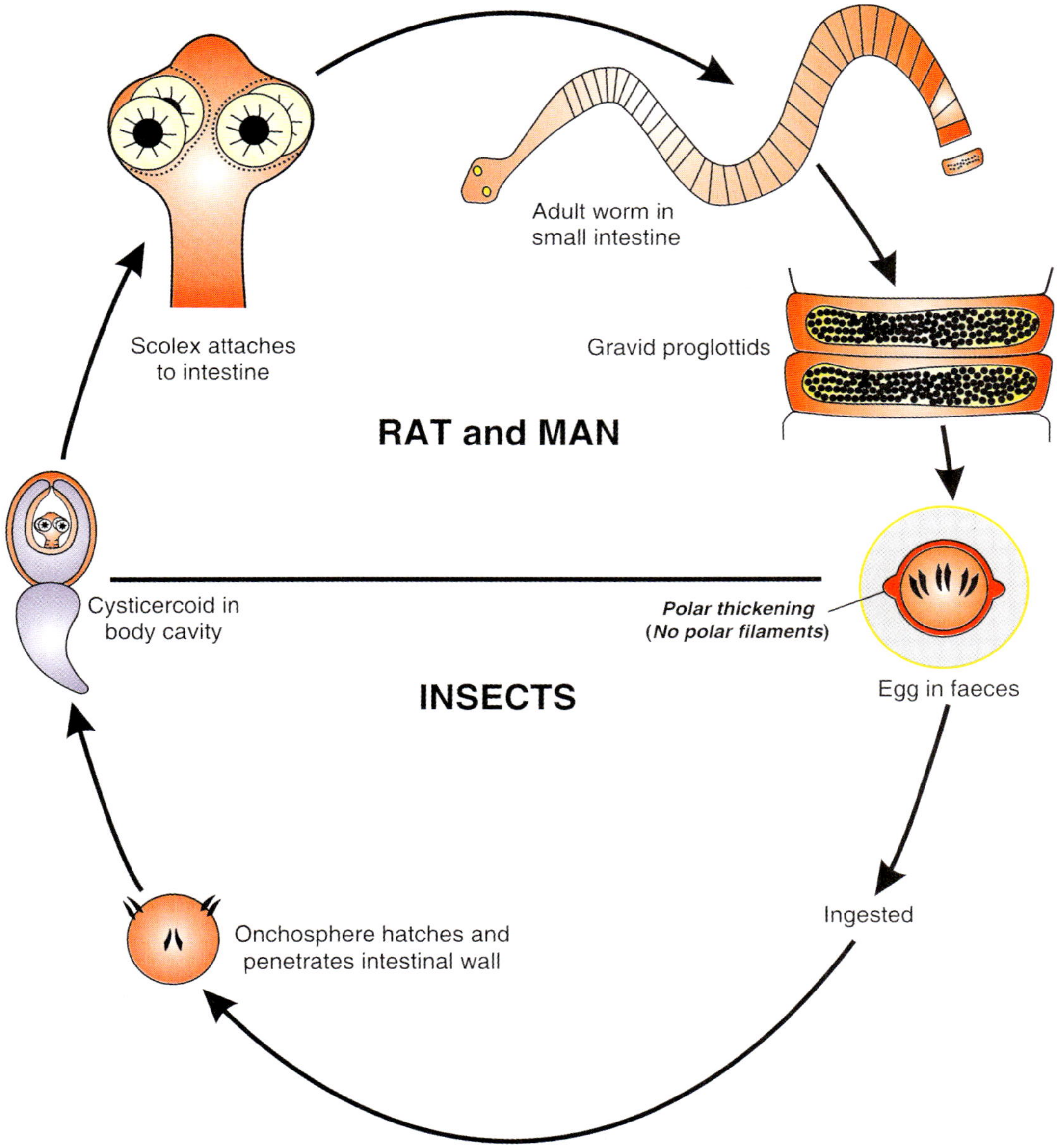

Fig. 9.15. Life cycle of *Hymenolepis diminuta*.

the oncosphere which has two polar thickenings but no polar filaments. Between the two membranes there is a colourless, gelatinous matrix (Figs. 9.15 and 9.16).

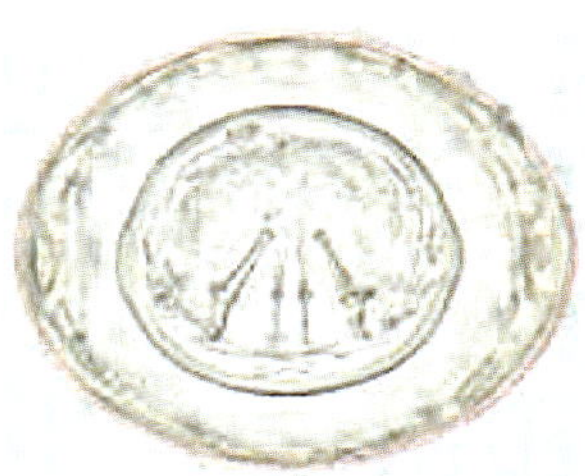

Fig. 9.16. Egg of *Hymenolepis diminuta* (saline wet mount, × 400).

Life cycle

The life cycle of *H. diminuta* is identical to the indirect life cycle of *H. nana* and always needs an intermediate host (Fig. 9.15). Therefore, **unlike *H. nana* eggs, the eggs of *H. diminuta* are not infectious from person to person**. Various arthropods (rat fleas, beetles, grain beetles) serve as obligatory intermediate hosts; these are all coprozoic or scavenger in their habits during their larval or adult stage. The cysticercoid (larval stage) is found in these arthropod hosts. The rodents become infected by ingestion of arthropod hosts.

Humans acquire infection accidentally by ingestion of these arthropods harbouring the cysticercoid larvae. In the human intestine, cysticercoid larva is released, which then develops into the adult worm.

Pathogenicity

Since infected rats and insects, functioning as final and intermediate hosts respectively are worldwide, therefore, *H. diminuta* infection is a **cosmopolitan zoonosis**. Like *H. nana*, *H. diminuta* is ordinarily well tolerated by the human host but the patient may develop diarrhoea, anorexia, nausea, headache, dizziness and eosinophilia.

Laboratory diagnosis

The diagnosis is based on recovery of the characteristic eggs and proglottids. *H. diminuta* can easily be differentiated from *H. nana* by the larger size of proglottids or the absence of polar filaments on the inner membrane of the eggs.

Treatment

Treatment is the same as for *H. nana*.

Prophylaxis

H. diminuta infection can be prevented by:

- Good sanitary conditions.
- Reduced rodent populations.
- Avoidance of close contact of rodents with humans or human food supplies.

DIPYLIDIUM CANINUM

Common name: The double-pored dog tapeworm.

Geographical distribution

D. caninum is a common tapeworm of the dog and cat throughout the world. Human infections have been reported from Europe, the Philippines, China, Japan, Argentina and the United States.

Morphology

Adult worm

The adult worm measures 10–70 cm in length. The scolex is small, rhomboidal, with a transverse diameter of 250–500 μm (Fig. 9.17). It has four deeply cupped, oval suckers and a median apical, club-shaped retractile rostellum armed with 1–7 rows of hooklets. The neck of the worm is short and slender. The strobila consists of about 200 proglottids. Mature and gravid proglottids are typically pumpkin-seed-shaped. Therefore, *D. caninum* is often called **pumpkin-seed tapeworm**. Each proglottid is provided with a double set of reproductive organs with genital pores on each lateral margin and has a maximum width of 3.2 mm. When gravid, the uterus is sac-like, breaks up into a number of egg-capsules, enclosed in an embryonic membrane, containing 8–15 eggs in each.

Egg

The eggs are spherical measuring 25–40 μm in diameter. They have thin, hyaline, **brick-red tinged shell**. Each egg contains an oncosphere with six hooklets.

Life cycle

Adult worms reside in the dog, cat and occasionally human intestine. Eggs in capsules or proglottids are ingested by the larval stages of the dog flea, the cat flea or the human flea (Fig. 9.17). The dog louse has also been incriminated as a suitable intermediate host of *D. caninum*. The oncospheres are liberated in the intestine of these insects and migrate into their body cavity, where they develop into **cysticercoid larvae**. When these insects are ingested by the definitive hosts (dogs, cats or humans), the larvae develop into adult worms which become sexually mature in 3–4 weeks. Gravid proglottids separate singly or in groups from the strobila and are passed out of anus. Disintegration of these proglottids does not commonly occur within the bowel and at times groups of eggs within the embryonic membrane are passed in the faeces, and the cycle is repeated.

Pathogenicity

Human infections are rare and normally restricted to young children. The infection results from accidental ingestion of insect hosts while fondling cats and dogs. Infected insect hosts may be crushed in the dog's mouth, thereby releasing the cysticercoids, and these may be transmitted to children in the dog's saliva. Usually, there is not more than a single worm. The symptoms are mild and consist of slight intestinal disturbances, including indigestion and loss of appetite. However, heavier worm burden may occur. It produces abdominal discomfort, anal pruritis, and diarrhoea. Anal pruritis results from the active migration of the motile proglottids.

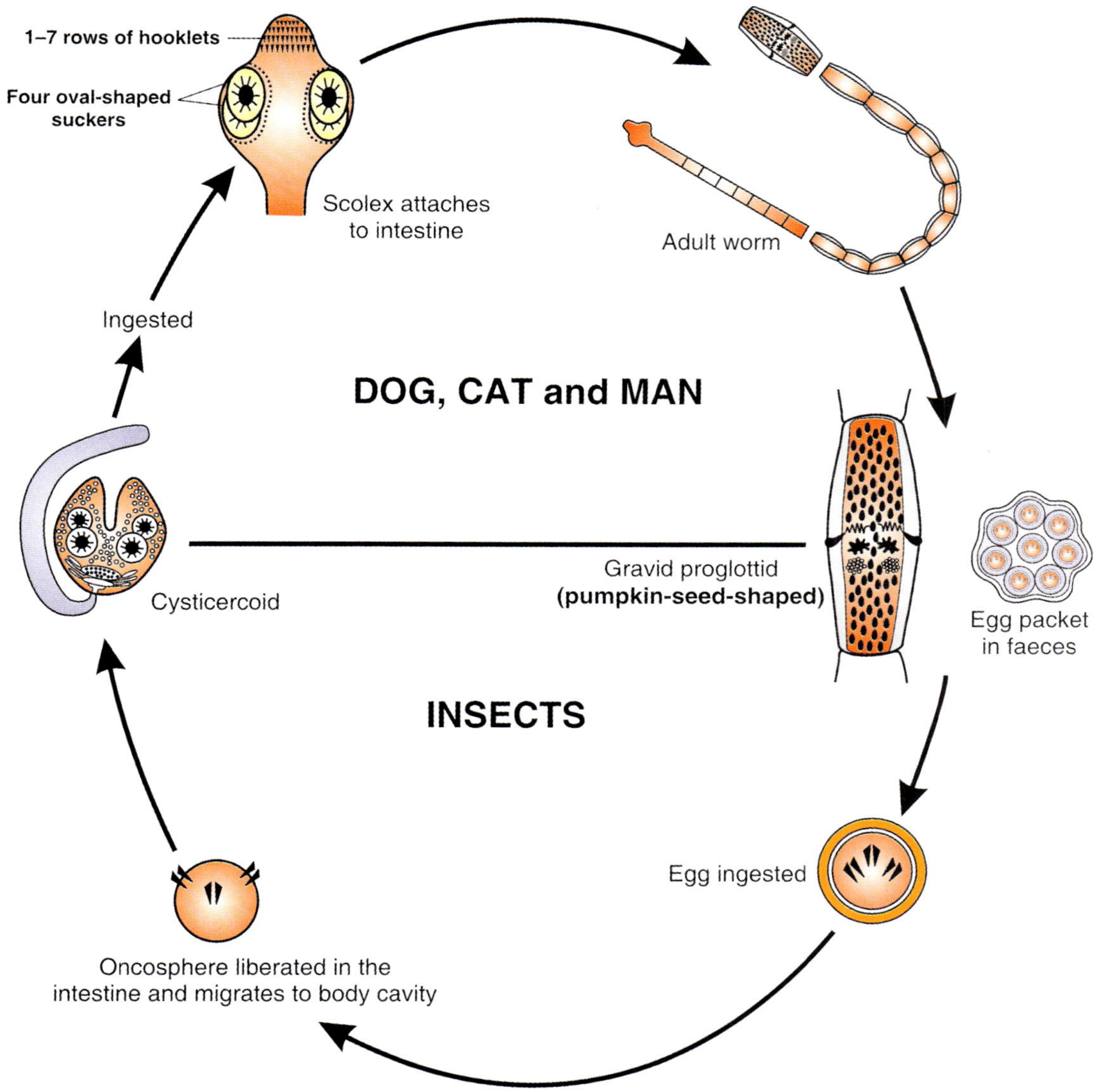

Fig. 9.17. Life cycle of *Dipylidium caninum*.

Laboratory diagnosis

Stool examination reveals the presence of pumpkin-seed-shaped proglottids. Furthermore, packets of 8–15 characteristic eggs can be seen microscopically enclosed in an embryonic membrane in the proglottids.

Treatment

Praziquantel and niclosamide can be used for the treatment of *D. caninum* infection.

Prevention

D. caninum infection can be prevented by:

- Insecticide dusting of pet dogs and cats to kill fleas.
- Periodic administration of taeniafuges to pet dogs and cats.

ECHINOCOCCUS GRANULOSUS

Common names

The dog tapeworm; the hydatid worm.

Morphology

Adult *E. granulosus* was described by Hartmann in the small intestine of dog in 1695 and the larval form (hydatid cyst) was subsequently described by Goeze in 1782. The life cycle of *Echinococcus* was demonstrated by von Siebold in 1853 when he infected dogs with hydatid cysts from sheep and 27 days later discovered intestinal worms consisting of a 'head' and three segments containing reproductive organs and eggs, which he called *Taenia echinococcus*. Naunyn in 1863 demonstrated that hydatid cyst in man is the bladder worm stage of *Echinococcus* found in the intestine of dog.

Geographical distribution

E. granulosus is worldwide, but it is more common in sheep and cattle-raising countries. It occurs mainly in South America, North Africa, Eastern Australia, Asia and also sporadically in the Middle East, Mongolia, Eastern Europe and the UK. It is a significant health problem in India and has been reported from Andhra Pradesh, Gujarat, Tamil Nadu, West Bengal, Orissa, Bihar, Punjab, Haryana, Himachal Pradesh, Uttar Pradesh, Kashmir, Delhi and Pondicherry.

Habitat

Adult worm resides in the small intestine of dog and other canine animals (wolf, fox and jackal). Larval form is seen in man and other intermediate hosts (sheep, goat, cattle, pig and horse). **The dog and sheep are optimum definitive and intermediate hosts respectively** and the cycle of transmission is maintained between them.

Morphology

Adult worm

It is a small tapeworm measuring 3–6 mm in length. It consists of a scolex, neck and strobila (Fig. 9.18).

Scolex

It is pyriform in shape and measures about 300 μm in

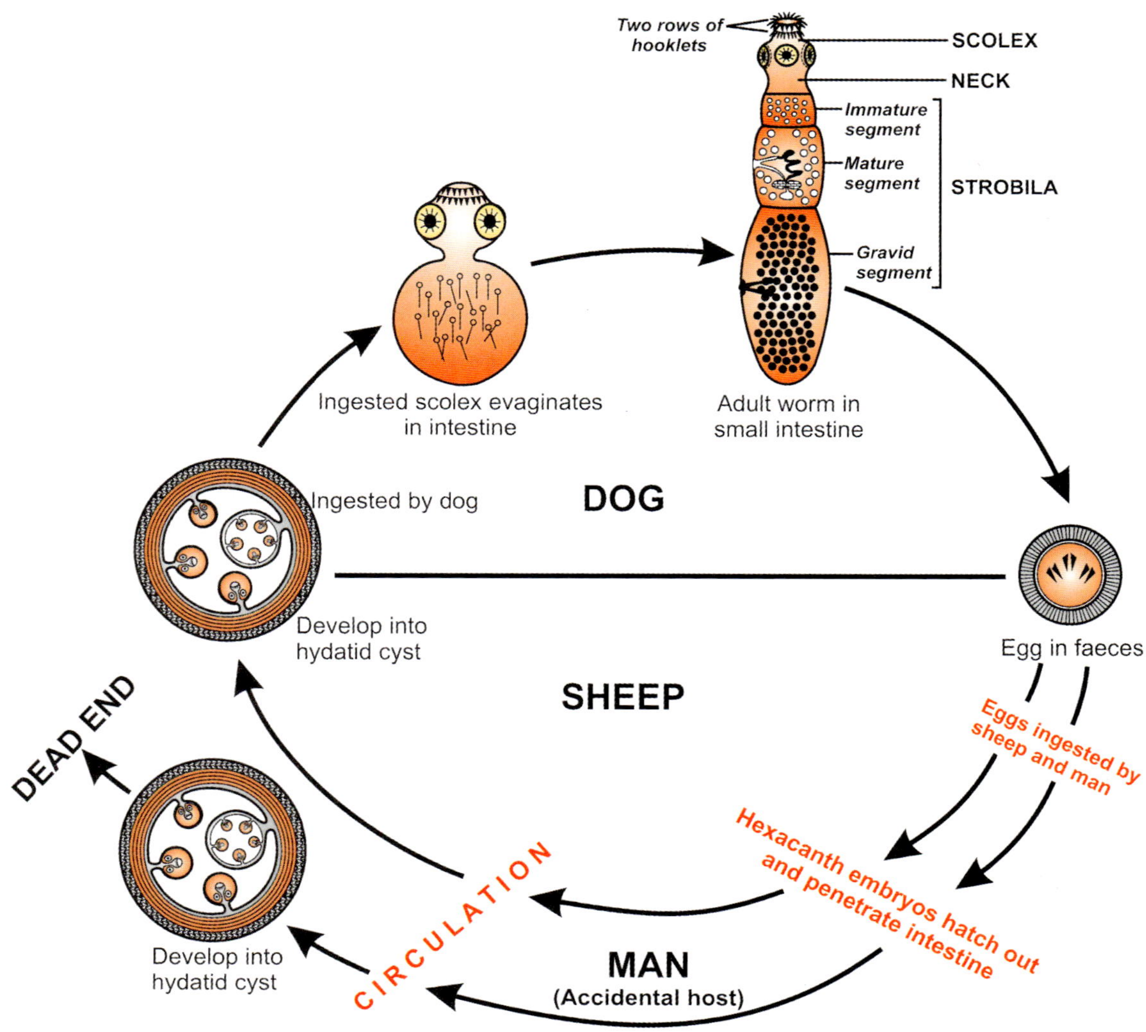

Fig. 9.18. Life cycle of *Echinococcus granulosus*.

diameter. It possesses four suckers and a protrusible rostellum with two circular rows of hooklets.

Neck

It is short and thick.

Strobila

It consists of three segments (occasionally four). The first segment is immature, the second is mature and the third (and the fourth when present) is gravid.

Eggs

These are indistinguishable from those of other *Taenia* species. These are spherical, brown in colour, and measure 31–43 μm in diameter, and contain hexacanth embryos with three pairs of hooklets.

Larval form

This is found within the hydatid cyst which develops in the intermediate host (see pathogenicity).

Life cycle

E. granulosus passes its life cycle in two hosts (Fig. 9.18). The adult worm lives attached to the mucosa of small intestine of dog and other canine animals. The eggs are discharged in the faeces. These are swallowed by the intermediate hosts while grazing in the fields. Man acquires infection by a direct contact with infected dog or by allowing the dog to feed from the same dish or by ingesting water or food contaminated with dog's faeces containing eggs of *E. granulosus*.

In the duodenum the hexacanth embryos called **oncospheres** hatch out. These penetrate the intestinal wall and enter into the radicles of portal vein and are carried to the liver. The liver acts as the first filter where 60–70% of human infections are located. Some embryos may pass through the hepatic capillaries and enter the pulmonary circulation. Lungs act as the second filter. A few of these embryos may pass pulmonary circulation too and enter general circulation and may lodge in various organs like brain, heart, spleen, kidneys, genital organs, muscles, bones, etc.

Wherever the embryos settle, an active cellular reaction consisting of monocytes, giant cells and eosinophils takes place around the parasite. A large number of the parasites may thus be destroyed by host defence mechanism. Some of the embryos, however, escape destruction and develop into hydatid cysts (Figs. 9.18–9.27). The cellular reaction in these cases gradually disappears, followed by the appearance of fibroblasts and the formation of new blood vessels.

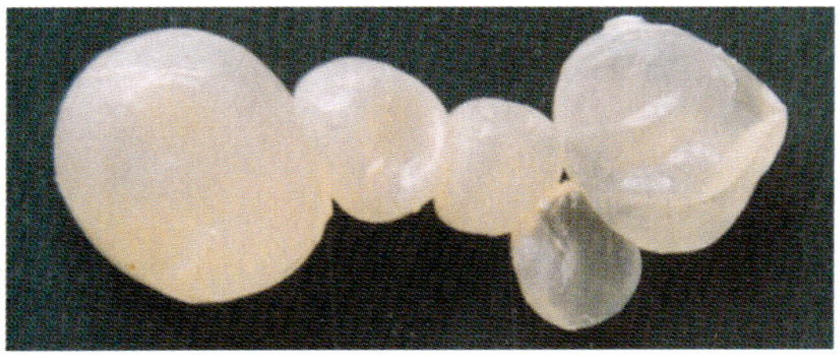

Fig. 9.19. Hydatid cysts.

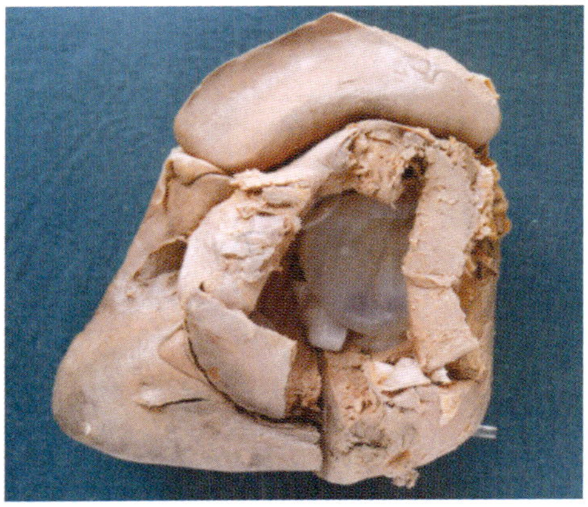

Fig. 9.20. Hydatid cysts of the liver.

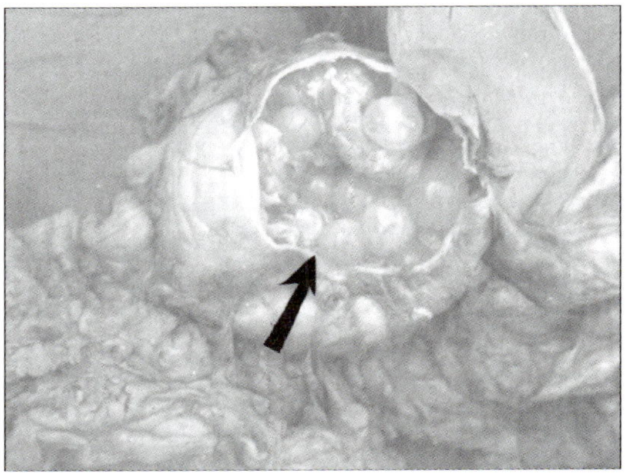

Fig. 9.21. Hydatid cyst of the liver showing numerous daughter cysts.

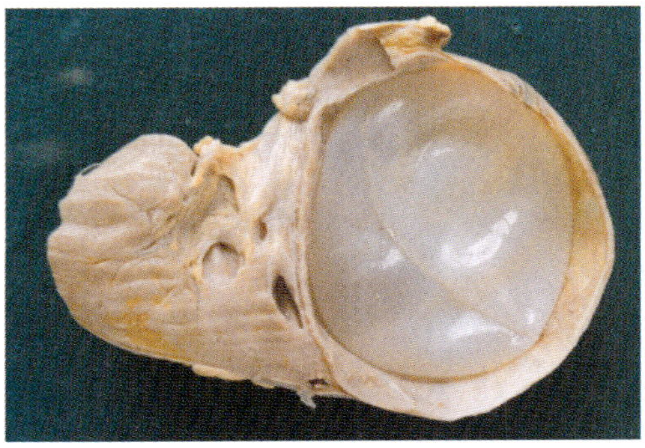

Fig. 9.22. Hydatid cyst of the kidney.

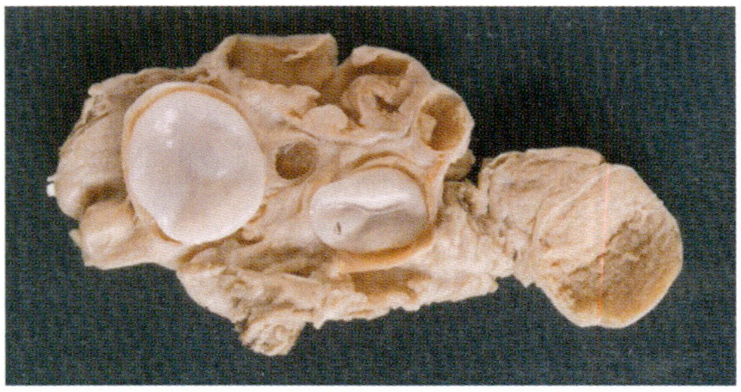

Fig. 9.23. Hydatid cysts of the spermatic cord.

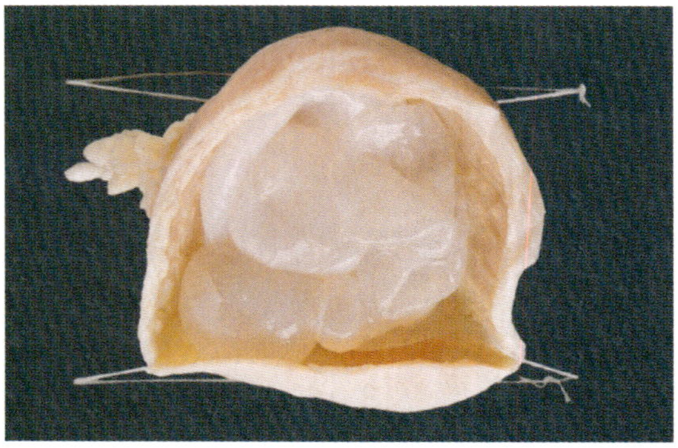

Fig. 9.24. Hydatid cyst ovary.

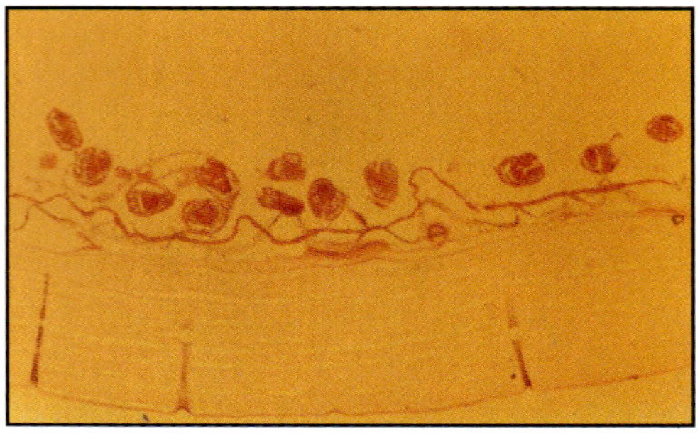

Fig. 9.25. Hydatid cyst showing laminated hyaline ectocyst and endocyst with scolices (haematoxylin and eosin stain, × 400).

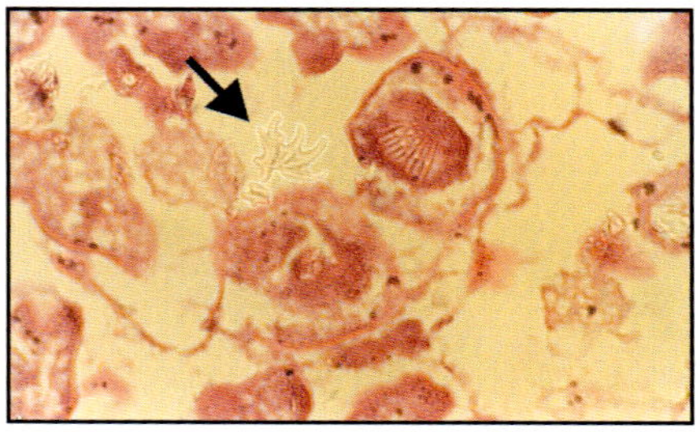

Fig. 9.26. Hydatid cyst showing armed scolices and free hooklets (haematoxylin and eosin stain, × 400).

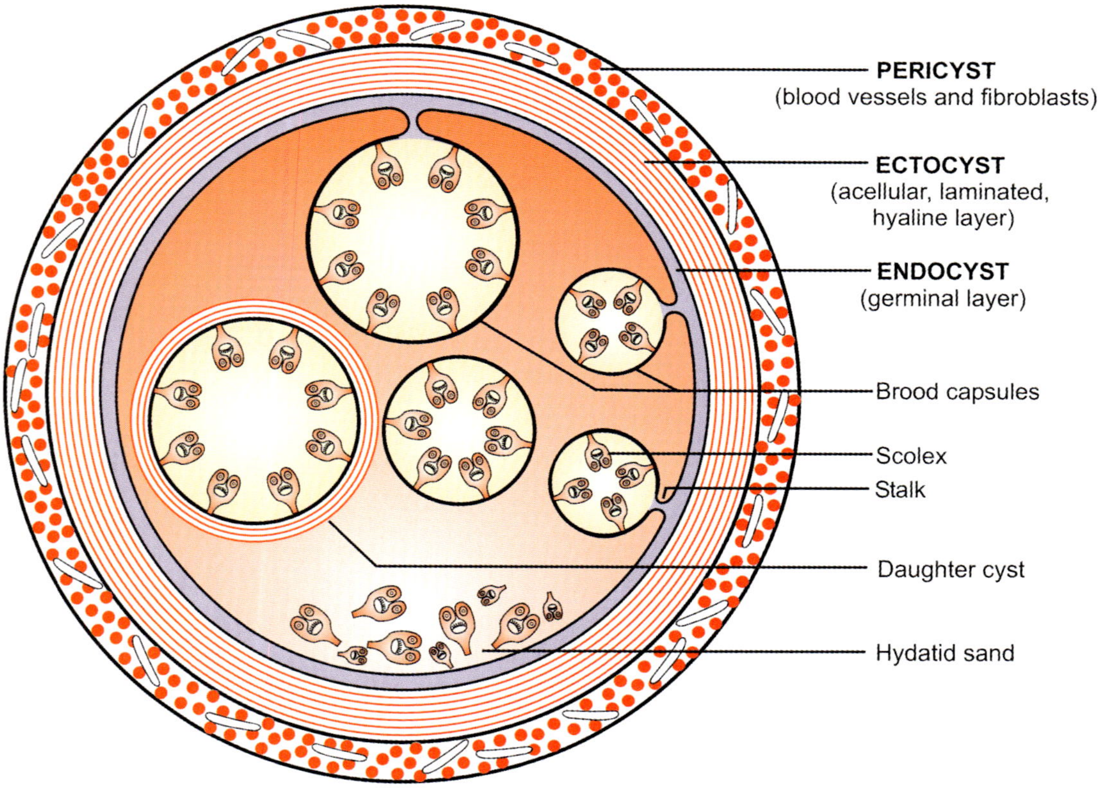

Fig. 9.27. Hydatid cyst.

Fibroblasts lay fibrous tissue, which envelops the growing embryo. This is known as **pericyst**. This merges with surrounding normal tissue. The parasite derives its nutrition through this layer. In old cysts the pericyst may become sclerosed or calcified and parasite within it may die.

Inside the pericyst, the embryo develops into a fluid-filled bladder known as **hydatid cyst**. From inner side of the cyst, **brood capsules** with a number of **scolices** are developed. When animals that serve as intermediate hosts are slaughtered, the viscera may not be disposed off properly and may be consumed by animals that serve as definitive hosts. The adult worms then develop in the intestine of definitive host. These lay eggs which are passed in the faeces of infected animals and the cycle is repeated. Since dog has no access to the hydatid cysts developed in viscera of man, therefore, the life cycle of the parasite comes to a dead end.

Pathogenicity

E. granulosus causes **cystic echinococcosis** or hydatidosis or **hydatid disease** or hydatid cyst in man. It represents larval form of the parasite. The disease is generally acquired during childhood though it does not manifest before adult life. The cyst wall secreted by the embryo consists of two layers (Figs. 9.25 and 9.27):

Ectocyst

It is outer layer. It is tough, acellular, laminated, hyaline membrane up to 1 mm in thickness. It resembles white of a hard-boiled egg. It is elastic, therefore, when excised or ruptured, it curls on itself thus exposing the inner layer containing brood capsules, scolices and daughter cysts.

Endocyst

It is inner or germinal layer. It consists of a number of nuclei embedded in a protoplasmic mass. It measures 22–25 μm in thickness. It gives rise to ectocyst on outside and brood capsules and scolices on inside. It also secretes hydatid fluid.

Hydatid fluid is clear, colourless or pale yellow. It has specific gravity of 1.005–1.010. It is slightly acidic (pH 6.7) and contains sodium chloride, sodium sulphate, sodium phosphate and sodium and calcium salts of succinic acid. It is antigenic, therefore, it is used for **Casoni's test** and when absorbed it leads to anaphylactic shock. Centrifuged deposit of the hydatid fluid shows **hydatid sand** which consists of brood capsules, free scolices and hooklets.

If the cyst ruptures, either spontaneously in the body or during surgery, the danger from death from anaphylactic shock is high. Metastatic cystic lesions can also develop in virtually any of the visceral organs if the primary cyst ruptures. If the cyst material seeds the peritoneal lining, massive proliferation can occur with vascular invasion and spread to other organs.

Acephalocysts

Some cysts are sterile and never produce brood capsules; some become sterile by bacterial invasion or calcification. In other cysts the brood capsules never produce scolices; hence they are called acephalocysts. If ingested by definitive host these cysts do not lead to infection.

Endogenous daughter cyst

Sometimes a fragment of the germinal layer may detach and develop into daughter cyst inside the mother cyst (Figs. 9.21 and 9.27). This is known as endogenous daughter cyst. It also has both ectocyst and endocyst with brood capsules and scolices. Grand daughter cysts may also be formed.

Exogenous cyst

In case of hydatid disease of bone, because of high intracystic pressure, herniation or rupture of germinal and laminated layer may occur through some weaker part of the bone resulting in formation of exogenous cyst.

Clinical disease

Hydatid disease in humans is potentially dangerous; however, cyst size and organ location will greatly influence the outcome. In untreated or in inadequately treated patients mortality is > 90% within 10–15 years of diagnosis.

Liver cysts

The majority of hydatid cysts occur in the liver, causing symptoms that may include chronic abdominal discomfort, occasionally with a palpable or visible abdominal mass. Liver cysts tend to occur more frequently in the right lobe. If a cyst becomes infected with bacteria, it resembles an abscess. If the cyst ruptures, either spontaneously, from trauma, or during surgery, there may be serious allergic reactions, including skin rash, anaphylactic shock, or death.

Lung cysts

Cysts in the lungs are usually asymptomatic until they

become large enough to cause cough, shortness of breath, or chest pain. Cyst rupture may lead to expectoration of hydatid fluid or membranes, followed by the development of infection and a lung abscess. If rupture occurs into the lung, it may cause pneumothorax and empyema, allergic reactions, and even anaphylactic shock.

Other sites

Other organs which may also be involved include spleen (3–5%), central nervous system and heart (1–1.5%), kidneys, bones, muscles, female genital tract, eyes, etc. leading to visible swelling and pressure effects.

Location of cyst in relation to age

It is well-known that hydatid cysts are most commonly found in liver and lungs; but lung, brain, spinal, and orbital cysts have been more commonly seen in younger patients.

Laboratory diagnosis

It can be carried out by the following methods:

1. Casoni's test

It is an immediate hypersensitivity skin test which was introduced by Casoni in 1911. Antigen for the Casoni's test is sterile hydatid fluid drawn from **unilocular hydatid cysts** from sheep, pig, cattle or man. The fluid is filtered, tested for sterility and stored in sealed ampoules under refrigeration. For the test, 0.2 ml of the antigen is injected intradermally in one arm. For control, an equal amount of sterile normal saline is injected intradermally on the other arm. The control fades almost immediately, while the tested site in positive case develops a large wheal measuring 5 cm or more in diameter with multiple pseudopodia within 30 minutes. This test has a low sensitivity (55–70%) and gives false positive reactions in patients suffering from other cestode infections.

2. Differential leucocyte count

Differential leucocyte count may reveal eosinophilia (20–25%).

3. Serological tests

Serodiagnosis of hydatid cyst may be carried out by enzyme-linked immunosorbent assay (ELISA), radioimmunoassay (RIA), complement fixation, indirect haemagglutination (IHA), bentonite flocculation and latex agglutination tests.

4. Examination of cyst fluid

Examination of cyst fluid reveals scolices,brood capsules and hooklets. Because leakage of fluid in the adjoining tissue may lead to anaphylactic shock, therefore, the fluid aspirated from surgically removed cyst should be examined and diagnostic puncture of cyst is not recommended.

5. Histological examination

Histological examination of surgically removed cyst reveals different layers of the hydatid cyst, i.e., pericyst, ectocyst and endocyst (Fig. 9.25).

6. Radiodiagnosis

X-ray, ultrasound and CT scan are also helpful in the diagnosis of hydatid cyst.

Treatment

Removal of the cysts by surgery is the preferred treatment, but leakage from ruptured cysts may spread disease to other organs. Prolonged regimens of albendazole, either alone or as an adjunct to surgery, are reportedly of some benefit. Benzimidazole treatment should be administered in the perioperative period.

Prophylaxis

E. granulosus infection can be prevented by:

- Strict personal hygiene.
- Dogs should not be allowed to eat the carcasses of slaughtered animals in endemic areas.
- Reduction of stray dog population.

ECHINOCOCCUS MULTILOCULARIS

Geographical distribution

E. multilocularis, the causative agent of alveolar echinococcosis, or alveolar or multilocular hydatid cyst, occurs in Europe, America, Canada, Russia, Central Asian Republics, and western China.

Morphology

E. multilocularis is smaller than *E. granulosus*. It measures 1.2–3.7 mm in length. The eggs are typically *Taenia*-like.

Life cycle

Foxes and wolves are definitive hosts and small wild rodents including squirrels, field mice, and voles are intermediate hosts. Domestic dogs and cats may also become infected and act as definitive hosts when they eat infected wild rodents. Man is an accidental intermediate host. The adult worm lives attached to the mucosa of the small intestine of the canine definitive hosts. The eggs are passed in the faeces and are infective to intermediate hosts. Man acquires infection by ingestion of vegetables, fruits, and salads contaminated wth faeces of foxes and dogs or from contaminated hands. Persons who work with fox fur are often exposed to alveolar or multilocular hydatid disease. In the duodenum hexacanth embryos hatch out and penetrate the intestinal wall. These forms enter the circulation and take up residence primarily in the liver and lungs but also possibly in the brain.

Pathogenicity

E. multilocularis causes **alveolar echinococcosis**, or **alveolar or multilocular hydatid cyst**. The organ most commonly involved is the liver. Cyst of *E. multilocularis*, as the species name implies, has multiple locules. The multilocular infiltrating lesion appears like a grossly invasive growth that may be mistaken for a malignant tumour. Destruction of liver parenchyma may lead to hepatic failure. The lesions tend to spread by direct extension into the surrounding tissues and can also be transported to other body sites via the lymphatic or haematogenous routes. In about 2% of cases, pieces of the germinal membrane can metastasize to other body sites, including the brain, lungs, and mediastinum.

It is among the most lethal of all helminthic infections of man. If untreated, 70% cases progress to death. Central necrosis and cavitation are the common findings. The cavity contains little or no fluid. The formation of hyaline layer is less conspicuous; the germinal layer is often hyperplastic and folded on itself and there is a tendency of persistent cellular reaction by eosinophils and endothelial cells in the surrounding tissue. Most of the alveolar or multilocular hydatid cysts, in man, are sterile.

Laboratory diagnosis

Diagnosis of alveolar or multilocular hydatid cyst is made by the biopsy of the affected organ. *E. multilocularis* rarely produces scolices, therefore, the identification depends on recognition of the characteristic germinal and laminated membranes. CT scan and ultrasound are helpful in ascertaining the site and shape of the cyst. Immunologic tests described for *E. granulosus* hydatid cyst are equally applicable to that caused by *E. multilocularis*.

Treatment

It is similar to that for the hydatid disease caused by *E. granulosus*. However, some patients are not cured despite multiple courses of therapy, where lifelong therapy with albendazole may be required. Benzimidazole treatment should be administered in the perioperative period.

Prophylaxis

Eliminating *E. multilocularis* from its wild animal hosts is impractical. Therefore, contact with dogs and foxes in areas where the infection is endemic should be avoided. Strict personal hygiene will also prevent infection in man.

ECHINOCOCCUS VOGELI

Echinococcus vogeli is the aetiological agent of polycystic disease in humans in areas such as Brazil, Colombia, Venezuela, Panama, and Ecuador. It is long and slender, measuring up to 5.6 mm in length. It has a scolex and three proglottids (immature, mature and gravid). The scolex possesses a large rostellum armed with 36 hooklets arranged in two rows. The gravid proglottid is 3–4 mm in length and 0.3 mm in width. The eggs measure about 35 μm in diameter.

The natural cycle of the parasite is passed in the bush dog (*Speothos venaticus*) and the paca (*Cuniculus paca*) as definitive and intermediate hosts respectively. Man acquires infection from the faeces of domestic dogs that have been fed on viscera of infected pacas. *E. vogeli* causes **polycystic echinococcosis** or **polycystic hydatid disease** formed by endogenous proliferation of the germinal laminated membranes forming folds and pockets within the primary vesicle.

The organ most commonly involved is liver followed by lungs, mesentery, spleen, and pancreas. The germinal membrane is delicate, covered by a relatively thick (20–400 μm), laminated membrane which, in turn, is surrounded by a connective tissue capsule (70–250 μm). The parasite is invasive and is spread by exogenous budding, producing a pathologic process similar to that of hepatic carcinoma. Patient develops abdominal pain, hepatomegaly, jaundice, weight loss, anaemia, fever, haemoptysis, palpable abdominal masses, and signs of portal hypertension. Diagnosis is usually made by examination of surgical specimens or tissues obtained at autopsy. The treatment is the same as in case of cystic echinococcosis.

Further Reading

1. Bartholomot, B., Vuiton, A., et al. 2002. Combined ultrasound and serologic screening for hepatic alveolar echinococcosis in central China. *Am J. Trop. Med. Hyg.*, **66**, 23–9.
2. Cosentino, C., Valez, M., et al., 2002. Cysticercosis lesions in basal ganglia are common but clinically silent. *Clin. Neurol. Neurosurg*, **104**, 57–60.
3. Del Brutto, O.H., Rajshekhar, V., et al. 2001. Proposed diagnostic criteria for neurocysticercosis. *Neurology*, **57**, 177–83.
4. Dorny, P., Brandt, J., et al. 2003. Immunodiagnostic tools for human and porcine cysticercosis. *Acta Trop.*, **87**, 79–86.
5. Ferrer, E., Cortez, M.M., et al. 2002. Serological evidence for recent exposure to *Taenia solium* in Venezuelan Amerindians, *Am J. Trop. Med. Hyg.*, **66**, 170–4.
6. Galan-Puchades, M.T. and Fuentes, M.V. 2000. Human cysticercosis and larval tropism of *Taenia asiatica*. *Parasitol. Today*, **12**, 123.
7. Garcia, H.H. and Del Brutto, O.H. 2000. *Taenia solium* cysticercosis. *Infect. Dis. Clin. N. Am.*, **14**, 97–119.
8. Gonzalez, L.M., Montero, E., et al. 2002. Differential diagnosis of *Taenia saginata* and *Taenia solium* infections: from DNA probes to polymerase chain reaction. *Trans. R. Soc. Trop. Med. Hyg.*, **96**, S1/243–50.
9. Lightowlers, M.W., Flisser, A., et al. 2000. Vaccination against cysticercosis and hydatid disease. *Parasitol. Today*, **16**, 191–6.
10. White, A.C. 2000. Neurocysticercosis: updates on epidemiology, pathogenesis, diagnosis and management. *Ann. Rev. Med.*, **51**, 187–206.

Important Questions

1. Describe morphology, life cycle, pathogenicity and laboratory diagnosis of:
   (a) *Diphyllobothrium latum*
   (b) *Taenia saginata*
   (c) *Taenia solium*
   (d) *Hymenolepis nana*
   (e) *Echinococcus granulosus*
2. Write short notes on:
   (a) General characters of cestodes
   (b) Classification of cestodes
   (c) *Spirometra* or sparganosis
   (d) *Taenia asiatica*
   (e) *Taenia multiceps*
   (f) *Hymenolepis diminuta*
   (g) *Dipylidium caninum*
   (h) *Echinococcus multilocularis*
   (i) *Echinococcus vogeli*

Multiple Choice Questions

1. In which of the following cestodes man can act as both definitive and intermediate host?
   (a) *Taenia saginata*.
   (b) *Taenia solium*.
   (c) *Diphyllobothrium latum*.
   (d) *Hymenolepis nana*.
2. Which of the following cestodes belongs to family Diphyllobothriidae?
   (a) *Diphyllobothrium latum*.
   (b) *Taenia solium*.
   (c) *Hymenolepis nana*.
   (d) *Echinococcus multilocularis*.
3. Adult worms of the following cestodes are seen in the intestine of man **except**:
   (a) *Taenia saginata*.
   (b) *Diphyllobothrium latum*.
   (c) *Hymenolepis nana*.
   (d) *Echinococcus granulosus*.
4. Common name for *Diphyllobothrium latum* is:
   (a) the fish tapeworm.
   (b) the beef tapeworm.
   (c) the pork tapeworm.
   (d) the rat tapeworm.
5. Which is the longest tapeworm found in man?
   (a) *Diphyllobothrium latum*.
   (b) *Taenia saginata*.
   (c) *Taenia solium*.
   (d) *Echinococcus granulosus*.
6. Parasite-induced pernicious anaemia is seen in infection with:
   (a) *Diphyllobothrium latum*.
   (b) *Spirometra mansoni*.
   (c) *Taenia saginata*.
   (d) *Taenia solium*.
7. Which form of *Spirometra* is seen in man?
   (a) Adult worm.
   (b) Coracidium larva.
   (c) Procercoid larva.
   (d) Plerocercoid larva.

8. Which is the intermediate host for *Taenia saginata*?
   (a) Man.
   (b) Cattle.
   (c) Pig.
   (d) Sheep.
9. Larval form of *Taenia solium* is seen in:
   (a) pig.
   (b) cattle.
   (c) dog.
   (d) cat.
10. Which is the drug of choice for *Taenia saginata* infection?
   (a) Praziquantel.
   (b) Niclosamide.
   (c) Albendazole.
   (d) Amphotericin B.
11. Which is the smallest tapeworm infecting man?
   (a) *Hymenolepis nana*.
   (b) *Taenia saginata*.
   (c) *Taenia solium*.
   (d) *Diphyllobothrium latum*.
12. Common name of *Hymenolepis nana* is:
   (a) the dwarf tapeworm.
   (b) the fish tapeworm.
   (c) the pork tapeworm.
   (d) the rat tapeworm.
13. Which of the following cestodes is capable of completing its life cycle in a single host?
   (a) *Taenia saginata*.
   (b) *Echinococcus granulosus*.
   (c) *Diphyllobothrium latum*.
   (d) *Hymenolepis nana*.
14. Which is the intermediate host in indirect life cycle of *Hymenolepis nana*?
   (a) House fly.
   (b) Head louse.
   (c) Body louse.
   (d) Rat flea.
15. Rat tapeworm is the common name of:
   (a) *Hymenolepis nana*.
   (b) *Hymenolepis diminuta*.
   (c) *Taenia saginata*.
   (d) *Diphyllobothrium latum*.
16. Coenurus is the larval form of:
   (a) *Taenia solium*.
   (b) *Taenia multiceps*.
   (c) *Echinococcus granulosus*.
   (d) *Echinococcus multilocularis*.
17. The common name of *Dipylidium caninum* is:
   (a) the fish tapeworm.
   (b) the beef tapeworm.
   (c) the double-pored dog tapeworm.
   (d) the dog tapeworm.
18. Common name of *Echinococcus granulosus* is:
   (a) the fish tapeworm.
   (b) the beef tapeworm.
   (c) the dwarf tapeworm.
   (d) the dog tapeworm.
19. Which is the definitive host for *Echinococcus granulosus?*
   (a) Dog.
   (b) Sheep.
   (c) Cattle.
   (d) Man.
20. Larval form of *Echinococcus granulosus* is seen in:
   (a) dog.
   (b) man.
   (c) wolf.
   (d) fox.
21. Which is the most common organ involved in hydatidosis?
   (a) Liver.
   (b) Lung.
   (c) Spleen.
   (d) Kidney.
22. Alveolar echinococcosis is caused by:
   (a) *Echinococcus granulosus*.
   (b) *Echinococcus multilocularis*.
   (c) *Echinococcus vogeli*.
   (d) *Taenia multiceps*.
23. Cyst of *Echinococcus multilocularis* differs from that of *Echinococcus granulosus* in having:
   (a) multiple locules.
   (b) little or no fluid.
   (c) hyperplastic germinal layer.
   (d) All of the above.
24. Which is/are the intermediate host/s of *Echinococcus multilocularis*?
   (a) Squirrels.
   (b) Field mice.
   (c) Man.
   (d) All of the above.

25. Polycystic echinococcosis is caused by:
    (a) *Echinococcus granulosus.*
    (b) *Echinococcus multilocularis.*
    (c) *Echinococcus vogeli.*
    (d) *Taenia multiceps.*
26. Liver is the most common organ involved in infection with:
    (a) *Echinococcus granulosus.*
    (b) *Echinococcus multilocularis.*
    (c) *Echinococcus vogeli.*
    (d) All of the above.
27. A 30-year-old patient reported in the medical outpatient department with chief complaints of fatigue, weakness, diarrhoea and numbness of extremities. The peripheral blood film revealed megaloblastic anaemia and stool examination showed yellowish-brown operculated eggs, 70 µm in length and 45 µm in breadth. Which of the following parasites is likely to be the cause of the disease?
    (a) *Fasciola hepatica.*
    (b) *Clonorchis sinensis.*
    (c) *Paragonimus westermani.*
    (d) *Diphyllobothrium latum.*
28. The parasite transmitted by inadequately cooked freshwater fish is:
    (a) *Diphyllobothrium latum.*
    (b) *Taenia solium.*
    (c) *Taenia saginata.*
    (d) *Echinococcus granulosus.*
29. Operculated eggs are produced by:
    (a) *Hymenolepis nana.*
    (b) *Taenia solium.*
    (c) *Echinococcus granulosus.*
    (d) *Diphyllobothrium latum.*
30. The egg containing hexacanth embryo with radially striated embryophore is seen in:
    (a) *Diphyllobothrium latum.*
    (b) *Taenia solium.*
    (c) *Hymenolepis nana.*
    (d) *Dipylidium caninum.*
31. Which of the following parasites requires two intermediate hosts?
    (a) *Taenia solium.*
    (b) *Diphyllobothrium latum.*
    (c) *Hymenolepis nana.*
    (d) *Echinococcus granulosus.*
32. Cysticercoid is the larval form of:
    (a) *Hymenolepis nana.*
    (b) *Echinococcus granulosus.*
    (c) *Taenia solium.*
    (d) *Taenia saginata.*
33. Which of the following parasites liberates eggs that are not bile-stained?
    (a) *Diphyllobothrium latum.*
    (b) *Taenia saginata.*
    (c) *Taenia solium.*
    (d) *Hymenolepis nana.*
34. Man serves as an intermediate host of:
    (a) *Echinococcus granulosus.*
    (b) *Taenia saginata.*
    (c) *Wuchereria bancrofti.*
    (d) *Diphyllobothrium latum.*
35. Larval form of *Taenia solium* is called:
    (a) cysticercus cellulosae.
    (b) cysticercus bovis.
    (c) cysticercoid.
    (d) hydatid cyst.
36. Larval form of *Taenia saginata* is called:
    (a) cysticercus cellulosae.
    (b) cysticercus bovis.
    (c) cysticercoid.
    (d) hydatid cyst.
37. Larval form of *Echinococcus granulosus* is called:
    (a) cysticercus cellulosae.
    (b) cysticercus bovis.
    (c) cysticercoid.
    (d) hydatid cyst.
38. Which of the following parasites does not possess rostellum?
    (a) *Taenia solium.*
    (b) *Taenia saginata.*
    (c) *Echinococcus granulosus.*
    (d) *Hymenolepis nana.*
39. The skin test used for the diagnosis of hydatid cyst is known as:
    (a) Casoni's test.
    (b) Dick test.
    (c) Schick test.
    (d) Montenegro test.
40. Which of the following tapeworms is acquired by eating raw or undercooked pork?
    (a) *Taenia saginata.*
    (b) *Taenia solium.*

(c) *Diphyllobothrium latum.*
(d) *Hymenolepis nana.*

41. Which of the following tapeworms is acquired by eating raw or undercooked beef?
(a) *Taenia saginata.*
(b) *Taenia solium.*
(c) *Diphyllobothrium latum.*
(d) *Hymenolepis nana.*

42. *Taenia solium*, a parasite that is transmitted to humans by eating undercooked pork, is classified as:
(a) fluke.
(b) flagellate.
(c) nematode.
(d) cestode.

43. Which of the following is a cestode?
(a) *Clonorchis sinensis.*
(b) *Toxocara canis.*
(c) *Schistosoma mansoni.*
(d) *Hymenolepis diminuta.*

44. Eggs of *Hymenolepis nana*:
(a) have 4–8 polar filaments emanating from polar thickenings at either end of embryophore.
(b) contain a hexacanth embryo.
(c) are spherical or oval, hyaline, 35–40 μm in diameter.
(d) All of the above.

45. Which of the following cestodes lays eggs in egg packets rather than single eggs?
(a) *Taenia solium.*
(b) *Hymenolepis diminuta.*
(c) *Hymenolepis nana.*
(d) *Dipylidium caninum.*

46. Which of the following genera produces eggs with a thick-walled shell and contain an embryo with 3 pairs of hooklets?
(a) *Taenia.*
(b) *Fasciola.*
(c) *Necator.*
(d) *Strongyloides.*

47. In the stool of an infant objects that look like pumpkin seeds have been noticed. The patient has not eaten this vegetable. What could these objects be?
(a) Proglottids of *Taenia solium.*
(c) Proglottids of *Taenia saginata.*
(c) Proglottids of *Dipylidium caninum.*
(d) Proglottids of *Hymenolepis nana.*

48. Which of the following parasites deprives the host of vitamin B_{12}, causing pernicious anaemia?
(a) *Taenia solium.*
(b) *Taenia saginata.*
(c) *Echinococcus granulosus.*
(d) *Diphyllobothrium latum.*

49. The most lethal of all helminthic infections of man is:
(a) *Echinococcus granulosus.*
(b) *Echinococcus multilocularis.*
(c) *Echinococcus vogeli.*
(d) *Taenia solium.*

50. A 40-year-old female patient is suffering from abdominal pain, megaloblastic anaemia and weight loss. She is habitual of tasting fish before cooking. Which of the following parasites is most likely cause of her illness?
(a) *Taenia solium.*
(b) *Echinococcus granulosus.*
(c) *Diphyllobothrium latum.*
(d) *Hymenolepis nana.*

51. Intradermal test of which of the following pathogens gives rise to an erythema and induration 5 cm or more in diameter with pseudopodia within 30 minutes of inoculation?
(a) *Mycobacterium tuberculosis.*
(b) *Mycobacterium leprae.*
(c) *Echinococcus granulosus.*
(d) *Leishmania donovani.*

ANSWERS TO MCQs

1 (b), 2 (a), 3 (d), 4 (a), 5 (a), 6 (a), 7 (d) 8 (b), 9 (a), 10 (a), 11 (a), 12 (a), 13 (d), 14 (d), 15 (b), 16 (b), 17 (c), 18 (d), 19 (a), 20 (b), 21 (a), 22 (b), 23 (d), 24 (d), 25 (c), 26 (d), 27 (d), 28 (a), 29 (d), 30 (b), 31 (b), 32 (a), 33 (d), 34 (a), 35 (a), 36 (b), 37 (d), 38 (b), 39 (a), 40 (b), 41 (a), 42 (d), 43 (d), 44 (d), 45 (d), 46 (a), 47 (c), 48 (d), 49 (b), 50 (c), 51 (c).

10

Trematodes or Flukes*

GENERAL CHARACTERISTICS

Trematodes or flukes belong to the kingdom Animalia, phylum Platyhelminthes and class Digenea (Table 1.6). They are leaf-like unsegmented flat worms. These vary in size from 1 mm to several centimeters in length. The most characteristic external structures are two suckers – one oral through which the digestive tract opens and the other ventral (acetabulum) for attachment. Each individual worm is hermaphrodite (monoecious) except the schistosomes which are unisexual (dioecious). The body is covered with integument, which often bears spines. Body cavity is absent. Alimentary canal is present but incomplete. It consists of a mouth surrounded by oral sucker, a muscular pharynx and the oesophagus which bifurcates in front of the ventral sucker into a pair of blind intestinal caeca. The anus is absent.

The excretory and nervous systems are present. Excretory system consists of flame cells and collecting tubules which lead to a median bladder opening at the posterior end of the body, usually on the dorsal aspect. The nervous system consists of a group of paired ganglion cells and nerve trunks. Reproductive system is highly developed. With the exception of schistosomes, the reproductive organs are hermaphroditic. The genital organs lie between the two branches of the intestine.

Trematodes are **oviparous** and lay eggs which, with the exception of schistosomes, are operculated. In case of *Fasciola hepatica, Fasciolopsis buski*, *Clonorchis sinensis*, *Schistosoma japonicum* and *S. mansoni*, the eggs are passed in the faeces and in case of *S. haematobium* and *Paragonimus westermani* they are passed in urine and sputum respectively.

Life cycle

Trematodes pass their life cycle in two different hosts. Man, who harbours the adult worm, is the definitive host and a freshwater snail or mollusc is the intermediate

* This chapter has been contributed by Dr. Paramjeet Singh Gill, Professor, Department of Microbiology, PGIMS, Rohtak.

host. A second intermediate host (fish or crab) is required for encystment in some trematodes. The eggs liberated by the definitive host gain access into the water and hatch either immediately (*S. haematobium, S. mansoni* and *S. japonicum*) or following a short period of embryonation (*F. hepatica, F. buski,* and *P. westermani*). Free-living **miracidia** are released, which are either ingested or penetrate into the flesh of the first intermediate host, a snail. Eggs of *C. sinensis* and *Opisthorchis* spp. hatch only after ingestion by the snail in its midgut. Within the snail, the miracidia transform into a second larval stage known as **sporocyst**.

The sporocysts develop either into second-generation sporocysts (schistosomes) or into somewhat more complex daughter organisms, known as **rediae** (hermaphroditic trematodes). Within the second-generation sporocysts or rediae develop tailed larvae, the **cercariae**. On maturity, the cercariae escape from the parent organism, and then leave the snail host and become free-living in the water. In schistosomes, cercariae have a forked tail and infect the definitive host by direct skin penetration.

In the hermaphroditic flukes, the cercariae have an unsplit tail, and they encyst on vegetables or within a second intermediate host, fish or crab, to form the **metacercariae**, which are the infective forms. Humans become infected by ingesting the metacercariae contained on raw or undercooked vegetables (*F. hepatica, F. buski* and *Watsonius watsoni*), in fish (*C. sinensis* and *Heterophyes heterophyes*) or in crabs (*P. westermani*). All encysted metacercariae excyst in the upper levels of the small intestine and migrate to the tissues or organs where they develop into mature worms.

Pathogenicity

The clinical picture of trematode infections depends upon size and number of worms present in the host and organs or tissues parasitized. The pathogenic lesions produced may be local or systemic, usually both. The former consists of ulceration, sloughing of tissue and abscess formation. Systemic manifestations are usually due to absorption of antigenic by-products of the worms which frequently provoke a generalized leucocytosis, hypereosinophilia and allergic manifestations.

CLASSIFICATION OF TREMATODES

Zoological classification and classification on the basis of the habitat of trematodes is given in Tables 10.1 and 10.2 respectively.

Table 10.1. Zoological classification of trematodes

Phylum: Platyhelminthes
Class: Digenea

Family	Genus	Species
Schistosomatidae	*Schistosoma*	*S. haematobium* *S. mansoni* *S. japonicum* S. mekongi *S. intercalatum*
Gastrodiscidae	*Gastrodiscoides*	*G. hominis*
	Watsonius	*W. watsoni*
Fasciolidae	*Fasciola*	*F. hepatica*
	Fasciolopsis	*F. buski*
Opisthorchiidae	*Opisthorchis*	*O. felineus* *O. viverrini*
	Clonorchis	*C. sinensis*
Heterophyidae	*Heterophyes*	*H. heterophyes*
	Metagonimus	*M. yokogawai*
Paragonimidae	*Paragonimus*	*P. westermani*

Table 10.2. Classification of trematodes on the basis of their habitat

Blood trematodes	
In vesical and pelvic venous plexus	*S. haematobium*
In rectal venous plexus and portal venous system	*S. mansoni, S. japonicum*
Hepatic trematodes	*F. hepatica, C. sinensis, O. felineus, O. viverrini*
Lung trematodes	*P. westermani*
Intestinal trematodes	
Small intestine	*F. buski, H. heterophyes, M. yokogawai, W. watsoni.*
Large intestine	*G. hominis*

SCHISTOSOMES OR BLOOD FLUKES

Schistosomes are the causative agents of the disease **schistosomiasis**, also known as **bilharziasis** or **snail fever**. It is the most important and prevalent of **water-borne parasitic diseases**. The three main species infecting humans are *Schistosoma haematobium, S. japonicum* and *S. mansoni*. Two other species, more localized geographically, are *S. mekongi* and *S. intercalatum*. In addition, other species of schistosomes, which parasitize birds and mammals, can cause **cercarial dermatitis** in humans. *S. haematobium* was first observed, in Cairo in 1851, by Theodor Bilharz in the blood of mesenteric veins of a young man on autopsy. After the name of its discoverer, it was named *Bilharzia*. The name was changed subsequently to *Schistosoma*.

The name *Schistosoma* is derived from the appearance of the adult male the body of which has a longitudinal genital groove or canal, known as gynaecophoric canal, that serves as a receptacle for the female during copulation. It appears as though the body of the male is split longitudinally to produce this canal, hence the name *Schistosoma* (*schisto*, split and *soma*, body).

General characters

1. Schistosomes are obligate intravascular parasites and are not found in cavities, ducts, and other tissues.
2. They are unisexual (dioecious) trematodes, i.e., the sexes are separate.
3. Males are shorter and stouter than females.
4. Males possess a gynaecophoric canal, which is formed by the infolding of the lateral margins ventrally, for holding the female during copulation (Fig. 10.1).
5. Suckers are armed with delicate spines.
6. Muscular pharynx is absent and intestinal caeca reunite behind the ventral sucker to form a single canal.
7. In females, Laurer's canal (vestigial vagina) is absent.
8. In males, the number of testes varies from 4–8.
9. Eggs are non-operculated and are fully embryonated when laid.
10. The infective forms of schistosomes are skin-penetrating **cercariae** liberated from snails, and these differ from other flukes in that they are not eaten on vegetation, in fish, or in crustaceans.
11. Cercariae have bifid tails. They can penetrate the unbroken skin of the definitive host.
12. Encysted metacercarial stage is absent.
13. Adult worms reside in venous plexuses in the body of the definitive host, the location varying with the species.
14. Three *Schistosoma* species, *S. haematobium*, *S. mansoni* and *S. japonicum*, cause the majority of human infections. *S.mekongi*, which resembles *S. japonicum*, and *S.intercalatum*, whose ova resemble those of *S. haematobium* but whose clinical illness mimics *S. mansoni* infection, are two other species with limited geographic distribution in Cambodia and Laos and in Central Africa, respectively. The geographical distribution, morphology, habitat, and definitive and intermediate hosts of three major species of schistosomes (*S. haematobium*, *S. mansoni* and *S. japonicum*) are given in Table 10.3.

Life cycle

The life cycle of all species follows a common pathway (Fig. 10.1). The adult worms of *S. japonicum* and *S. mansoni* inhabit the mesenteric veins draining ileo-caecal and sigmoido-rectal regions respectively, whereas *S. haematobium* lives primarily in the veins of vesical and pelvic plexuses, less commonly in the portal vein and its mesenteric branches. The female, held in the gynaecophoric canal of the male, extends its anterior end far into the smallest venules and deposits the eggs one at a time. Each time an egg is laid, the worm withdraws a short distance and lays another egg immediately behind the first. In this way the venules are filled with eggs.

The eggs then work their way through the vessels and the mucosa of urinary bladder (*S. haematobium*), sigmoido-rectal region (*S. mansoni*) and ileo-caecal region (*S. japonicum*) and enter into the lumen of these organs. These eggs are then discharged in urine (*S. haematobium*) and faeces (*S. mansoni* and *S. japonicum*). Embryonated eggs that are passed in the urine or faeces into freshwater (lakes, canals and the like), hatch quickly, releasing free-swimming larvae (**miracidia**) which move freely in water in search of their intermediate hosts, the snails of the genera *Bulinus* (*S. haematobium*), *Biomphalaria* (*S. mansoni*) and *Oncomelania* (*S. japonicum*).

The miracidia on entering their proper larval hosts, penetrate into the soft tissues of the snails and ultimately make their way into the liver. Inside the snail, the miracidia lose their cilia and in the course of 4–8 weeks, successively pass through the **first- and second-generation sporocysts**. Within the second-generation sporocysts, hundreds of **fork-tailed cercariae** are produced by asexual reproduction. These are infective to man. The cercariae break off from the sporocysts and escape from the snail into water.

The free-swimming cercariae released from infected snails have the capability of directly penetrating the water-softened skin of human beings bathing or wading in this water. On entering the skin, the cercariae shed

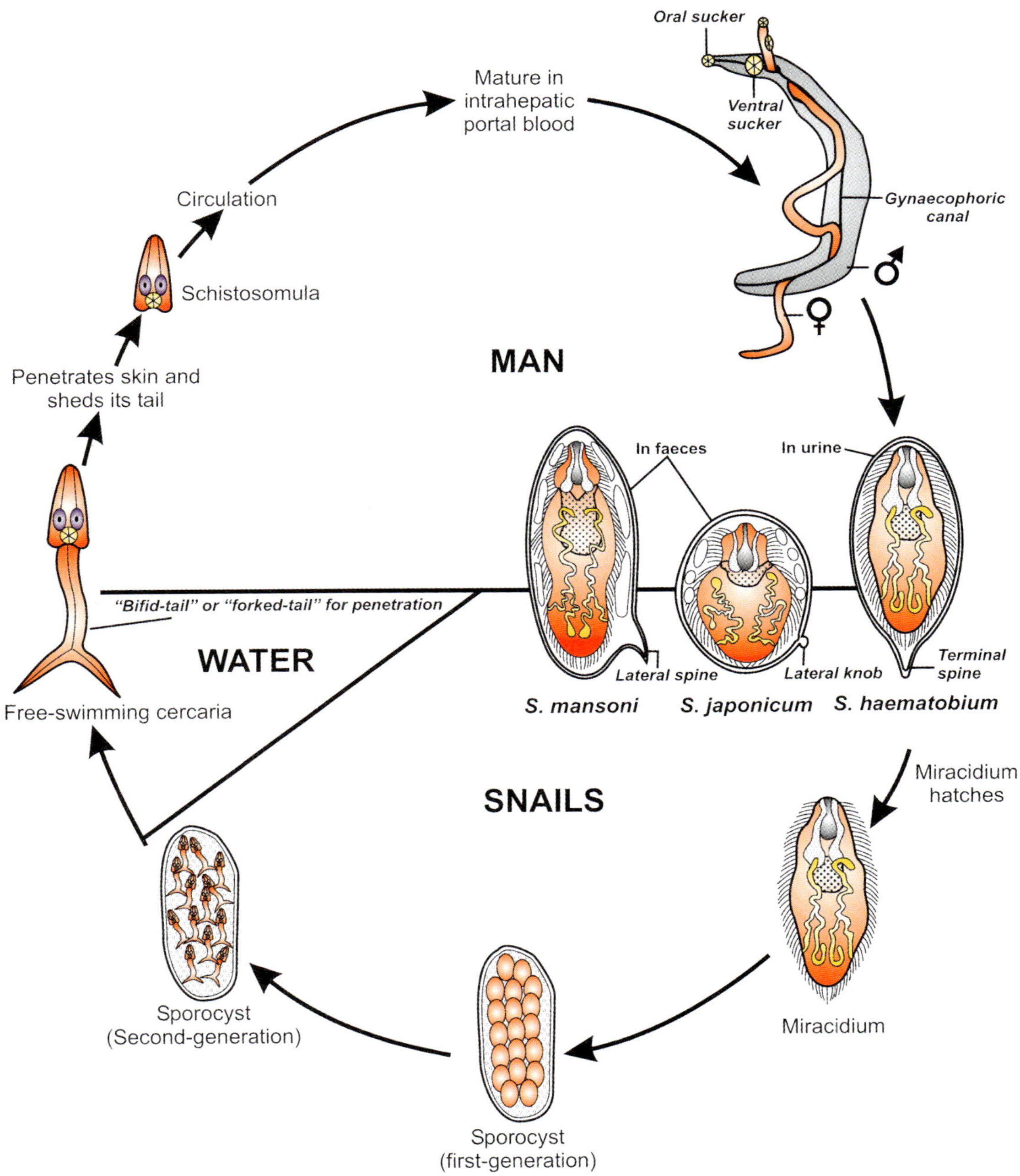

Fig. 10.1. Life cycle of *Schistosoma* species.

their tails and become **schistosomulae** which enter into peripheral venules. From here they are carried through the vena cava into the right heart, the pulmonary circulation, the left heart and the systemic circulation. The majority of the schistosomulae, from the systemic circulation, are shunted in the abdominal aorta and gain access to the mesenteric artery, pass through capillary bed in the intestine and enter portal circulation and reach the liver.

In the intrahepatic portal veins the schistosomulae grow, pairing of worms take place on sexual maturation, and they migrate against the blood current into the portal system venules, primarily those of the urinary bladder (*S. haematobium*), sigmoido-rectal region (*S. mansoni*) and ileo-caecal region (*S. japonicum*). Female worms lay the eggs which depending upon the species, are discharged in faeces or urine and the cycles are repeated.

Table 10.3. Differentiating features of *S. haematobium, S. mansoni* and *S. japonicum*

	S. haematobium	*S. mansoni*	*S. japonicum*
1. **Geographical distribution**	51 eastern Mediterranean and African countries, India and Turkey	36 countries in Africa, 9 in the Americas and 7 in the East Mediterranean	China, Indonesia, the Philippines and Thailand
2. **Morphology**			
Male			
• Size	10–15 mm in length and 0.8 mm in breadth	6.4–12 mm in length and 1 mm in breadth	12–20 mm in length and 0.5 mm in breadth
• Integument	Covered with minute tuberculations	Covered with more conspicuous tuberculations	Smooth
• Number of testes	4–5	6–9	7
Female			
• Size	20 mm in length and 0.25 mm in breadth	7.2–17 mm in length and 0.25 mm in breadth	26 mm in length and 0.3 mm in breadth
• Ovary	In the posterior one-third of the body	In the anterior half of the body	In the middle of the body
• Uterus	Contains 20–200 eggs	Contains 1–3 eggs	Contains 50 or more eggs
• Egg	Elongated, 110–170 μm long and 40–70 μm wide; has a thin, smooth shell, a rounded anterior end and a characteristic terminal spine from the tapered posterior end	Elongated, 115–180 μm long and 40–70 μm wide; has a thin, smooth shell with a prominent lateral spine near the more rounded posterior end; anterior end tends to be somewhat pointed and curved	Oval or subspherical, 70–100 μm long and 55–65 μm wide; has a smooth, relatively thick shell; a small lateral knob may be seen; because it is often located in a depression in the shell, this is often difficult to see
• Egg discharged in	Urine	Faeces	Faeces
• Infective form	Fork-tailed cercariae that penetrate skin of humans wading in fresh-water canals	As in case of *S. haematobium*	As in case of *S. haematobium*
• Cephalic glands in cercariae	Two pairs oxyphilic and three pairs basophilic	Two pairs oxyphilic and four pairs basophilic	Five pairs oxyphilic (no basophilic)
3. **Habitat**	Veins of the vesical and pelvic plexuses, less commonly in portal vein and its mesenteric branches	Mesenteric veins draining sigmoido-rectal region (inferior mesenteric vein and its branches)	Mesenteric veins draining ileo-caecal region (superior mesenteric vein and its branches)
4. **Definitive host**	Man	Man	Man and domestic animals
5. **Intermediate snail host**	*Bulinus* spp.	*Biomphalaria* spp.	*Oncomelania* spp.

Pathogenicity

Pathological lesions of various *Schistosoma* spp. are caused mainly by the eggs deposited in various tissues. Host immune response to antigens excreted from embryonated eggs results in the formation of granulomas that in chronic infections lead to fibrotic changes. Cercariae may induce **dermatitis** with itching and pruritic papular lesion in the skin within 24 hours of invasion by the cercariae. It disappears within a week. Migration of schistosomulae into lungs provoke cough and mild fever. In some patients anaemia may be observed.

Acute schistosomiasis or **Katayama fever** occurs in about a month after infection with *S. japonicum* and *S. mansoni* and rarely with *S. haematobium*. Characteristic symptoms include high fever, hepatosplenomegaly, lymphadenopathy, eosinophilia, and dysentery. This corresponds with the start of oviposition by mature female worms.

S. mansoni and *S. japonicum* female worms lay eggs in the mesenteric branches of the portal vein along the intestinal wall. By the blood flow a large number of eggs are carried into the liver and other organs. The remainder eggs stay in small venules. The eggs elicit acute inflammation in the surrounding tissues and the formation of granulomas and pseudotubercles around them. Acute inflammation results in the rupture of the vascular wall and escape of eggs from the venules through the intestinal submucosa and mucosa into the intestinal lumen. The inflammation leads to recurrent daily fever, pain abdomen, enlarged tender liver and spleen, and discharge of eggs into the intestinal canal accompanied by dysentery or diarrhoea. Eosinophilia and increased serum levels of IgE antibodies is observed in most of the patients.

The *Schistosoma* eggs secrete soluble substances which pass through the microscopic pores in the **egg shell** and provoke a granulomatous inflammation. **Egg granuloma** is composed of egg at the centre, surrounded by mononuclear phagocytes, neutrophils, lymphocytes, plasma cells, giant cells and fibroblasts. The chronic phase of manifestations in *S. mansoni* and *S. japonicum* infections is characterized by hepatosplenomegaly and may therefore be called **hepatosplenic schistosomiasis**, although development of polyps or mucosal proliferation of the intestine may also be observed in most cases.

The enlarged spleen may reach the level of the umbilicus and even at times expand to fill most of the abdomen. Liver gradually decreases in size but increases in hardness as fibrosis gradually extends into the parenchyma, resulting eventually in liver cirrhosis in several cases. Patient may develop **ascites** due to portal hypertension and hypoalbuminaemia. In advanced cases dilatation of abdominal collateral veins and oesophagogastric varices are seen. Bleeding from the varices may cause sudden death. In case of infection with *S. japonicum*, acute or chronic cerebral involvement may occur due to embolism of eggs or heterotopic parasitism of female worms leading to headache, Jacksonian epileptic seizures, paraesthesia and poor vision.

In *S. haematobium* infection, Katayama fever is much less common. The main complaint is recurrent painless haematuria resulting from ulcers of the bladder. A burning sensation on micturition, frequency and suprapubic discomfort or pain may precede or be associated. The bladder wall may be thickened, with a papillary proliferation of mucosa. *S. haematobium* infection may be complicated by urinary tract infection, hydronephrosis due to obstruction of urinary tract, urinary calculi due to obstructive uropathy and schistosomal cor pulmonale.

The International Agency for Research on Cancer (IARC) considers *S. haematobium* infection a definitive cause of urinary bladder cancer with an associated 5-fold risk. Bladder cancer associated with *S. haematobium* is histologically and pathologically distinct from non-*S. haematobium* associated bladder cancer occurring in North America and Europe, the former being a squamous cell carcinoma, with an early age of onset and generally sparing the trigone of bladder while the latter is of transitional cell type occurring in the older age group. Fibrosis induced by schistosome eggs may induce proliferation, hyperplasia and metaplasia all of which are possible precancerous changes.

The evidence supporting role of *S. japonicum* in cancer occurrence is weaker, although it has been associated with both liver and anorectal cancer. *S. haematobium* may also cause infection of vulva, vagina, cervix, ovaries, fallopian tubes and uterus. Like other sexually transmitted diseases, **female genital schistosomiasis** may be an important risk factor for transmission of human immunodeficiency virus, presumably through lesions in the genital mucosa.

Laboratory diagnosis

Specific diagnosis of schistosomiasis can be made by detection of the characteristic ova in the:

- Stool (*S. mansoni* and *S. japonicum*) or urine (*S. haematobium*) under microscopic examination (Fig. 10.2).
- Biopsy material obtaine7d through the proctoscope (*S. mansoni* and *S. japonicum*) and cystoscope (*S. haematobium*) and examined microscopically after compression or sectioning.

Immunodiagnostic techniques such as immunofluorescent antibody test, ELISA, RIA and complement fixation test may be used as indirect methods for the diagnosis.

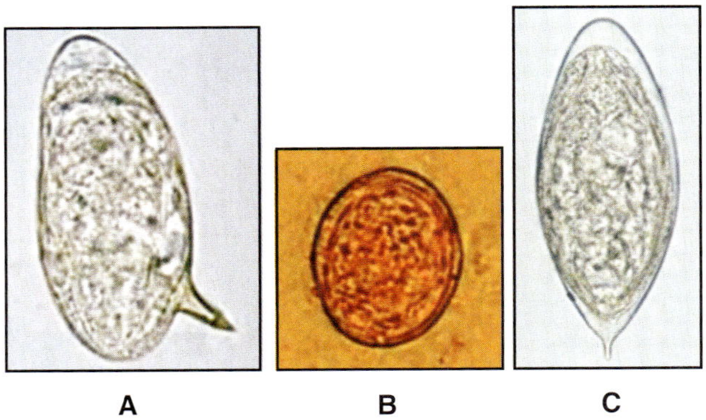

Fig. 10.2. Egg of *Schistosoma mansoni* (A) and *S. japonicum* (B) in stool, and that of *S. haematobium* in urine (C) (saline wet mount, × 400).

Treatment

Praziquantel is the drug of choice for the treatment of schistosomiasis.

Prophylaxis

Preventive measures include the following:

- Prevention of pollution of water with human excreta.
- Eradication of the molluscan hosts in endemic areas by molluscicidal campaigns.
- Avoidance of swimming, bathing, wading or washing in infected water.
- Effective treatment of infected persons to lessen the likelihood of water pollution.

Paddy field (farmers') dermatitis

Paddy field dermatitis among farmers is an occupational public health problem in rice growing regions of Asia. It is caused by cercariae of a number of *Schistosoma* species. In Assam, cercariae of *S. spindale*, which is a mammalian schistosome, have been incriminated as causative agents of farmers' dermatitis. Dermatitis among rice farmers caused by *S. spindale* has also been reported from Malaysia and Thailand. In India, the definitive hosts of *S. spindale* are cattle, sheep, goat and rarely equines and dogs. The other mammalian schistosomes which have also been incriminated as the causative agents of dermatitis among rice farmers are *S. bovis* in Italy and *Orientobilharzia turkistanicum* in Iran and Thailand, *Trichobilharzia brevis* in Malaysia and *Trichobilharzia maegraithi* in Thailand. More severe form of dermatitis among rice farmers has been reported due to *Gigantobilharzia sturniae*.

Control of schistosome cercarial dermatitis can be achieved by eliminating the intermediate snail hosts, which are present in large numbers in the affected paddy fields. This can be achieved using appropriate molluscicides, thus interrupting the life cycle of the parasite. Currently niclosamide is the only safe and acceptable molluscicide according to WHO Pesticide Evaluation Scheme.

SCHISTOSOMA MEKONGI

Adult worms of *S. mekongi* closely resemble those of *S. japonicum* in all aspects of size, shape, internal structure, and body surface, except that the ovary is larger. The adults are normally found in mesenteric veins. Eggs of *S. mekongi* are also quite similar in shape and structure to *S. japonicum*, but are smaller, measuring 61.7 × 51.2 µm. It is found in Thailand and Cambodia, along the Mekong river. Humans and dogs are the definitive hosts. An aquatic snail, *Tricula aperta*, is the intermediate host. Humans acquire infection in the same way as in *S. japonicum*. It causes schistosomiasis resembling the disease caused by *S. japonicum*.

SCHISTOSOMA INTERCALATUM

The parasite is found in West and Central Africa. The life cycle is similar to that of other schistosomes. Adult worms are found in the mesenteric veins, and eggs are shed in the faeces. Eggs resemble those of *S. haematobium*, having a terminal spine. These can be differentiated from those of *S. haematobium* eggs in that they are acid-fast. Clinical manifestations are similar to those of *S. mansoni* infection.

FASCIOLA HEPATICA

Common names

The sheep liver fluke; the common liver fluke.

F. hepatica was the first trematode to be described. It was reported by de Brie in 1379 in sheep with 'liver rot'. It was named by Linnaeus in 1758.

Geographical distribution

Fascioliasis occurs worldwide. Human infections with *F. hepatica* are found in areas where sheep and cattle are raised, and where humans consume raw watercress. The largest number of infections have been reported from Bolivia, Equador, Egypt, France, Iran, Peru, and Portugal.

Habitat

Adult worms reside in the biliary passages of the liver of sheep, goat, cattle and man.

Morphology

Adult worm

It is a large leaf-shaped fluke, measuring 30 mm × 13 mm and brown to pale grey in colour (Fig. 10.3). It is bilaterally symmetrical with three body layers, but has no true body cavity. At the anterior end there is a distinct conical projection. The posterior end is broadly pointed. The oral sucker measures 1 mm in diameter and is situated in the conical projection at the anterior end. The ventral sucker is 1.6 mm in diameter and is situated nearby in a line with two shoulders. The intestinal

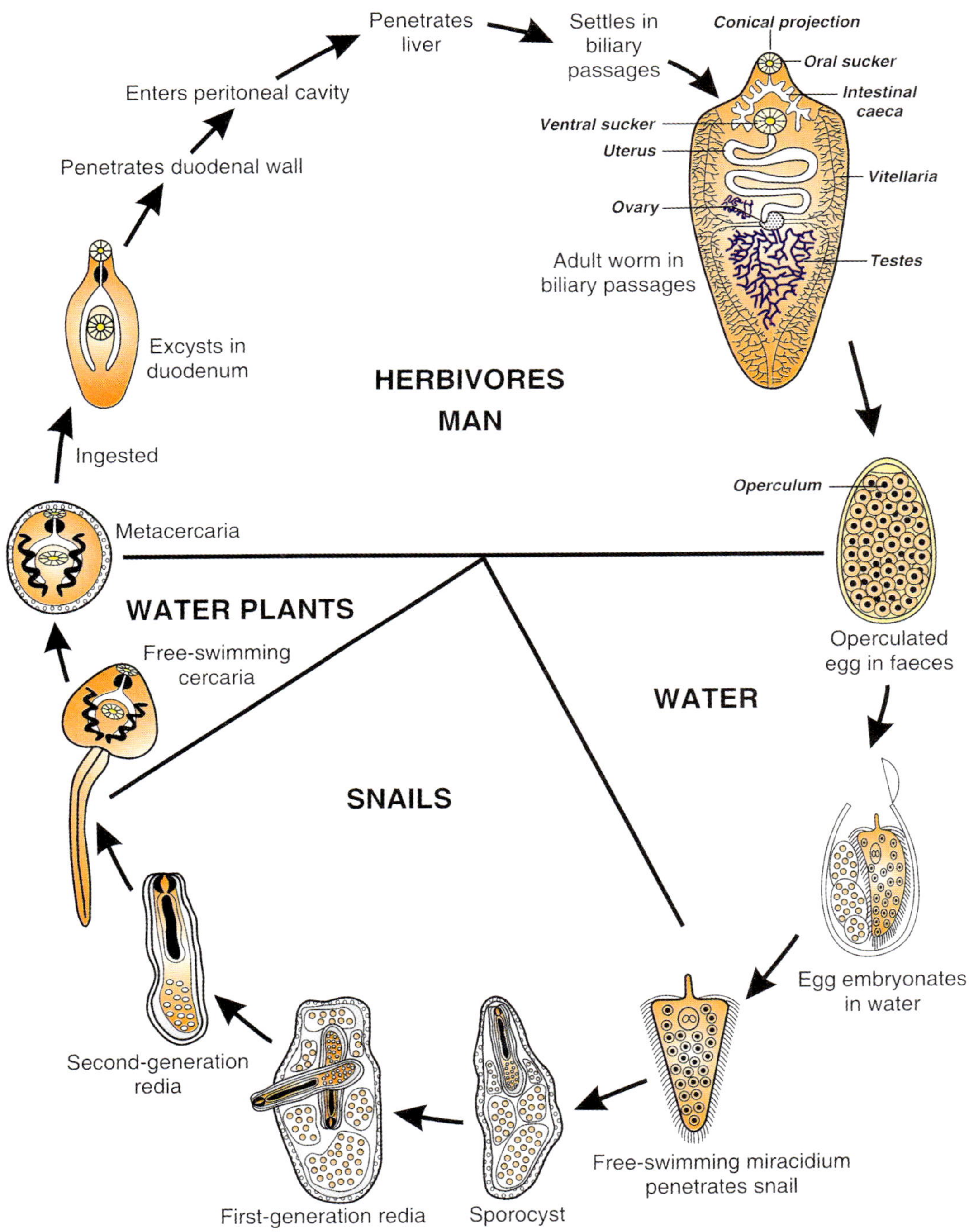

Fig. 10.3. Life cycle of *Fasciola hepatica*.

caeca, testes and vitelline follicles of the parasite are extensively branched. Life span of the adult worm is around 10 years.

Eggs

Eggs are large, elliptical to oval, operculate, **light yellowish-brown (bile-stained)** and measure 140 μm × 80 μm. The shell is thin with a smooth surface. Each egg contains a large unsegmented ovum in a mass of yolk cells (Figs. 10.3 and 10.4). It is excreted with the bile into the duodenum and then passed out along with the faeces. **It does not float in saturated solution of common salt.** Further development of the eggs takes place only in water.

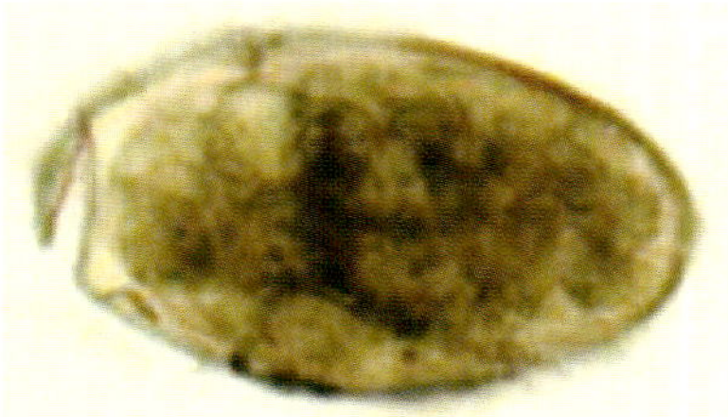

Fig. 10.4. Egg of *Fasciola hepatica* (saline wet mount, × 400).

Infective form

Metacercariae encysted on water plants that are ingested by humans.

Life cycle

F. hepatica passes its life cycle in one definitive and two intermediate hosts (Fig. 10.3).

Definitive hosts

Sheep, goat, cattle and man. The first three are the reservoir hosts of *F. hepatica*.

Intermediate hosts

- ***First intermediate host:*** Snails of the genus *Lymnae*.
- ***Second intermediate host:*** Aquatic vegetation, e.g., watercress.

The adult worms reside in the biliary passages of the liver of the definitive host. Eggs are laid in the biliary passages of the host, reach the intestine and are passed out in the faeces. Eggs that are passed in the faeces into freshwater (lakes, canals and the like), hatch under suitable conditions (22–25°C for 9–15 days), releasing a free-swimming **miracidium**, which burrows into the flesh of an appropriate snail within 8 hours.

As it penetrates the snail's tissues, the miracidium sheds its ciliated cover. Within 3 weeks after penetration, the miracidium passes through the stages of **sporocyst**, **first-generation (mother) rediae**, **second-generation (daughter) rediae**, and finally lead to the release of hundreds of free-swimming, straight-tailed **cercariae**. The cercariae escape from the snail into water, attach to aquatic vegetation and encyst as infective **metacercariae**. Herbivorous animals and occasionally humans acquire infection by ingesting uncooked aquatic plants. The consumption of water-cress has been implicated in most human *F. hepatica* infections especially in Europe.

The metacercariae excyst in the duodenum and migrate through the duodenal wall into the peritoneal cavity, penetrate the capsule of the liver, traverse its parenchyma and ultimately settle in the biliary passages and grow to sexual maturity. The migration takes 6–7 weeks. The adult worms begin producing eggs which exit in the faeces 3–4 months after ingestion of metacercariae. The cycle is then repeated.

Pathogenicity

F. hepatica infection (**fascioliasis**) occurs mainly in rural areas and is most common among sheep and cattle herders.

Pathogenicity of the larvae

The metacercarial larvae of *F. hepatica* that excyst in the duodenum normally produce no significant damage as they migrate through the duodenal wall into the peritoneal cavity, but traumatic and necrotic lesions, 1 cm or more in diameter and heavily infiltrated with eosinophils are formed in the liver parenchyma by the young migrating flukes. These are accompanied by fever, mild to severe abdominal pain, urticaria, hepato-splenomegaly, ascites containing eosinophils and other leucocytes, and jaundice.

Larvae migrating through the peritoneal cavity may become lodged in ectopic foci, where abscesses or fibrotic lesions may develop. These sites include blood vessels, lungs, subcutaneous tissue, ventricles of the brain, and the orbit.

Pathogenicity of adult worms

After arrival in the bile ducts, the larvae develop into adult worms. At this stage the patient is generally asymptomatic or may develop gastrointestinal symptoms. However, some patients develop chronic cholecystitis, cholangitis and cholelithiasis which may be accompanied by biliary colic, epigastric pain, jaundice, nausea, pruritus and upper right quadrant pain. In heavy infections the young worms may wander back into the liver parenchyma producing abscesses.

Laboratory diagnosis

Laboratory diagnosis of fascioliasis can be made by:

- Detection of eggs in stool or in bile obtained by duodenal intubation. Formalin-ether sedimentation is the most appropriate method to concentrate eggs in the stools. The eggs of *F. hepatica* and *Fasciolopsis buski* are indistinguishable.
- Moderate to high eosinophilia.
- Immunodiagnostic tests based on antibody detection. A variety of immunological tests have been used. ELISA is a sensitive and practical method. It becomes positive within 2 weeks of infection and becomes negative after treatment.

Treatment

Triclabendazole, given as a single oral dose of 10 mg/kg or in cases of severe infection 20 mg/kg divided into 2 doses, is the drug of choice for treatment of fascioliasis.

Prophylaxis

Fascioliasis can be prevented by:

- Sanitation improvement and health education.
- Avoidance of eating raw or undercooked aquatic vegetation.
- Eradication of the disease in animals by treatment of infected animals and destruction of molluscan hosts by use of molluscicides.

FASCIOLA GIGANTICA

F. gigantica is the **largest of the human liver and lung flukes**. It measures up to 75 mm in length and 12 mm in width. It tends to be more oblong with a longer rounded posterior end as compared to broadly pointed posterior end of *F. hepatica*. It has a shorter cephalic cone, a larger ventral sucker and a more anterior position of the testes. The eggs of *F. gigantica* are larger (180 µm × 80 µm) than those of *F. hepatica* (140 µm × 80 µm). It resides in the bile duct of sheep, goat, cow, and zebra. It can also cause infection in humans.

It has been reported from Africa, Asia, Hawaii, Russia, Vietnam and Iraq. The life cycle is similar to that of *F. hepatica*, but *F. gigantica* employs different snails as intermediate hosts, development is slower, and metacercariae are more susceptible to desiccation. Pathology and clinical features are similar to those of *F. hepatica*. Like *F. hepatica*, *F. gigantica* may also be found in ectopic locations.

FASCIOLOPSIS BUSKI

Common name

The large or giant intestinal fluke.

This fluke was first discovered by Busk, in 1843, in the duodenum of an East Indian who died in London.

Geographical distribution

F. buski is a common parasite of man and pig in Asia and the Indian subcontinent, especially in areas where humans raise pigs and consume freshwater plants.

Habitat

The adult worm lives attached to the mucosa of the duodenum and jejunum of man and pig. Pig serves as reservoir of infection for man.

Morphology

Adult worm

It is the **largest intestinal trematode parasitising man**. It is fleshy, dark red, and elongate-ovoid, the anterior end being narrower than the posterior (Fig. 10.5). It measures 20–75 mm in length, 8–20 mm in breadth, and 0.5–3 mm in thickness. There is no cephalic cone. The ventral sucker measures 2–3 mm in diameter and lies close to oral sucker which measures 0.5 mm in diameter. The two intestinal caeca do not bear any branches. Life span of adult worm is about 6 months.

Eggs

The eggs are almost identical with those of *F. hepatica*. Each worm lays about 25,000 eggs per day.

Infective forms

Metacercariae encysted on aquatic vegetations that are ingested by humans.

Life cycle

Definitive hosts

Man and pig.

Intermediate hosts

- ***First intermediate host:*** Snails of the genera *Segmentina*, *Hippeutis* and *Polypylis*.
- ***Second intermediate host:*** Aquatic vegetations especially the seed pods of the water caltrop, the bulb of the water chestnut, and the roots of the lotus and water bamboo.

The life cycle of *F. buski* closely parallels that of *F. hepatica* (Fig. 10.5). The adult worms live attached to the mucosa of duodenum and jejunum of man and pig. The immature eggs are discharged in faeces and reach freshwater. The **miracidia** develop inside the eggs in 3–7 weeks at summer temperatures, after which they come out of the eggs and swim about in water. On contact with an appropriate snail, they burrow into the soft tissues and within a period of a few weeks **sporocysts**, **first- and second-generation rediae** and **cercariae** are produced in succession.

The cercariae, on coming out of the snail, encyst on the seed pods of the water caltrop, the bulb of the water chestnut and the roots of the lotus, water bamboo,

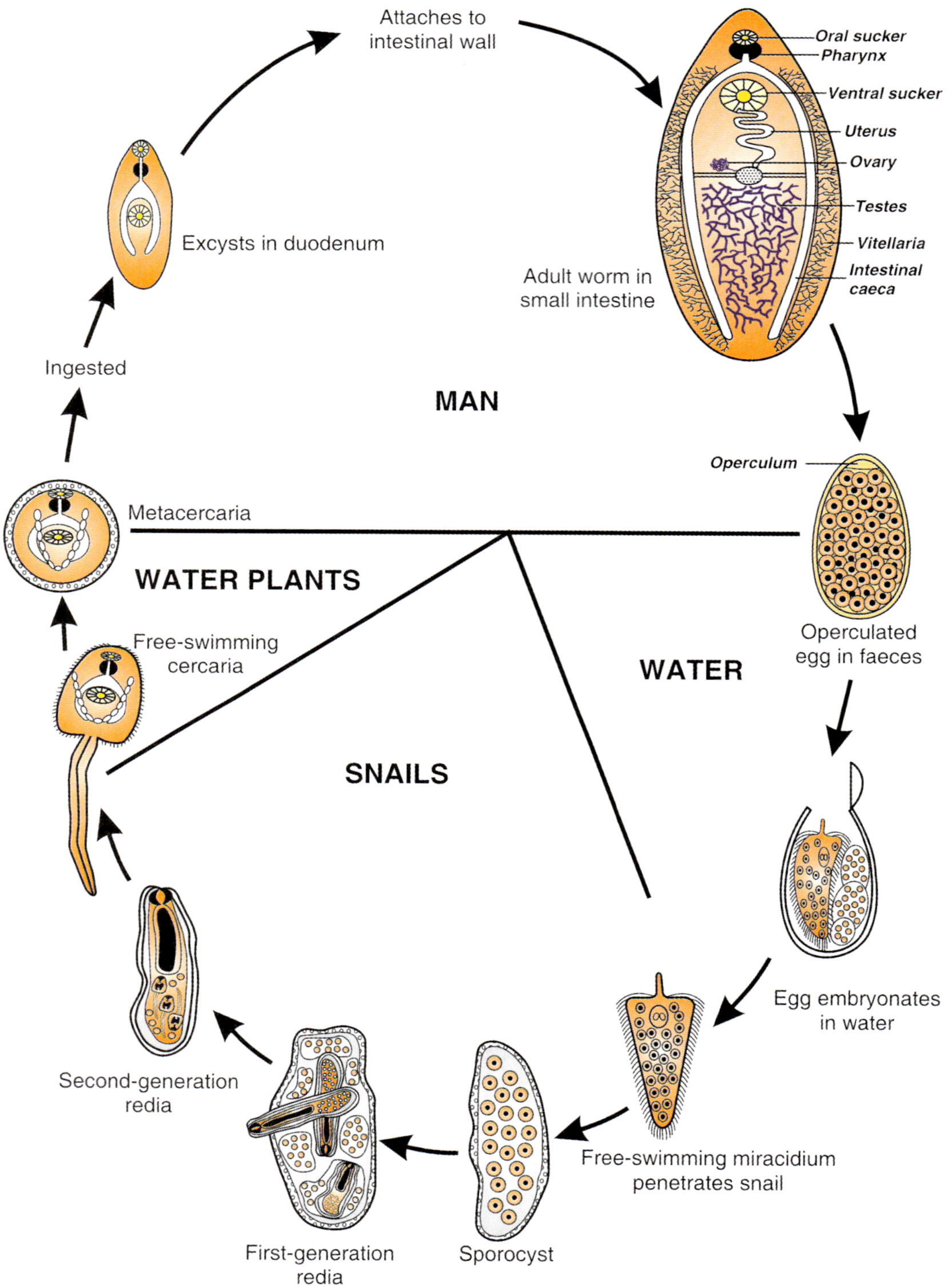

Fig. 10.5. Life cycle of *Fasciolopsis buski*.

and other aquatic vegetation becoming **metacercariae** or **infective forms**. Man acquires infection from peeling off the skin of these infested plants between the teeth and lips before swallowing the raw nut. The metacercariae excyst in the duodenum, become attached to the intestinal wall and develop into adult worms in about 3 months. Eggs are then liberated which exit in the faeces and the cycle is repeated.

Pathogenicity

Infection caused by *F. buski* is known as **fasciolopsiasis**. The damage caused by *F. buski*, which lives attached to the mucosa of duodenum and jejunum, may be traumatic, obstructive, and toxic. At the site of attachment the worms cause inflammation and ulceration of the mucosa. Large number of worms provoke increased secretions of mucus and may lead to partial obstruction of the bowel. In massive infections patient develops profound intoxication and sensitization that result from absorption of the worm's metabolites into the system. Occasionally, vitamin B_{12} absorption is impaired, with resulting low vitamin B_{12} levels.

Patient complains of diarrhoea, initially alternating with constipation and persistent thereafter, abdominal pain, anorexia, nausea, vomiting, generalized toxic and allergic symptoms usually in the form of oedema particularly of the face, abdominal wall, and lower limbs. Ascites, anaemia, and asthenia are common and patient may die of profound toxaemia.

Laboratory diagnosis

Diagnosis of fasciolopsiasis can be made by:

- Detection of large, golden (**bile-stained**) operculated eggs in the faeces. The eggs of *F. buski* and *F. hepatica* are indistinguishable.
- Exact identification is a therapeutic problem because treatment is not the same for both infections. Whereas *Fasciolopsis buski* responds favourably to praziquantel, *E. hepatica* does not. Examination of a sample of the patient's bile differentiates the species; if the eggs are present in bile, they are *F. hepatica* not *F. buski*, which is limited to the small intestine.
- Adult worms may be recovered and identified after a purgative or an anthelmintic.
- A marked eosinophilia and leucocytosis are commonly seen.

Treatment

Infection with *F. buski* responds well to single-day therapy with praziquantel.

Prophylaxis

Fasciolopsiasis can be prevented by:

- Avoidance of eating raw aquatic vegetations like the seed pods of the water caltrop and the bulb of the water chestnut. Before consumption these should be immersed in boiling water for a few seconds or these should be peeled off and washed in clean water.
- Prohibition of use of night soil as fertilizer or sterilization of night soil being used as a fertilizer.
- Destruction of molluscan hosts by use of molluscicides.

CLONORCHIS SINENSIS

Common names

The Chinese liver fluke; Oriental liver fluke.

This fluke was first described in 1875 by McConnell in the bile passages of a Chinese carpenter in Calcutta (now Kolkata). However, it was not clear whether he had got the infection in India or elsewhere. Details of life cycle were worked out by Faust and Khaw in 1927. Mahanta et al., 1995 reported a case of human clonorchiasis from Assam (India).

Geographical distribution

This parasite is endemic in Japan, Korea, China, Taiwan and Vietnam.

Habitat

Adult worms are located in the biliary tract and occasionally in the pancreatic duct of man, dog, cat and rat.

Morphology

Adult worm

Clonorchis sinensis is narrow, oblong, flat worm with pointed anterior and somewhat rounded posterior end (Fig. 10.6). It measures 10–25 mm in length by 3–5 mm in breadth. The oral sucker is slightly larger than the ventral sucker. The latter is situated at the junction of the anterior and the middle third of the body just anterior to a loosely coiled uterus. The anterior sucker leads to an oesophagus that branches into blind intestinal caeca that extend laterally to the posterior end. It has two large deeply lobulated or branched testes. These are situated one behind the other in the posterior third of the body.

Eggs

The eggs are broadly ovoid, have a moderately thick, light **yellowish-brown shell** (**bile-stained**) and are provided with a distinct convex operculum resting on shoulders. A small knob is often seen at the posterior end. They measure 28–35 μm × 12–19 μm (average 29 μm × 16 μm). They contain ciliated embryos (**miracidia**) when discharged into the bile ducts (Figs.

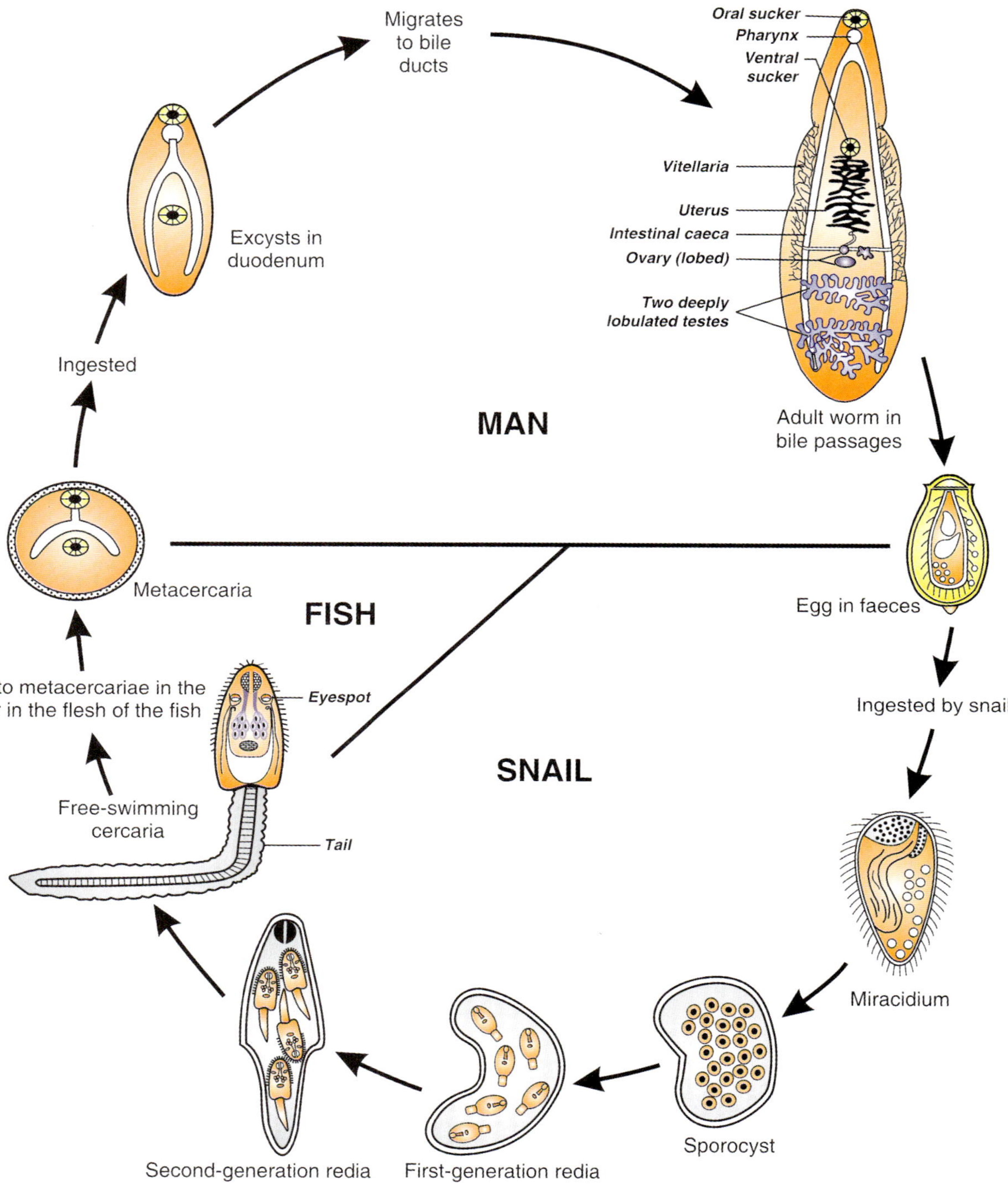

Fig. 10.6. Life cycle of *Clonorchis sinensis*.

10.6 and 10.7). They hatch only after ingestion by suitable molluscan hosts. **They do not float in saturated solution of common salt.** This egg is morphologically similar to those of *Heterophyes heterophyes*, *Opisthorchis felineus* and *Metagonimus yokogawai*.

Infective form

Metacercariae encysted in flesh of freshwater fish.

Life cycle

C. sinensis passes its life cycle in three hosts, one definitive host and two intermediate hosts (Fig. 10.5).

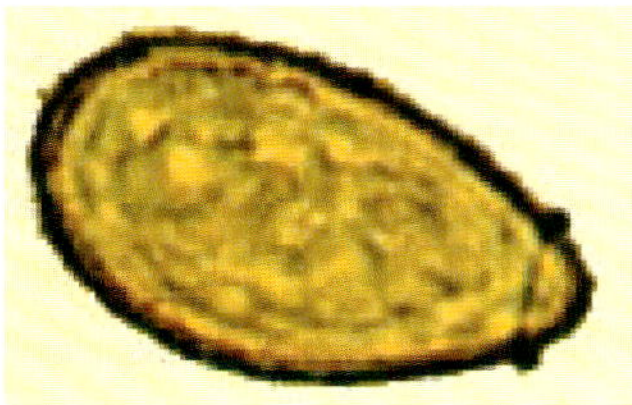

Fig. 10.7. Egg of *Clonorchis sinensis* (saline wet mount, ×400).

Definitive hosts

Man, pig, dog, cat and rat.

Intermediate hosts

- ***First intermediate host:*** Suitable species of operculate snails (*Bulimus*, *Parafossarulus*, *Semisulcospira*, *Alocinma*, and *Melanoides*).
- ***Second intermediate host:*** Freshwater fish of the family Cyprinidae.

Adult worms are located in the biliary tract and occasionally in the pancreatic duct of man, pig, dog, cat and rat. Eggs containing miracidia are discharged with the bile fluid into the faeces of definitive hosts and on entering into water, are ingested by the appropriate molluscan host. The **miracidium** hatches in the midgut of the snail, penetrates its intestinal wall and enters the vascular spaces where it passes through the stages of **sporocyst**, **first-generation rediae**, **second-generation rediae** and **finally cercariae**.

The cercariae escape from the snail into water. After escape from the snail and a brief free-swimming existence, attack certain freshwater fish of the family Cyprinidae. The cercariae cast off their tails and encyst to metacercariae in the scale or in the flesh of the fish. The period of development in fish host, during summer, is 23 days.

Man acquires infection by eating raw, undercooked, salted or pickled freshwater fish harbouring metacercariae of *C. sinensis*. The metacercariae excyst in the duodenum, and usually enter the common bile duct through the ampulla of Vater and migrate to the distal bile capillaries, where they mature in about 1 month. Attachment and detachment of its two suckers, together with a collar of spines on the immature worm, combined with extension and contraction of the body are presumably used, by *C. sinensis*, to migrate up the biliary tract, against the flow of bile. Mature worms probably move short distances within the ducts. Attachment is secured by the ventral sucker adhering to the biliary epithelium, leaving the oral sucker free for feeding. Adult worms produce an average of 10,000 eggs per day which exit the bile ducts and are excreted in the faeces. The cycle is then repeated.

Pathogenicity

C. sinensis causes proliferative and inflammatory reactions in the biliary epithelium of the bile ducts with which it makes contact. This is followed by encapsulating fibrosis of the ducts. Bile ducts are dilated particularly at the points where the flukes are attached to the inner lining and biliary obstruction is rare except in extreme heavy infections. In most cases, the disease tends to remain low grade and chronic, with organisms persisting for three decades or more, producing only minor symptoms of abdominal distress, intermittent diarrhoea, and liver pain or tenderness.

C. sinensis has been linked to ***cholangiocarcinoma****. It is most frequently observed in areas where clonorchiasis is endemic. This cancer has a very poor prognosis, and few patients live longer than 6 months after diagnosis.*

Laboratory diagnosis

The diagnosis of clonorchiasis is based on:

- **Demonstration of eggs** by microscopical examination of faeces or aspirated bile by duodenal aspiration. It is difficult to distinguish the eggs of *C. sinensis* from those of *Heterophyes heterophyes*, *Opisthorchis* spp. and *Metagonimus yokogawai*.
- **Differential leucocyte count** with eosinophilia (10–40%).
- Demonstration of antibodies against *C. sinensis* by ELISA, complement fixation test and indirect haemagglutination test.
- Skin test using extracts of adult *C. sinensis* as antigen.

Treatment

Praziquantel 25 mg/kg orally for three doses, spaced 8 hours apart, is the recommended treatment.

Prophylaxis

Clonorchiasis can be prevented by:

- Sanitation improvement and health education.
- Avoidance of eating raw or undercooked fish.
- Temporary storage of night soil. Eggs of *C. sinensis* in night soil die within 1 week.
- Destruction of molluscan hosts by use of molluscicides.

PARAGONIMUS WESTERMANI

Common name

The Oriental lung fluke.

Paragonimus westermani was discovered by Kerbert in 1878 in the lungs of two Bengal tigers that died in the Hamburg and Amsterdam Zoological Gardens. A year later Ringer reported this parasite at the autopsy of Portuguese patient who died of this infection. In 1880, Manson found eggs in rusty-brown sputum of a Chinese patient residing in Formosa (Taiwan).

Geographical distribution

P. westermani is endemic in eastern and southern Asia, western and central Africa and central and south America. In India, it has been reported from Assam, Bengal, Tamil Nadu and Kerala.

Habitat

The adult worms reside usually in pairs, in the parenchyma of lung, close to the bronchioles of man and other definitive hosts.

Morphology

Adult worm

It is thick, fleshy, oval-shaped and reddish-brown in colour with an integument covered with scale-like spines (Fig. 10.8). Its anterior end is slightly broader than the posterior end. It measures up to 16 mm in length, 8 mm in width and 5 mm in thickness. The ventral sucker is located towards the middle of the body and is of similar size to the oral sucker on the anterior end. The fluke possesses a large excretory bladder extending from the posterior extremity to the level of pharynx in the anterior region. The two blind intestinal caeca are unbranched and extend to the caudal region.

Life span of adult worm is about 6–7 years.

Eggs

The eggs of *P. westermani* are oval, **yellowish-brown**, measure 90 × 50 μm and have a prominent 'shouldered' operculum. The shoulder serves to distinguish the *Paragonimus* ova from those of *Diphyllobothrium latum*, the opercula of which are devoid of shoulders. *P. westermani* eggs also do not possess knoblike protrusion at the other end which is characteristic of *Diphyllobothrium* eggs. *P. westermani* eggs are unembryonated when laid.

Infective form

Metacercariae encysted in flesh of various crustaceans (crayfish, crab).

Life cycle

Life cycle is passed in three hosts, one definitive host and two intermediate hosts (Fig. 10.8).

Definitive hosts

Man, wolf, fox, tiger, leopard, cat, dog and monkey.

Intermediate hosts

- ***First intermediate host:*** A freshwater snail of the genera *Semisulcospira* and *Brotia*.
- ***Second intermediate host:*** A freshwater crayfish or a crab (Crustacea).

The adult worms reside, usually in pairs, in the parenchyma of lung and lay eggs. Eggs escape into the bronchi and are coughed up and voided in sputum, or swallowed and passed in faeces. Freshwater bodies (lakes, canals, small ponds, rivers, flooded rice fields and other reservoirs of water) become contaminated with eggs from sputum and faeces. They develop and hatch in water after approximately 3 weeks, releasing a free-swimming **miracidium**, which burrows into the flesh of an appropriate snail.

Inside the snail, the miracidium passes through the stages of **sporocyst**, **first-generation rediae**, **second-generation rediae**, finally giving birth to **cercariae**. The mature cercariae escape from the snail into water and penetrate gills and muscles of its second intermediate host, a freshwater crab or a crayfish. Crabs and crayfish can also become infected by eating the infected snail. Inside the crustacean host, the cercariae transform into **metacercariae** in the viscera, muscles and gills.

Humans become infected following ingestion of raw or poorly cooked or salted crab or crayfish, flesh of which contains encysted metacercariae. Ingested metacercariae excyst in the duodenum releasing larvae that attach to the duodenal mucosa. These larvae penetrate the intestine and enter into abdominal cavity. Then they migrate upwards, piercing through or around the diaphragm to the pleural cavity and lungs, finally arriving in the vicinity of the bronchioles, where they develop into adult worms usually in pairs encapsulated by host's inflammatory response and produce eggs. The time required for completion of their development in the definitive host is 65–90 days. Eggs are expelled in the sputum or may be dislodged by coughing,

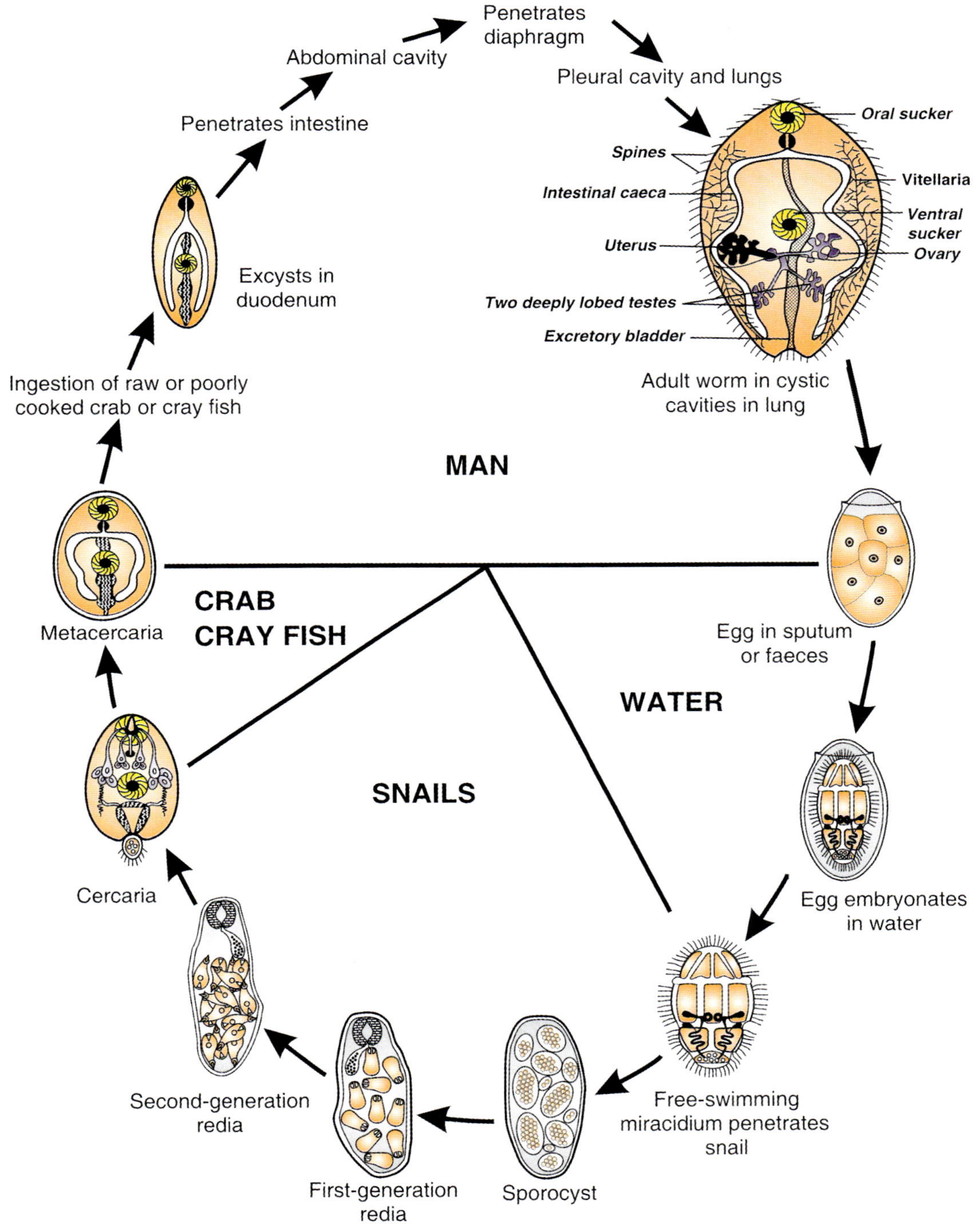

Fig. 10.8. Life cycle of *Paragonimus westermani*.

swallowed and excreted in faeces. The cycle is thus repeated.

Pathogenicity

During the migratory phase of *P. westermani* nonspecific symptoms, e.g., chills, fever, marked eosinophilia, diarrhoea, abdominal and chest pain may be present. The adult worms in the lungs provoke granuloma formation consisting mainly of eosinophils and neutrophils, followed by development of a broad layer of fibrous tissue outside, thus producing a thick cystic encapsulation of the parasite. The cyst enlarges as the adult fluke grows, reaching up to 1.5–5 cm in diameter, and may break into an adjacent bronchiole.

Leakage of fluid into the bronchioles causes paroxysmal **coughing and haemoptysis**. Up to 50 ml of gelatinous, **rusty-brown sputum containing traces of blood and yellowish-brown parasite eggs** may be expectorated daily during paroxysmal coughing. It is often misdiagnosed as tuberculosis because of overlapping clinical manifestations including chest pain, cough and haemoptysis and confusing radiological findings in chest X-ray.

In addition to the usual migratory routes, ***P. westermani*** **may become lodged in ectopic sites**. These include liver, intestinal wall, peritoneum, pleura, mesenteric lymph nodes, brain, heart, muscles and subcutaneous tissue of the groin. *When this occurs completion of the life cycle is not achieved, because the eggs laid cannot exit from these sites*. Flukes which lodge in ectopic sites invoke inflammatory response, similar to that seen in lungs, leading to ulcerations and abscesses. The clinical manifestations in these cases depend on the organ involved. Dull abdominal tenderness and bloody diarrhoea are the chief complaints of abdominal paragonimiasis. If parasites lodge in brain or spinal cord, patient develops headache, fever, paralysis, visual disturbances and convulsive seizures.

Laboratory diagnosis

Laboratory diagnosis of paragonimiasis can be made by:

1. Demonstration of eggs

Characteristic, **yellowish-brown, operculated eggs in the sputum**, aspirated pleural effusion or faeces. The sputum is blood-tinged and is peppered with rusty-brown flecks, consisting of clumps of yellowish-brown eggs.

2. Serological tests

A variety of serological tests, of which ELISA is sensitive and practical, are available.

3. Skin test

Skin test using extracts of adult *P. westermani* as antigen.

4. Biopsy

Parasite fragments and eggs can sometimes be seen in biopsy.

5. X-ray chest

It shows patchy foci of fibrotic change, with a characteristic 'ring shadow'.

Prophylaxis

Paragonimiasis can be prevented by:

- Sanitation improvement and health education. Sanitation interrupts transmission from sputum and faeces and health education stops people from eating raw, freshly salted or undercooked crab or crayfish.
- Anthelmintic treatment of infected persons to eliminate long-lived parasites, thus interrupting transmission of infection.
- Destruction of molluscan hosts by the use of molluscicides.

Treatment

Praziquantel 25 mg/kg 3 times a day for 3 days is effective for the treatment of paragonimiasis. Alternatively, bithionol can be administered orally in a dose of 30 mg/kg body weight, every other day, for a total period of 10–15 days.

TREMATODES OF MINOR IMPORTANCE

GASTRODISCOIDES HOMINIS

This trematode was discovered by Lewis and McConnell in 1876 from the caecum of an Indian patient suffering from diarrhoea. It has been reported from India (Assam, Bengal, Bihar and Orissa), Vietnam, the Philippines and Malaya.

Morphology

Adult worm

The adult worm is pyriform in shape with conical anterior and hemispherical posterior portion. It measures 5–10 mm in length and 4–6 mm in width at its widest part. The living worm has a bright pinkish colour. The ventral surface has a deep concavity which has a prominent ventral sucker that bears a characteristic notch.

Egg

The eggs are greenish-brown, ovoid, operculated, measure 150 μm × 60–70 μm and are immature when laid (Fig. 10.9).

Life cycle

The adult worms reside in the caecum and ascending colon of man, pigs, monkeys, rats and other rodents. Some birds may also harbour adult worms. Pigs and

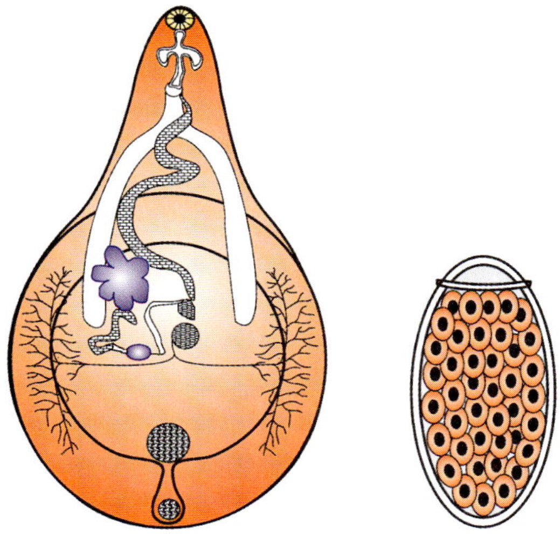

Fig. 10.9. *Gastrodiscoides hominis.*

monkeys are common reservoir hosts. When eggs passed in faeces reach water, they hatch and the released larva, the **miracidium**, penetrates aquatic gastropod mollusc. Within the mollusc the miracidium transforms into **sporocyst**, **first-generation rediae**, **second-generation rediae and finally cercariae**. Cercariae are released from the mollusc and encyst as metacercariae on vegetation and the snail host. Man, animals and birds become infected by feeding upon vegetation or snails harbouring the metacercariae.

Pathogenicity

The presence of *G. hominis* in man, attached to the caecum and ascending colon with the help of its large posterior sucker, may cause oedema of the intestinal wall and mucous diarrhoea.

Laboratory diagnosis

It can be established by demonstration of characteristic eggs in stool.

Prophylaxis

Human infection with *G. hominis* can be prevented by avoiding the consumption of uncooked vegetation which has originated from or close to water bodies.

WATSONIUS WATSONI

Various species of primates in eastern Asia and Africa are natural hosts of *Watsonius watsoni*. It was found only once in a human subject, at the autopsy of an emaciated West African Negro who died of a severe diarrhoea. The worms were found attached to duodenal and jejunal wall as well as free in the lumen of the colon. Adult worm is pear-shaped, flattened dorso-ventrally and measures 8–10 mm in length by 4–5 mm in breadth. The living worm has a reddish-yellow colour. The eggs are ovoid, operculated, light yellow, measure 122–130 μm × 75–80 μm and are immature when laid. The life cycle and prophylaxis are probably similar to those of *G. hominis*. The diagnosis depends upon finding the characteristic eggs in the faeces.

OPISTHORCHIS FELINEUS

Common name

The cat liver fluke.

Opisthorchis felineus occurs in the Russian Federation, eastern Europe and India. The adult worm lives attached by its two suckers in the biliary and pancreatic passages of man, dog and other animals that consume raw fish. They are thin, transparent, lancet-shaped and measure 7–12 mm in length by 2–3 mm in breadth. The living worm in the biliary tract is reddish-bile coloured. Unlike *C. sinensis*, the two testes are not branched but are lobed and are situated in the posterior part of the body. The small, oval or slightly lobed ovary is median in position. Eggs of *O. felineus* resemble those of *C. sinensis* and measure 30 μm × 11 μm (Fig. 10.10). The life cycle of *O. felineus* is also similar to that of *C. sinensis*.

Acute infection, with *O. felineus* is characterized by chills and high fever, abdominal pain and distension, hepatitis-like symptoms and eosinophilia. In heavy

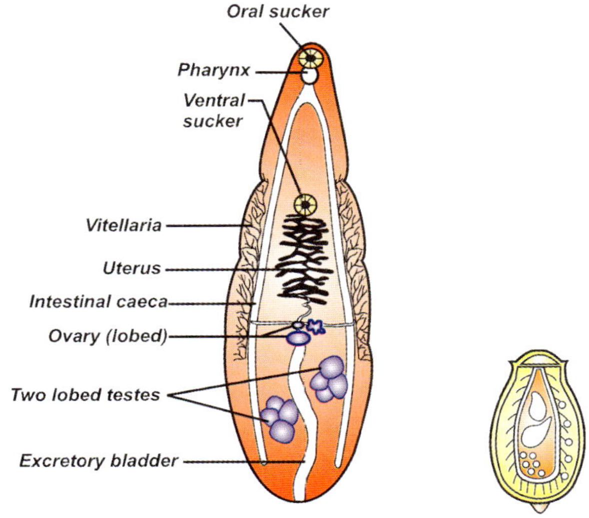

Fig. 10.10. *Opisthorchis felineus.*

infections the worms invade the pancreas, with digestive disturbances. Bile stones may form around eggs as nuclei and cause cholecystitis with colic. The diagnostic and preventive measures are similar to those of *C. sinensis*.

OPISTHORCHIS VIVERRINI

Opisthorchis viverrini (**Southeast Asian liver fluke**) occurs in Thailand and Laos. It can be differentiated from *O. felineus* by the greater proximity of its ovary and testes, and the aggregation of its vitellaria into a few clusters of glandular material. The eggs of *O. viverrini* resemble those of *Clonorchis*, *Heterophyes*, and *Metagonimus*. The life cycle, pathogenicity, laboratory diagnosis and preventive measures are similar to those of *C. sinensis*. Fish-eating animals especially cats and dogs serve as reservoir hosts. **The very important clinical aspect of *O. viverrini* (and also *C. sinensis*) infection is the extreme susceptibility of infected people to cholangiocarcinoma.**

O. noverca and *O. guayaguilensis* are other species of this genus which may cause occasional human infection.

HETEROPHYES HETEROPHYES

Common name

Von Siebold's fluke.

Heterophyes heterophyes occurs relatively commonly in humans in China, Korea, Japan, Taiwan and the Philippines.

Morphology

Adult worm

It is an elongate, pyriform, small fluke measuring 1–1.7 mm in length by 0.3–0.4 mm in breadth. The integumentary scales are narrow and closely set. They are most numerous in the anterior portion of the body. At the anterior end it has an oral sucker. It is smaller than the ventral sucker. The latter is thick-walled, muscular, and lies in the anterior part of the middle third of the body. A sucker surrounds the genital pore which opens posterolaterally near the ventral sucker.

Egg

Eggs of *H. heterophyes* resemble those of *C. sinensis*. They are small, operculated, ovoid, light brown, and measure 30 μm × 16 μm. When laid, the egg contains a fully developed miracidium (Fig. 10.11).

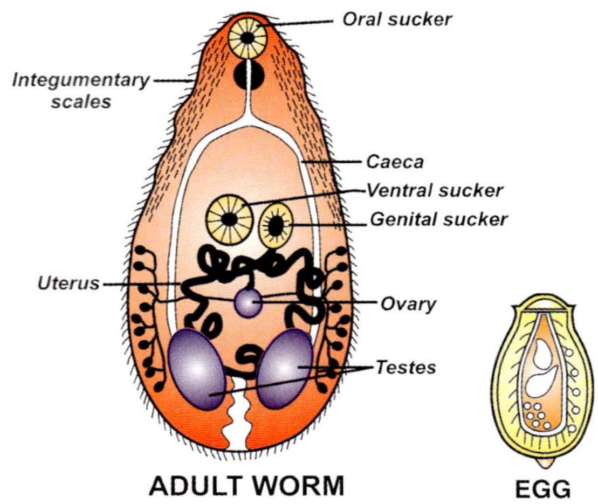

Fig. 10.11. *Heterophyes heterophyes.*

Life cycle

The adult worms reside, attached to the mucosa or burrowed into the mucosa, in the small intestine of cat, dog, fox, wolf and man. Their eggs are passed with the faeces and hatch to release **miracidia** which penetrate freshwater snails in which a **sporocyst**, **two generations of rediae** and **cercariae** are produced in succession. Cercariae leave the mollusc and encyst (**metacercariae**) under the scales and in superficial muscles of freshwater fishes. Humans and other fish-eating mammals acquire the infection by eating raw, poorly cooked or pickled fish harbouring the metacercariae.

Pathogenicity

H. heterophyes causes mild inflammatory reaction at the sites where the worms become attached to the intestinal mucosa or burrow into the mucosa of the small intestine and lead to colicky pain and mucous diarrhoea. Eggs of *H. heterophyes*, in the intestinal wall, may be carried by the mesenteric lymphatics, and be filtered out in various parts of the body, including the heart and brain.

Laboratory diagnosis

The diagnosis of heterophyiasis is based on the finding of eggs in the stool.

Prophylaxis and treatment

The infection can be prevented by ensuring that fish intended as food are well cooked or frozen prior to ingestion. For the treatment praziquantel is the drug of choice.

METAGONIMUS YOKOGAWAI

Common name

Yokogawa's fluke.

Metagonimus yokogawai is the **smallest fluke** which parasitizes humans. It is prevalent in southern Japan, Korea, China, Taiwan and Siberia. In its habitat, size, and shape, it resembles *H. heterophyes*. However, in *M. yokogawai* the ventral sucker is situated to the right of the midline. There is no genital sucker present and the genital pore is anterior to the ventral sucker. The eggs also resemble those of *H. heterophyes*. They measure 26–28 µm × 15–17 µm in size (Fig. 10.12). Life cycle is similar to that of *H. heterophyes*.

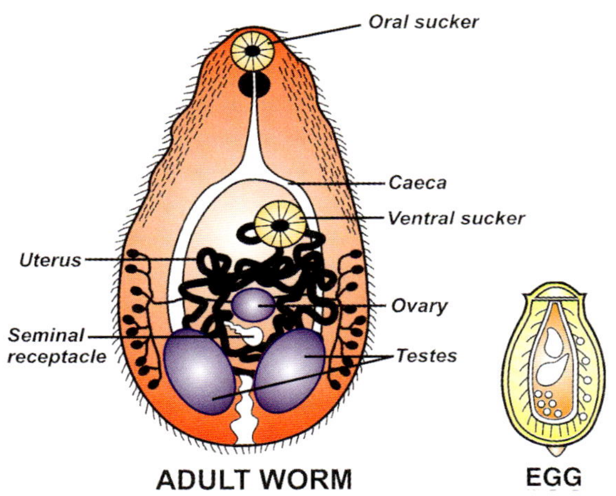

Fig. 10.12. *Metagonimus yokogawai.*

The parasite causes diarrhoea and colicky abdominal pain in man. At times it causes eosinophilic and neutrophilic infiltration of the intestinal wall, particularly around eggs that are deposited in the tissues or they may enter into intestinal capillaries and lymphatics and are carried to the myocardium, brain, spinal cord and other tissues. The diagnosis is based on the finding of characteristic eggs in stools. Prophylaxis and treatment are similar to that of *H. heterophyes*.

Further Reading

1. Chan, H.H., Lai, K.H., et al. 2002. The clinical and cholangiographic picture of hepatic clonorchiasis. *J. Clin. Gastroenterol.*, **34**, 183–6.
2. Engels, D., Chitsulo, L., et al. 2002. The global epidemiological situation of schistosomiasis and new approaches to control and research. *Acta Trop.*, **82**, 139–46.
3. Haseeb, A.N., el-Shazly, A.M., et al. 2002. A review on fascioliasis in Egypt. *J. Egypt Soc. Parasitol.*, **32**, 317–54.
4. Kim, Y.H. 2003. Carcinoma of the gall bladder associated with clonorchiasis: Clinicopathologic and CT evaluation. *Abdom. Imaging*, **28**, 83–6.
5. Kobayashi, J., Vannachone, B., et al. 2000. An epidemiological study on *Opisthorchis viverrini* infection in Laos villages. *Southeast Asian J. Trop. Med. Pub. Health*, **31**, 128–32.
6. Pearce, E.J. 2003. Progress towards a vaccine for schistosomiasis. *Acta Trop.*, **86**, 309–13.
7. Pearce, E.J. and MacDonald, A.S. 2002. The immunobiology of schistosomiasis. *Nat. Rev. Immunol.*, **2**, 499–511.
8. Stripa, B. and Kaewkes, S. 2002. Gall bladder and extrahepatic bile duct changes in *Opisthorchis viverrini*-infected hamsters. *Acta Tropica*, **83**, 29–36.
9. Uppal, B. and Wadhwa, V. 2005. Rare case of *Metagonimus yokogawai*. *Indian J. Med. Microbiol.*, **23**, 61–2.
10. Watanapa, P. and Watanapa, W.B. 2002. Liver fluke-associated cholangiocarcinoma. *Br. J. Surg.*, **89**, 962–70, review.

Important Questions

1. Discuss general characteristics and classification of trematodes.
2. Discuss general characters, life cycle, pathogenicity and laboratory diagnosis of:
   (a) *Schistosoma haematobium*
   (b) *Schistosoma mansoni*
   (c) *Schistosoma japonicum*
3. Tabulate differences between *Schistosoma haematobium*, *Schistosoma mansoni* and *Schistosoma japonicum*.
4. Discuss geographical distribution, habitat, morphology, life cycle, pathogenicity and laboratory diagnosis of:
   (a) *Fasciola hepatica*
   (b) *Fasciolopsis buski*
   (c) *Clonorchis sinensis*
   (d) *Paragonimus westermani*
5. Write short notes on:
   (a) *Fasciola gigantica*
   (b) *Gastrodiscoides hominis*
   (c) *Watsonius watsoni*
   (d) *Opisthorchis felineus*
   (e) *Opisthorchis viverrini*
   (f) *Heterophyes heterophyes*
   (g) *Metagonimus yokogawai*

Multiple Choice Questions

1. In which of the following parasites sexes are separate?
   (a) *Schistosoma haematobium.*
   (b) *Clonorchis sinensis.*
   (c) *Taenia solium.*
   (d) *Paragonimus westermani.*
2. Operculated eggs are seen in the following **except**:
   (a) *Fasciola hepatica.*
   (b) *Schistosoma japonicum.*
   (c) *Clonorchis sinensis.*
   (d) *Diphyllobothrium latum.*
3. Eggs are passed in urine in case of infection with:
   (a) *Schistosoma mansoni.*
   (b) *Schistosoma haematobium.*
   (c) *Schistosoma japonicum.*
   (d) *Clonorchis sinensis.*
4. Eggs are passed in sputum in case of infection with:
   (a) *Clonorchis sinensis.*
   (b) *Ascaris lumbricoides.*
   (c) *Strongyloides stercoralis.*
   (d) *Paragonimus westermani.*
5. Which of the following is **not** a hepatic trematode?
   (a) *Fasciola hepatica.*
   (b) *Fasciolopsis buski.*
   (c) *Clonorchis sinensis.*
   (d) *Opisthorchis felineus.*
6. Largest trematode is:
   (a) *Fasciola hepatica.*
   (b) *Fasciolopsis buski.*
   (c) *Clonorchis sinensis.*
   (d) *Metagonimus yokogawai.*
7. Gynaecophoric canal is seen in case of male worm of:
   (a) *Ascaris lumbricoides.*
   (b) *Trichinella spiralis.*
   (c) *Schistosoma mansoni.*
   (d) *Clonorchis sinensis.*
8. Pseudotubercles may be formed around the eggs of:
   (a) *Schistosoma haematobium.*
   (b) *Fasciola hepatica.*
   (c) *Clonorchis sinensis.*
   (d) *Fasciolopsis buski.*
9. Katayama fever is produced by:
   (a) *Schistosoma japonicum.*
   (b) *Clonorchis sinensis.*
   (c) *Fasciola hepatica.*
   (d) *Fasciolopsis buski.*
10. Carcinoma of urinary bladder is associated with which of the following parasites?
    (a) *Schistosoma japonicum.*
    (b) *Schistosoma haematobium.*
    (c) *Schistosoma mansoni.*
    (d) *Schistosoma intercalatum.*
11. Sheep liver fluke is the common name of:
    (a) *Fasciola hepatica.*
    (b) *Fasciola gigantica.*
    (c) *Clonorchis sinensis.*
    (d) *Fasciolopsis buski.*
12. Chinese liver fluke is the common name of:
    (a) *Fasciola hepatica.*
    (b) *Fasciola gigantica.*
    (c) *Clonorchis sinensis.*
    (d) *Fasciolopsis buski.*
13. Cholangiocarcinoma is associated with which of the following trematodes?
    (a) *Clonorchis sinensis.*
    (b) *Fasciola hepatica.*
    (c) *Fasciola gigantica.*
    (d) *Schistosoma haematobium.*
14. Which of the following parasites is **not** transmitted by eating raw or undercooked fish?
    (a) *Clonorchis sinensis.*
    (b) *Schistosoma japonicum.*
    (c) *Diphyllobothrium latum.*
    (d) *Paragonimus westermani.*
15. All of the following worms lay bile-stained eggs **except**:
    (a) *Ascaris lumbricoides.*
    (b) *Fasciola hepatica.*
    (c) *Ancylostoma duodenale.*
    (d) *Taenia solium.*
16. All of the following parasites reside in small intestine **except**:
    (a) *Gastrodiscoides hominis.*
    (b) *Watsonius watsoni.*
    (c) *Heterophyes heterophyes.*
    (d) *Metagonimus yokogawai.*

17. Cercaria is the infective stage of:
   (a) *Schistosoma haematobium.*
   (b) *Paragonimus westermani.*
   (c) *Clonorchis sinensis.*
   (d) *Fasciola hepatica.*
18. Which of the following parasites lays elongate eggs with lateral spines?
   (a) *Schistosoma haematobium.*
   (b) *Schistosoma japonicum.*
   (c) *Schistosoma mansoni.*
   (d) *Schistosoma intercalatum.*
19. Rusty-brown sputum containing traces of blood and yellowish brown eggs are seen in infection with:
   (a) *Taenia solium.*
   (b) *Paragonimus westermani.*
   (c) *Ascaris lumbricoides.*
   (d) *Diphyllobothrium latum.*
20. Which of the following parasites is located in the biliary tract?
   (a) *Fasciolopsis buski.*
   (b) *Paragonimus westermani.*
   (c) *Clonorchis sinensis.*
   (d) *Schistosoma haematobium.*
21. Which of the following parasites **does not** reside in the biliary tract?
   (a) *Fasciola hepatica.*
   (b) *Fasciolopsis buski.*
   (c) *Clonorchis sinensis.*
   (d) *Opisthorchis felineus.*
22. Which of the following schistosomes can lodge in the veins of vesical and pelvic plexuses and can cause haematuria?
   (a) *Schistosoma haematobium.*
   (b) *Schistosoma japonicum.*
   (c) *Schistosoma mekongi.*
   (d) *Schistosoma mansoni.*
23. Freshwater crayfish is the second intermediate host of:
   (a) *Paragonimus westermani.*
   (b) *Schistosoma mansoni*
   (c) *Fasciola hepatica.*
   (d) *Fasciolopsis buski.*
24. Which of the following parasites infects by the penetration of skin?
   (a) *Fasciolopsis buski.*
   (b) *Schistosoma haematobium.*
   (c) *Paragonimus westermani.*
   (d) *Heterophyes heterophyes.*
25. Which of the following parasites resides in human small intestine?
   (a) *Fasciolopsis buski.*
   (b) *Schistosoma haematobium.*
   (c) *Paragonimus westermani.*
   (d) *Opisthorchis felineus.*
26. Which of the following parasites resides in human lungs?
   (a) *Heterophyes heterophyes.*
   (b) *Paragonimus westermani.*
   (c) *Fasciola hepatica.*
   (d) *Schistosoma haematobium.*
27. Snail is **not** the intermediate host of:
   (a) *Trichinella spiralis.*
   (b) *Schistosoma haematobium.*
   (c) *Clonorchis sinensis.*
   (d) *Fasciola hepatica.*
28. In life cycle of schistosomes:
   (a) transmission is direct.
   (b) transmission involves an aquatic snail.
   (c) transmission involves an insect vector.
   (d) humans are infected by swallowing eggs.
29. The parasitic helminths that are most likely to be found in bile ducts, lungs and blood are the:
   (a) tapeworms.
   (b) roundworms.
   (c) flatworms.
   (d) flukes.
30. All of the following are trematodes **except**:
   (a) *Naegleria fowleri.*
   (b) *Schistosoma haematobium.*
   (c) *Paragonimus westermani.*
   (d) *Fasciola hepatica.*
31. Examination of a fresh faecal sample shows operculated eggs. Which of the following can be ruled out?
   (a) *Schistosoma haematobium.*
   (b) *Heterophyes heterophyes.*
   (c) *Clonorchis sinensis.*
   (d) *Metagonimus yokogawai.*
32. Eggs of which of the following parasites can be seen in the sputum?

(a) *Strongyloides stercoralis.*
(b) *Paragonimus westermani.*
(c) *Ancylostoma duodenale.*
(d) *Ascaris lumbricoides.*

33. Which of the following infections is acquired by eating raw or improperly cooked fish?
(a) *Heterophyes heterophyes.*
(b) *Fasciolopsis buski.*
(c) *Schistosoma haematobium.*
(d) *Trichinella spiralis.*

34. Which of the following parasites is **not** acquired by ingestion of infective eggs?
(a) *Enterobius vermicularis.*
(b) *Schistosoma japonicum.*
(c) *Trichuris trichiura.*
(d) *Taenia solium.*

ANSWERS TO MCQs

1 (a), 2 (b), 3 (b), 4 (d), 5 (b), 6 (b), 7 (c), 8 (a), 9 (a), 10 (b), 11 (a), 12 (c), 13 (a), 14 (b), 15 (c), 16 (a), 17 (a), 18 (c), 19 (b), 20 (c), 21 (b), 22 (a), 23 (a), 24 (b), 25 (a), 26 (b), 27 (a), 28 (b), 29 (d), 30 (a), 31 (a), 32 (b), 33 (a), 34 (b).

11

Nematodes

GENERAL CHARACTERISTICS

Nematodes belong to the kingdom Animalia, phylum Nemathelminthes, and class Adenophorea and Secernentea (Table 1.6). They are the most abundant and widespread animal group. Many species of nematodes are free-living in fresh or salt water, mud or soil and others are parasites of both animals and plants. They are elongated, cylindrical, bilaterally symmetrical, unsegmented worms with tapering ends. The name 'nematode' means thread-like (*nema*, thread). The body is covered with a tough cuticle which may be smooth, striated, bossed or spiny.

The adults vary greatly in size from less than 5 mm (*Trichinella spiralis* and *Strongyloides stercoralis*) to 50–80 cm (*Dracunculus medinensis*). The male is generally smaller than female and its posterior end is curved or coiled ventrally. They have a body cavity with a high hydrostatic pressure, a straight digestive tract with an anteriorly terminal mouth and posteriorly subterminal anus. Excretory and nervous systems are rudimentary, circulatory system is absent and the body wall consists of an outer layer of cuticle and an inner layer of longitudinal muscles.

The sexes are separate (dioecious). The male reproductive system consists of a long convoluted tube which can be differentiated into testis, vas deferens, seminal vesicle and ejaculatory duct which opens into the cloaca. The female reproductive system consists of the ovary, oviduct, seminal receptacle, uterus and vagina. The female nematodes may be divided as follows:

1. Oviparous (nematodes which lay eggs)

Laying unsegmented eggs

- *Ascaris lumbricoides*
- *Trichuris trichiura*

Laying eggs with segmented ova

- *Ancylostoma duodenale*
- *Necator americanus*

Laying eggs containing larvae

- *Enterobius vermicularis*

2. Viviparous (nematodes which give birth to larvae)

- *Dracunculus medinensis*
- *Wuchereria bancrofti*
- *Brugia malayi*
- *Trichinella spiralis*

3. Ovo-viviparous (nematodes laying eggs containing larvae which are immediately hatched out)

- *Strongyloides stercoralis*

The daily output of eggs for each female worm varies widely among different species. *S. stercoralis*, for example, lays only a few eggs daily, on the other hand *A. lumbricoides* may produce about 200,000 eggs per female worm per day. Nematodes have five life history stages, four larval and one adult, which are separated by a moult of the cuticle. It is common for the first one or two moults to occur within the egg. The infective stage of the nematode is usually third-stage larva.

Man is the optimum host for all the nematode parasites. They pass their life cycle in one host except the superfamilies Filarioidea and Dracunculoidea, where two hosts are required. Insect vectors and *Cyclops* constitute the second hosts in these superfamilies respectively. In cases where the nematodes choose one host they localise in the intestinal tract and the eggs reach the outside world in the faeces of the host. They undergo certain developmental changes before they can enter a new host.

In case of *T. spiralis,* pig is the optimum host and man represents the alternative host. It passes both its adult and larval stages in the same host.

MODES OF INFECTION WITH NEMATODE PARASITES

Infection with nematode parasites is acquired by:

1. Ingestion of:
   - Food and water contaminated with embryonated eggs, e.g., *A. lumbricoides*, *E. vermicularis* and *T. trichiura*.
   - Growing embryos in the intermediate host (infected *Cyclops*), e.g., *D. medinensis*.
   - Encysted embryos in infected pork, e.g., *T. spiralis*.
2. Penetration of skin, e.g., filariform larvae of *A. duodenale*, *N. americanus* and *S. stercoralis*.
3. Blood-sucking insects, e.g., parasites belonging to the superfamily Filarioidea.

CLASSIFICATION OF NEMATODES

Nematodes can be classified on the basis of the habitat of the adult worms (Table 11.1) and systematic classification (Table 1.6).

Table 11.1. Classification of nematodes on the basis of the habitat of adult worms

INTESTINAL	
Small intestine	
• *A. lumbricoides*	• *A. duodenale*
• *N. americanus*	• *S. stercoralis*
• *T. spiralis*	• *Capillaria philippinensis*
• *Trichostrongylus* spp.	
Large intestine (caecum and vermiform appendix)	
• *E. vermicularis*	
• *T. trichiura*	
SOMATIC	
Lymphatic system	
• *W. bancrofti*	
• *B. malayi*	
Subcutaneous tissues	
• *Loa loa*	
• *Onchocerca volvulus*	
• *D. medinensis*	
Body cavity	
• *Mansonella perstans*	
• *M. ozzardi*	
Conjunctiva	
• *Loa loa*	
Orbit, conjunctival sac, lacrimal gland	
• *Thelazia hepatica*	
Right heart and large blood vessels	
• *Dirofilaria immitis*	
Pulmonary artery	
• *Angiostrongylus cantonensis*	
Anterior mesenteric artery	
• *Angiostrongylus costaricensis*	
Stomach wall	
• *Gnathostoma spinigerum*	
• *Anisakis simplex*	
Liver	
• *Capillaria hepatica*	

TRICHINELLA SPIRALIS

Common name

The trichina worm.

Trichinella spiralis, the causative agent of trichinosis, was first discovered by Paget and Owen in 1835, in the encysted larval stage in the muscles of a 51-year-old patient who died of tuberculosis, but who had also been infected with *T. spiralis* some years before his death. Virchow discovered its life cycle in 1859. It occurs in humans both as an adult in the intestine and as a larval stage in the tissues (usually muscles).

Geographical distribution

T. spiralis has cosmopolitan distribution, but it is more prevalent in Europe and the United States than in Tropics and the Orient.

Habitat

Adult worms live buried in the duodenal or jejunal mucosa of pig, rat or man. The encysted larvae are present in the striated muscles of these hosts.

Morphology

Adult worm

It is **one of the smallest nematodes infecting man** (Fig. 11.1). The females measure approximately 3–4 mm in length by 0.06 mm in diameter. They are viviparous and release first-stage larvae into the intestinal mucosa. The male measures 1.4–1.6 mm in length by 0.04 mm in diameter. At its tail end, it bears a pair of conspicuous papillae, termed claspers, that it uses to hold onto the female worm during mating.

Larvae

These measure 80 µm in length × 7–8 µm in diameter. The infective larva becomes encysted in the striated muscle fibre and measures 1 mm in length by 36 µm in diameter. The larva in the cyst is coiled and hence, the species name *spiralis*.

The life span of the adult worm is very short. The male, after fertilizing the female, dies and the female dies after about 16 weeks, the period required for discharging larvae.

Life cycle

The whole life cycle is passed in one host (pig, rat or man) only (Fig. 11.1). However, for the preservation of the species the transference of the host is essential. **Man is the dead end of the parasite.** The continuance of the species is maintained by other animals. Pig is the optimum host and man represents alternative host. Infection normally passes from pig-to-pig, pig-to-rat and rat-to-rat. Infection of the new host is acquired by the ingestion of raw flesh of the animal containing viable encysted larvae.

Man acquires infection by ingestion of raw or inadequately cooked pork containing the viable larvae. Smoking, salting or drying the meat does not destroy the infective larval forms, however, prolonged freezing (20 days in the average home freezer or freezing at –20°C for 3 days) decontaminates the meat. The larvae are released in the stomach by the action of digestive enzymes and the freed larvae are transported by peristalsis to the duodenum and jejunum. They invade the intestinal mucosa, and after undergoing four moults during a period of 30 hours, mature to adults. Within 5 days they become sexually mature. The male, after fertilizing the female, dies.

The fertilized female (five days after infection) discharges a large number of first-stage larvae into the intestinal mucosa. The larvae are born continuously throughout the next five days. Intestinal trichinellosis can last up to 2–3 weeks. These larvae enter the lamina propria and from there penetrate the mesenteric lymphatics and blood stream. The larvae ultimately find the general circulation and become distributed to various tissues including striated skeletal muscles.

They kill all cells they enter except striated skeletal muscle cells which alone provide the proper conditions to support the growth and development of the parasites. Within 20 days after entering the muscle cell, the larvae undergo encystment in a coiled form. The muscles invaded most frequently include the extraocular muscles of the eye, the tongue, the deltoid, pectoral, and intercostal muscles, the diaphragm, and the gastrocnemius muscles. A muscle cell carrying larva of *T. spiralis* is known as **Nurse cell**. Encysted larvae can survive for months to years, but eventually most become calcified and die. In man the cycle ends here.

Immune responses

T. spiralis infection elicits both humoral and cellular immune responses. The latter is regulated by T helper lymphocytes (both Th 1 and Th 2). Intestinal infection can last up to 2–3 weeks, after which adult worms are expelled by immune responses of which inflammatory response plays a central role.

Pathogenicity

The infection caused by *T. spiralis* is known as **trichinellosis** or **trichinosis**. Most infections are subclinical. The minimum number of ingested larvae required to produce symptoms is about 100, and a fatal dose is estimated to be 300,000. The pathologic changes and the symptomatology are divided into three successive stages:

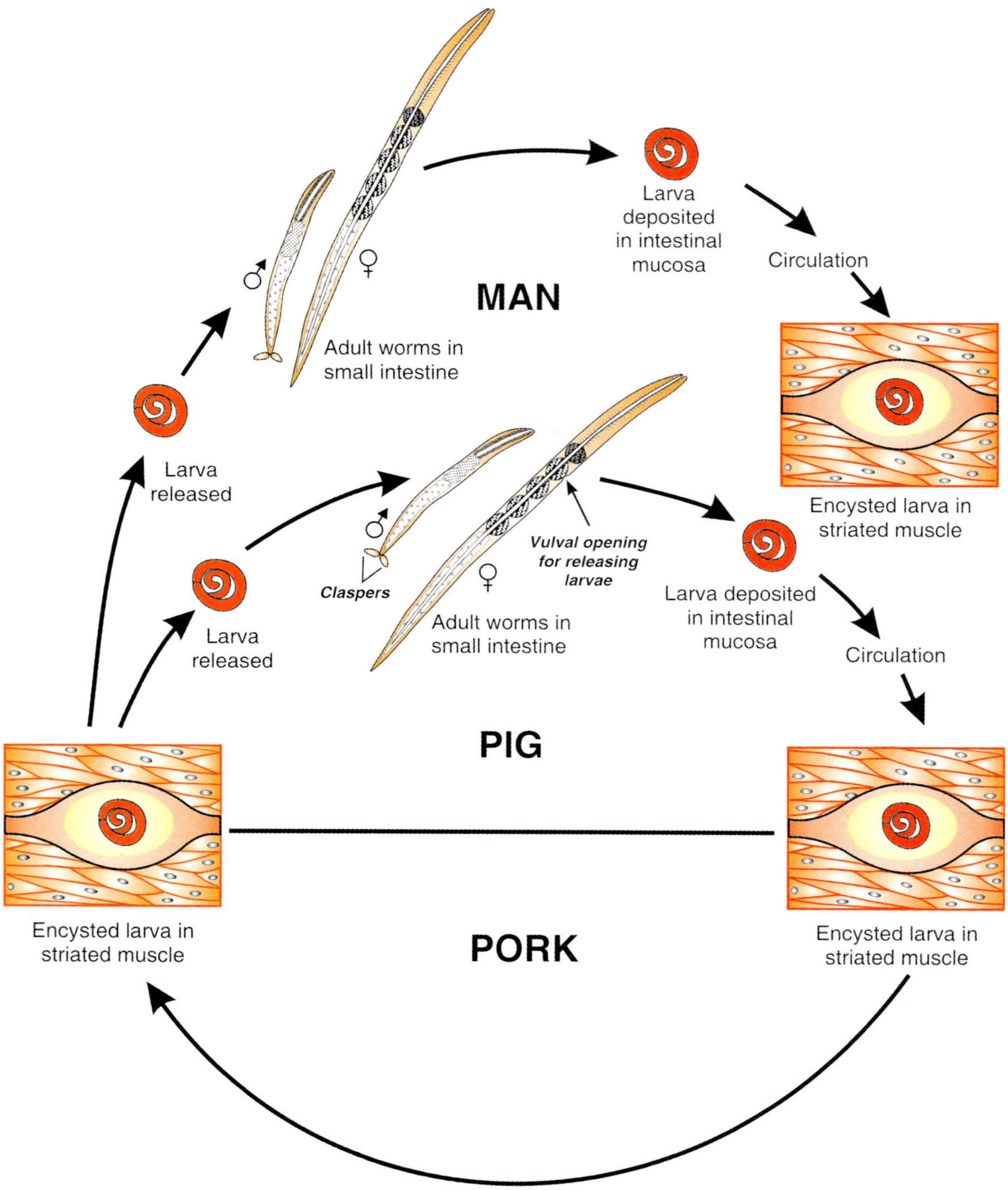

Fig. 11.1. Life cycle of *Trichinella spiralis*.

Stage of intestinal invasion

For a period of 2–3 weeks of the intestinal infection, the penetration and the development of the adult worms lead to inflammation of duodenal and jejunal mucosa. As newborn larvae are shed (i.e. 5–21 days after infection), mucosal inflammation intensifies with inflammation consisting of eosinophils, neutrophils and lymphocytes. Patient may develop malaise, nausea, vomiting, diarrhoea and abdominal cramps.

Stage of larval migration

The invasion of the muscles leads to fever, myalgia, periorbital oedema and haemorrhages in the nail beds, sclera of the eye and in the mucous membranes. Eosinophilia appears during or at the end of the second week of infection, reaches a peak in the third or fourth week, then gradually declines over a period of months. Relative eosinophilia varies from 20–95%.

Damage caused by larvae penetrating cells becomes serious when this occurs in cardiac and central nervous system tissues. Myocarditis, sometimes severe enough to cause death, is transient as Nurse cells cannot form in heart tissue. In the CNS, larvae tend to stay and wander about. Therefore, they frequently cause significant damage even in mild infection.

Stage of encystation

This occurs only in striated muscles while in other tissues they degenerate and are absorbed. Eventually all symptoms subside and, finally, the larvae calcify. The calcified cysts can be seen grossly in exposed muscle fibres.

Laboratory diagnosis

Diagnosis of trichinellosis can be made by:

1. *Detection of spiral larvae* in muscle tissue. Deltoid, biceps, gastrocnemius or pectoralis muscles are usually selected for biopsy. The specimen may be examined by:
   - First digesting the muscle fibres with trypsin and then mounting some of the digested tissue on a microscope slide. However, young larvae may be digested and thus are missed during microscopic examination.
   - Preparing a tease preparation of the muscle tissue in a drop of saline solution and squeezing it between two microscope slides.
   - Staining the pressed muscle tissue or tissue sections with safranin.
2. *Detection of adult worms and larvae* in the stool during the diarrhoeic stage. It is only occasionally positive.
3. *Blood examination*: It shows eosinophilia (20–95%). However, the total white blood cell count is slightly elevated (12,000–15,000/μl).
4. *Detection of T. spiralis antibody* by ELISA test using antigens obtained from the infective stage larvae of *T. spiralis*.
5. *History* of having eaten raw or inadequately cooked or improperly processed pork or pork products about two weeks earlier, accompanied by a bout of recent 'gastroenteritis'.
6. *Bachman intradermal test*: Intradermal injection of 0.1 ml of 1 in 1,000 dilution of Bachman antigen (prepared from *Trichinella* larvae obtained from infected rabbit's muscle) causes an immediate small white swelling around the site of injection. It is surrounded by an unraised, irregular, erythematous wheal 5 cm in diameter. The reading is made within 15–20 minutes, after which the reaction begins to fade. A positive test persists for 10–20 years.
7. *X-ray examination*: Calcified cysts may be detected on X-ray examination.

Treatment

Albendazole and mebendazole are effective against the intestinal forms of *T. spiralis* that are present in early infection. The efficacy of these agents or any anthelmintic agent on larvae that have migrated to muscle is questionable.

Prophylaxis

Trichinellosis can be prevented by:

- Properly cooking pork or freezing it at –20°C for 3 days.
- Inspection of slaughtered pigs.
- Preventing pigs from eating raw meat and offal.

TRICHURIS TRICHIURA

Common name

Whipworm.

This worm was first described by Linnaeus in 1771.

Geographical distribution

Trichuris trichiura is cosmopolitan in distribution but is more common in the warm, moist regions of the world. It is also seen in India.

Habitat

T. trichiura lives in the large intestine, particularly in the caecum and less commonly in the vermiform appendix and colon of man.

Morphology

Adult worm

Adult worms are characteristically whip-shaped (Fig. 11.2). The anterior three-fifth is very thin and hair-like and the posterior two-fifth is thick and stout, resembling the handle of the whip. The worm lives in the large intestine with the long, thin anterior end buried in the

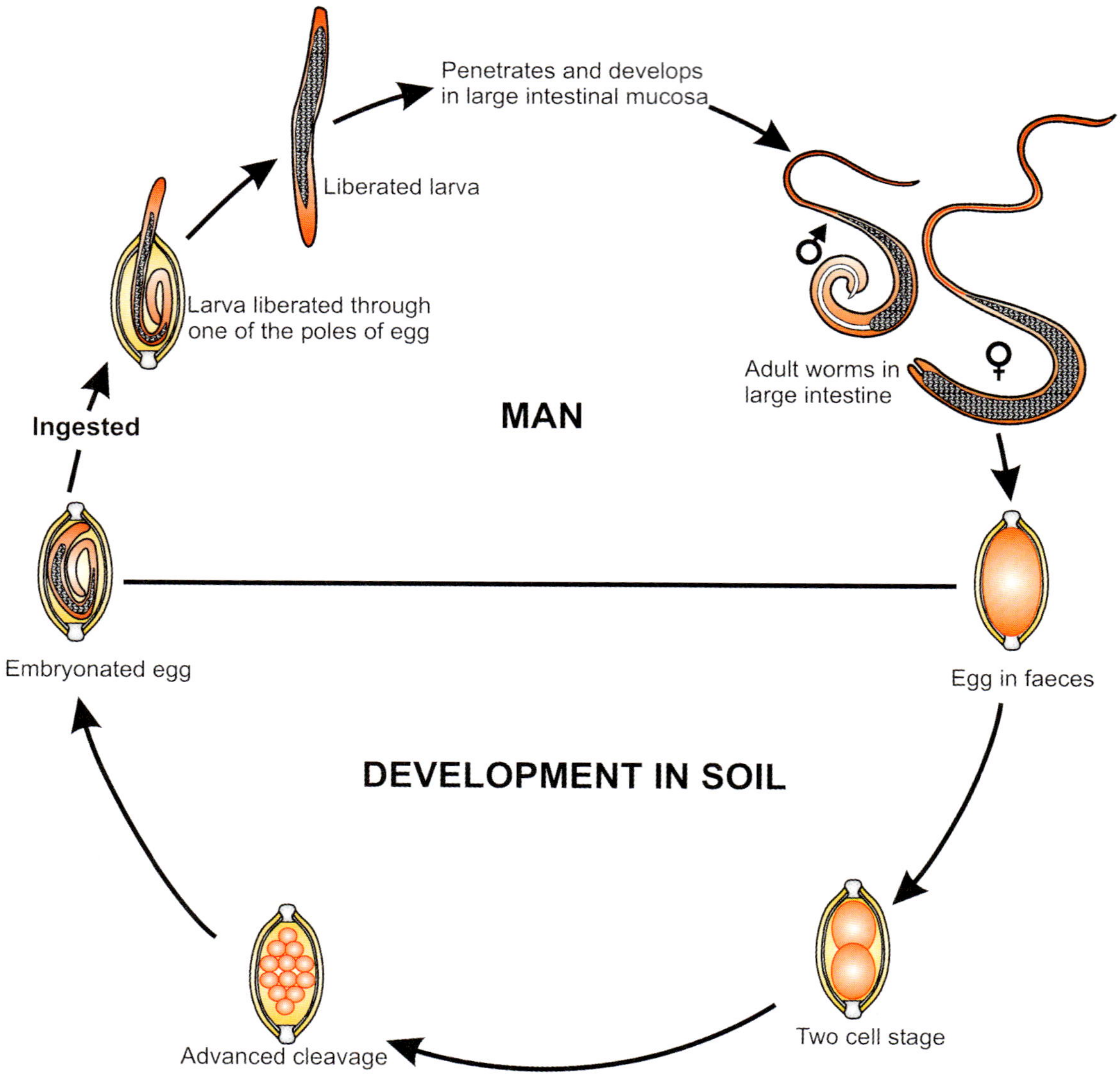

Fig. 11.2. Life cycle of *Trichuris trichiura*.

mucosa while the thicker posterior end, which contains the reproductive tract, extends into the intestinal lumen. The worms are white in colour. The male worms measure 30–45 mm in length and have coiled posterior end. The female worms are longer, measure 35–50 mm in length and their posterior extremity is comma- or arc-shaped.

Eggs

The eggs are barrel-shaped with a mucous plug at each pole. Shell is yellow to brown (bile-stained) and plugs are colourless. They measure 50–54 μm × 22–23 μm in size. **They float in saturated solution of common salt.** When freshly passed, they contain unsegmented ova and are not infective to man (Figs. 11.2 and 11.3).

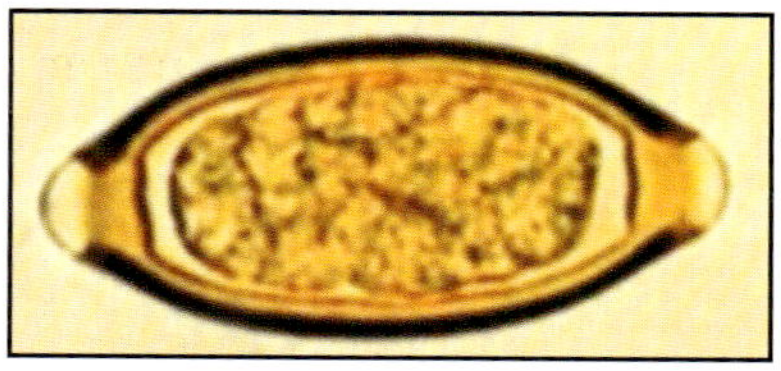

Fig. 11.3. Egg of *Trichuris trichiura* (saline wet mount, × 400).

Life cycle

No intermediate host is required. Its life cycle is completed in a single host, man. But for the continuance of the species a change of host is necessary. In contrast to *Ascaris* and hookworms, no tissue migratory phase occurs. Adult worms live in the large intestine of man. Eggs passed in faeces develop in water or damp soil.

Moisture is essential for their development. Within the egg shell develops a rhabditiform larva. In tropical climate, rhabditiform larva develops in 3–4 weeks and in temperate climate, the larva takes 6–12 months to complete its development. These embryonated eggs are infective to man.

Man acquires infection by ingesting embryonated eggs with contaminated food or water. The egg shells are dissolved by the digestive juices and the larvae emerge through one of the poles of the eggs in the small intestine. The liberated larvae pass down and penetrate the mucosa of the caecum and other parts of the large intestine. They grow into adult worms and sexually mature in about 3 months. Gravid female lays 3,000–10,000 eggs per day which are discharged in the faeces. The cycle is then repeated. Female worms can live for as long as 8 years.

Pathogenicity

The immature *T. trichiura* buries its entire body in the mucosa of the large intestine forming a tunnel. As the worm matures, its posterior portion is extruded or ruptures from the tunnel and hangs in the intestinal lumen, available for functions of copulation and oviposition.

Intimate contact of *T. trichiura* with the mucosa of large intestine leads to the inflammation of mucosa. Depending upon the intensity of infection, the inflammation may extend from the distal part of small intestine to the rectum. The mucosa may be oedematous and friable. The surface tissue of the rectum becomes extremely oedematous and when the patient strains to defecate, rectal prolapse may occur. **Rectal bleeding (whipworm dysentery)** with abdominal cramps and severe rectal tenesmus are seen in massive infections. The worms inhabiting the vermiform appendix may give rise to symptoms of **acute appendicitis**.

Prolonged massive infections lead to **iron deficiency anaemia**. This is due to the general malnutrition and **blood loss from the friable colon** and is not related to blood ingestion by the parasite. Anaemia does not occur in light infections, nor even in symptomatic infections, when there is adequate intake and assimilation of iron and protein.

Laboratory diagnosis

Specific diagnosis of trichuriasis can be made by the demonstration of the characteristic barrel-shaped eggs (Fig. 11.3) in the patient's faeces. Stool concentration methods such as simple salt floatation or formalin-ether sedimentation may be required to detect the light infection. Since the anterior end of the worm is buried in the mucosa of large intestine, therefore, adult worms are rarely seen in stool specimens. Heavy infections can be diagnosed clinically by examining the rectum for worms using a proctoscope.

Although dysentery with *T. trichiura* and dysentery with *Entamoeba histolytica* are very similar, whipworm dysentery is usually more chronic, associated with malnutrition, and likely to cause rectal prolapse. Recovery and identification of the eggs or protozoan trophozoites would differentiate the two infections.

Treatment

Mebendazole and albendazole are the most effective agents for treatment of whipworm infection. Both drugs provide significant reductions in host worm burdens even when used in a single dose. However, a cure (i.e., total worm burden removal) typically requires a 3-day course of therapy.

Prophylaxis

Trichuriasis may be prevented by:

- Sanitary disposal of faeces.
- Avoiding consumption of raw vegetables.
- Treatment of infected persons.

STRONGYLOIDES STERCORALIS

Strongyloides stercoralis, also known as dwarf threadworm, was first identified by Normand in 1876, in the faeces of French troops who had been suffering from uncontrollable diarrhoea in Cochin-China.

Geographical distribution

Strongyloides stercoralis is worldwide in distribution, however, it is more common in tropics and subtropics including those of Africa, South America and Asia including India. It is an important opportunistic pathogen in immunocompromised host. Infection with *S. stercoralis* in patients with HIV infection and other immunosuppressed hosts is being increasingly reported from Mumbai, Tamil Nadu and other parts of India.

Habitat

Adult fertilized female lives buried under the mucosa of small intestine especially in the duodenum and jejunum.

Morphology

Adult worms

Strongyloides stercoralis is the **smallest nematode known to cause infection in man**. Parasitic females measure 2–3 mm in length and 30–50 μm in width (Fig. 11.4). The cylindrical oesophagus extends through the anterior third of the body and the intestine extends through the posterior two-thirds. The caudal extremity is pointed, and the anal opening is situated mid-ventrally, a short distance in front of the caudal tip. The reproductive system contains vulva, which opens at the junction of the middle and posterior thirds of the body, and paired uteri extend anteriorly and posteriorly from vagina. The free-living adult female measures approximately 1 mm in length and 80 μm in width. The females are ovo-viviparous.

The existence of parasitic males has been debated over many years. It is believed that parasitic males exist, they are shorter and broader than the females and they do not have penetrating power, therefore, they do not invade the intestinal wall. The free-living male is slightly smaller than free-living female, measuring 0.7–1 mm in length by 40–50 μm in width. The copulatory spicules, which penetrate the female during copulation, are located on each side of the gubernaculum.

Eggs

In gravid female, the eggs are conspicuous within its body, lying antero-posteriorly in a single file (5–10 eggs in each uterus). The eggs measure 50–58 μm × 30–34 μm. They are thin-shelled, transparent and oval. They contain larvae ready to hatch. As soon as the eggs are laid, the rhabditiform larvae start hatching and bore their way out of the mucous membrane into the lumen from where they are passed in the faeces. As a result, it is the larvae which are excreted in faeces and the eggs are not routinely detected.

Rhabditiform larvae

This is the form most commonly seen in the stool specimens. They measure 200–250 μm in length × 16 μm in width. They have short mouth and double-bulb oesophagus.

Filariform larvae

These are longer and more slender than the rhabditiform larvae. They measure 630 μm in length × 10 μm in width. They possess short mouth, long cylindrical oesophagus and notched tail. They are highly infectious.

Life cycle

The life cycle of *S. stercoralis* differs from that of hookworms in three aspects:

1. Eggs hatch into larvae in the intestine before they are passed in faeces.
2. Larvae can mature into filariforms in the intestine and cause autoinfection.
3. A free-living, nonparasitic cycle can be established outside the human host.

Adult female *S. stercoralis* lives buried under the mucosa of small intestine especially in the duodenum and jejunum (Fig. 11.4). As soon as the eggs are laid the rhabditiform larvae hatch and bore their way out of the mucous membrane into the lumen from where they are passed in the faeces. The rhabditiform larvae may metamorphose into filariform larvae during passage through the bowel. These may penetrate colonic mucosa or perianal skin without leaving the host and going through a soil phase again, thus providing a source of **autoinfection (hyperinfection)**. *This provides a means by which the parasite can multiply within the host and explains how infection can be maintained for years after an individual leaves an endemic area.*

Rhabditiform larvae may be voided with the faeces and may undergo two types of development in the moist, warm soil:

1. Direct development
2. Indirect development

Direct development

The rhabditiform larvae metamorphose, in 3–4 days, into filariform larvae. In this case each rhabditiform larva gives rise to one filariform larva.

Indirect development

The rhabditiform larvae develop into free-living adult males and females in the course of 24–30 hours. Male fertilizes female and the latter lays a second batch of rhabditiform larvae which are indistinguishable from those produced by the parasitic females. In 3–4 days' time they are transformed into filariform larvae. It has been observed that the free-living cycle develops most frequently in tropical climates with moist soil, while the parasitic cycle may predominate in temperate regions.

The worm passes its life cycle in one host, man. No intermediate host is required. *Unlike other nematodes the change of host is not essential as it can*

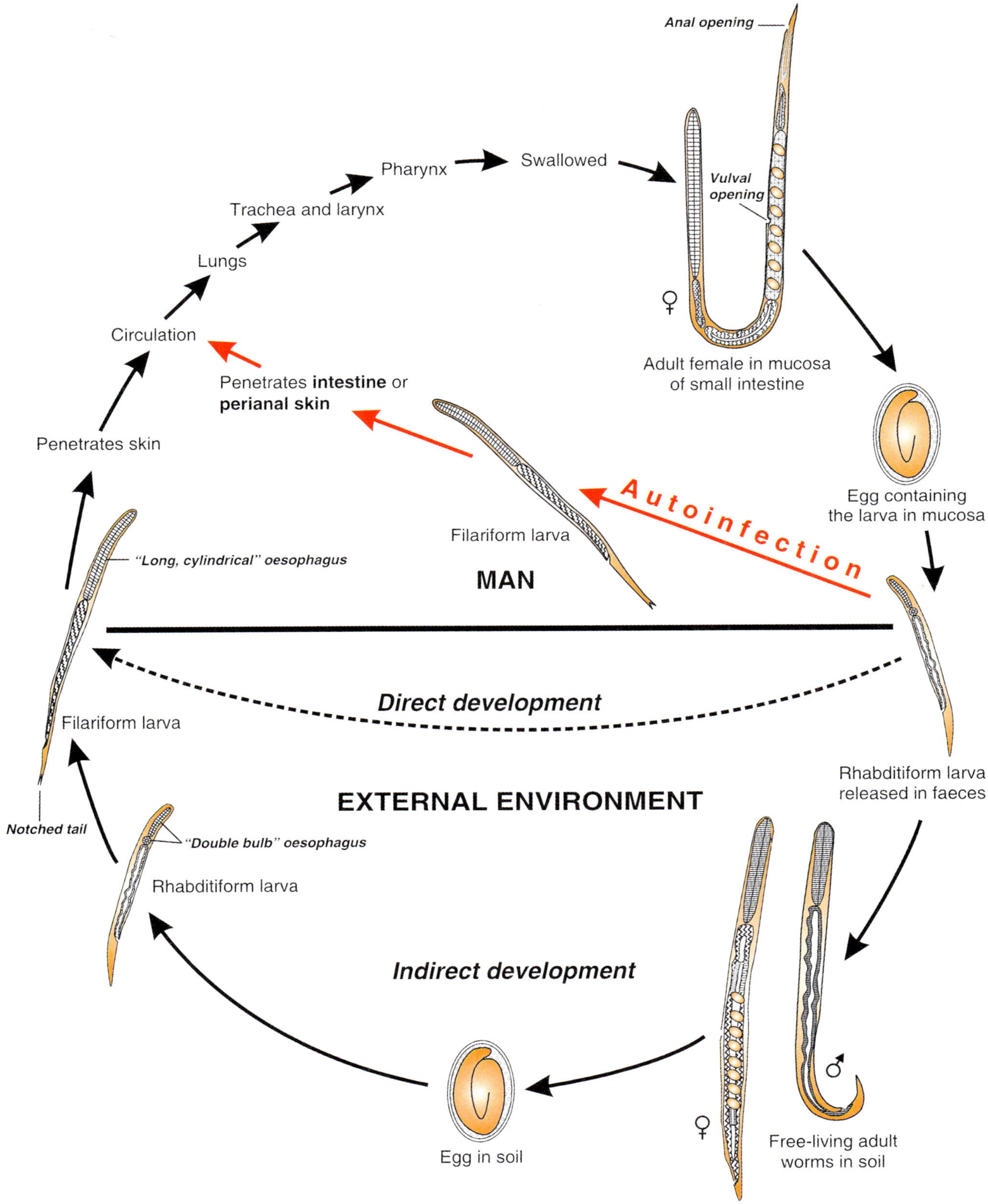

Fig. 11.4. Life cycle of *Strongyloides stercoralis*.

undergo a hyperinfective form of development. Man is the optimum host. Filariform larvae, developed in the soil or faeces, are the infective form of the parasite. Man acquires infection by walking barefoot on the faecally contaminated soil. The filariform larvae penetrate the skin coming in contact with soil.

Once within the dermis, larvae invade the venous circulation and are carried by the blood stream to the right heart and then to the lungs, where they become trapped within capillaries and break through to the lung alveoli. They then migrate up the respiratory tree i.e. the bronchi, trachea, larynx, crawl over the epiglottis to the pharynx and are swallowed. They travel to the small intestine especially the duodenum and jejunum. Here they develop into adult parasitic females. The parasitic female then burrows into the mucous membrane and lays eggs by **parthenogenesis** (reproduction by means of an unfertilized ovum). Each female produces about a dozen eggs daily. The rhabditiform larvae hatch out immediately and enter into lumen of the bowel. The cycle is then repeated.

Pathogenicity

Infection caused by *S. stercoralis* is known as **strongyloidiasis**. It is most frequently asymptomatic. In symptomatic cases the following lesions may be observed:

Skin lesions

On invading the skin, the filariform larvae produce petechial haemorrhage at each site of invasion, accompanied by intense pruritus followed by congestion and oedema around the invaded area. Pruritus and urticaria, particularly involving the perianal skin and buttocks, are common symptoms of chronic strongyloidiasis. A serpigenous, pruritic eruption usually found on the trunk or buttocks, may represent skin penetration by autoinfective filariform larvae of *S. stercoralis* in this area. This condition is known as **larva currens** (meaning racing larva).

Pulmonary lesions

When the larvae of *S. stercoralis* migrate through the lungs, they break out of the pulmonary capillaries into the alveoli leading to **haemorrhages in the lung alveoli and bronchopneumonia**. These areas are often infiltrated with eosinophils. Occasionally, larvae may lodge in the bronchial epithelium and develop to maturity there. This leads to chronic bronchitis or asthmatic symptoms. **Eggs and rhabditiform larvae of *S. stercoralis* may be seen in the patient's sputum.**

Intestinal lesions

The intestinal manifestations of *S. stercoralis* infection vary from few symptoms in light infections, to severe necrotizing bowel disease in heavy infections. Patient develops intermittent abdominal pain, distension, bloating and diarrhoea alternating with constipation. Children may develop malabsorption syndrome. Microscopically, duodenal and jejunal mucosa shows small tunnels through which parasitic females have burrowed their ways, congestion, haemorrhages, round cell infiltration and desquamation of epithelial cells.

Hyperinfection

Patients with *S. stercoralis* hyperinfection generally experience a worsening in abdominal symptoms, often accompanied by paralytic ileus, gastrointestinal bleeding and perforation. The increase in number of worms migrating through the lungs results in wheezing, dyspnoea and pulmonary haemorrhage. During hyperinfection, filariform larvae may enter into arterial circulation and lodge in various organs, e.g., lymph nodes, endocardium, pancreas, liver, kidneys and brain. The signs and symptoms will depend upon the organ involved.

Disseminated *S. stercoralis* infection has been reported in immunocompromised states like organ-transplant or cancer patients on chemotherapy and more so in acquired immunodeficiency syndrome. Satyanarayana et al., 2005 reported a case of disseminated *S. stercoralis* infection in an AIDS case in India.

Laboratory diagnosis

The diagnosis of strongyloidiasis can be made by:

- Demonstration of **rhabditiform larvae, filariform larvae and parasitic adult females of *S. stercoralis*** in Papanicolaou-stained smears of faeces, sputum or duodenal aspirates either by endoscopy or by use of Enterotest. Sometimes unhatched eggs are found which cause confusion with the hookworm eggs. During hyperinfection with dissemination, *Strongyloides* larvae can be detected in a variety of body fluids and tissues.
- **Baermann technique:** Use of Baermann technique (by which motile larvae are extracted from stool specimens) may increase the diagnostic yield of faecal examination:
  1. Set up a clamp supporting 6 inch glass funnel. Attach rubber tubing and a pinch clamp to the bottom of the funnel. Place a collection beaker underneath.

2. Place a wire gauze or nylon filter over the top of the funnel, followed by a pad consisting of two layers of gauze.
3. Close the pinch clamp at the bottom of the tubing and fill the funnel with tap water until it just soaks the gauze padding.
4. Spread a large amount of faecal material on the gauze padding so that it is covered with water. If the faecal material is very firm, first emulsify it in water.
5. Allow the apparatus to stand for 2 hours or longer. The larvae in the stool migrate through the gauze into the water and then sediment into the neck of the funnel.
6. Draw 10 ml of fluid into the beaker by releasing the pinch clamp, centrifuge the fluid for 2 minutes at 500 *g*, and examine the sediment under the microscope (magnification ×100 and ×400) for the presence of motile larvae.

- **Agar plate culture** tends to be more sensitive. Stool is placed onto agar plate, and it is sealed and held for 2 days at room temperature. As larvae crawl over the agar, they carry bacteria with them, thus creating visible tracks over the agar. The plates are examined under the microscope for confirmation of the presence of larvae, the surface of the agar is then washed with 10% formalin, and final confirmation of larval identification is made via wet examination of the sediment from the formalin washing.
- **Serological tests** such as enzyme-linked immunosorbent assay, indirect haemagglutination, and indirect immunofluorescence antibody test can be used for the diagnosis of strongyloidiasis.
- **Eosinophilia** may be present but its absence does not exclude the diagnosis.

Treatment

Ivermectin is the drug of choice for treatment of strongyloidiasis.

Prophylaxis

Strongyloidiasis can be prevented by:

- Proper disposal of human waste.
- Avoidance of contact with faecally contaminated soil.
- Treatment of all diagnosed cases.

HOOKWORMS

Human hookworms include two nematode species, *Ancylostoma duodenale* (the Old World hookworm) and *Necator americanus* (the New World hookworm). These hookworms differ only in geographic distribution, structure of mouthparts, and relative size. Both species have mouthparts designed for sucking blood from injured intestinal tissue. *A. duodenale* has chitinous teeth and *N. americanus* has shearing chitinous plates. A smaller group of hookworms infecting animals can invade and parasitize humans (*A. ceylanicum*) or can penetrate the human skin (causing cutaneous larva migrans), but do not develop any further (*A. braziliense*, *A. caninum* and *Uncinaria stenocephala*). Occasionally, *A. caninum* larva may migrate to the human intestine causing eosinophilic enteritis; this may happen when larva is ingested rather than through skin invasion.

Human hookworm infection is the second most common human helminthic infection (after ascariasis). It has worldwide distribution, mostly in areas with moist, warm climate. An estimated more than 900 million people worldwide are infected with hookworm (mostly *A. duodenale*), 0.2% of whom suffer from severe anaemia. Both *A. duodenale* and *N. americanus* are found in Africa, Asia and the Americas. *N. americanus* predominates in the Americas and Australia, *A. duodenale* is found in Middle East, North Africa, and southern Europe. In India, about 20 million people are infected by both *A. duodenale* and *N. americanus*.

ANCYLOSTOMA DUODENALE

Common name

The Old World hookworm.

The first accurate description of this parasite was given by Dubini in 1843. Mode of infection and the pathogenesis in man was first worked out by Arther Looss in 1897.

Habitat

The adult worm lives in the small intestine of man, particularly in the jejunum, less often in the duodenum and rarely in the ileum.

Morphology

Adult worms

They are small, pinkish and fusiform in shape (Fig. 11.5). The anterior end is curved dorsally, hence the name hookworm. This curve is in the same direction as the general body curvature. The oral aperture is not terminal but directed towards the dorsal surface (Fig.

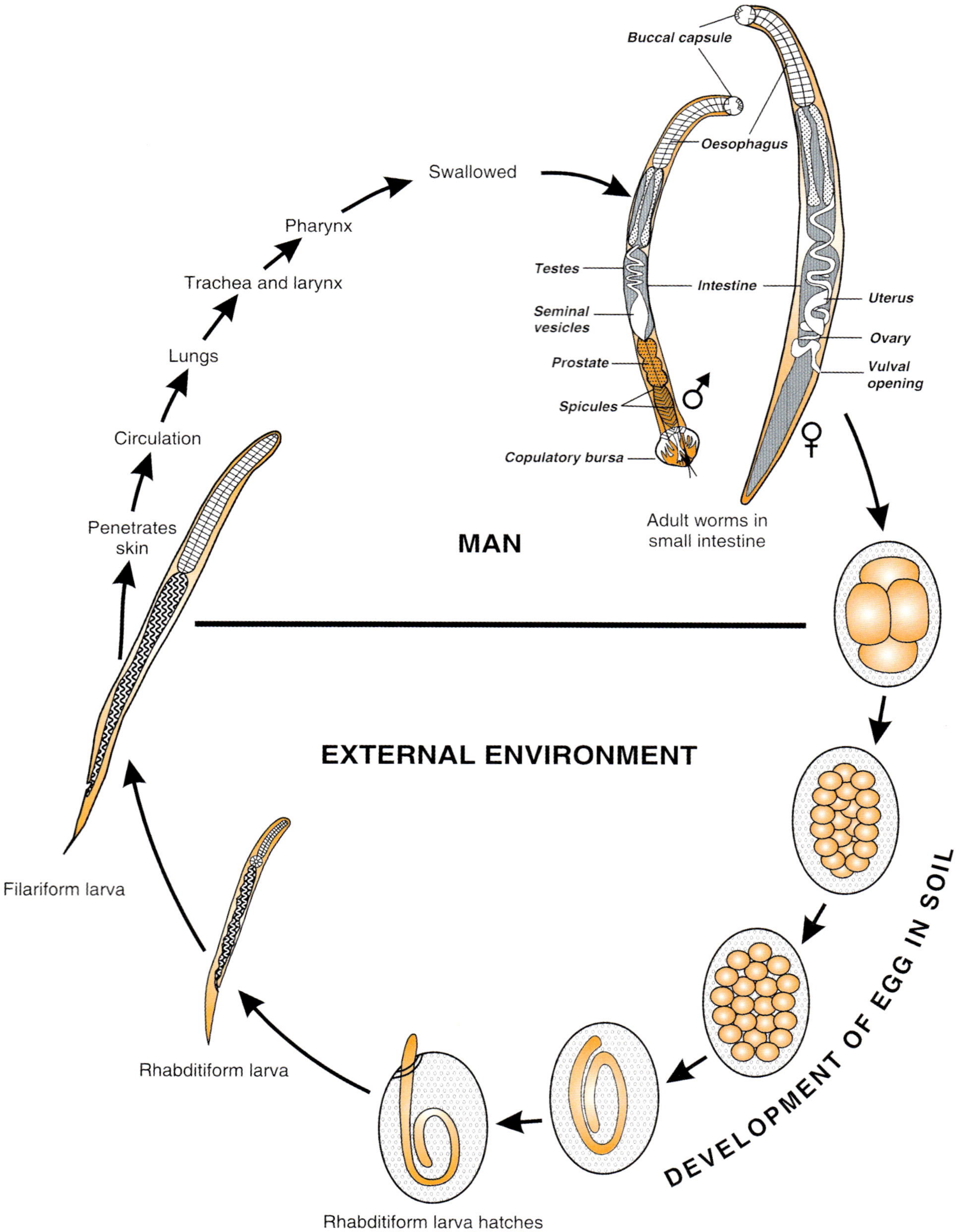

Fig. 11.5. Life cycle of *Ancylostoma duodenale*.

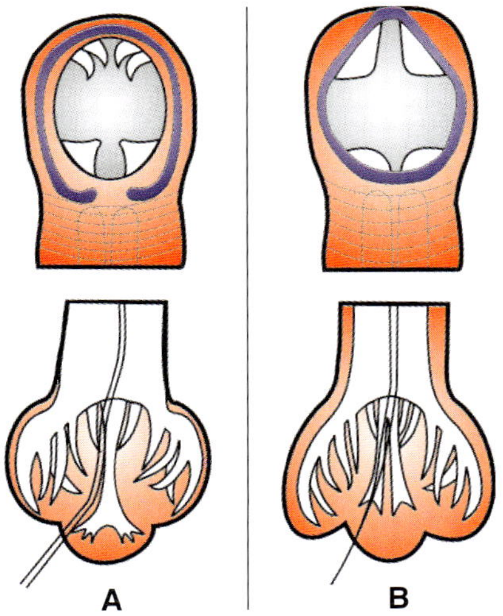

Fig. 11.6. Buccal capsule and copulatory bursa of (A) *Ancylostoma duodenale* and (B) *Necator americanus*.

11.6). The oral cavity is provided with four hook-like teeth on ventral surface and two knob-like teeth on dorsal surface. The differences between male and female *A. duodenale* are given in Table 11.2. Owing to the position of genital openings of male and female worms they assume a Y-shaped figure during copulation. Adult worms are rarely seen, since they remain firmly attached to the intestinal mucosa by means of well-developed mouth parts.

Copulatory bursa

Copulatory bursa (Fig. 11.6) is present in the male worm for attachment with the female during copulation. This consists of three lobes – one dorsal and two lateral. These lobes are supported by 13 chitinous rays, five each in lateral lobes and three in dorsal lobe – one dorsal and two externodorsal rays. The dorsal ray is partially divided at the tip and each division is tripartite. The life span of the adult worms in the human intestine is about 3–4 years.

Eggs

Eggs are oval or elliptical measuring 60 μm in length and 40 μm in width. They are **colourless (not bile-stained)** and are surrounded by a thin transparent hyaline shell. They possess a segmented ovum with usually four blastomeres. **There is a clear space between the segmented ovum and the egg shell** (Figs. 11.5 and 11.7). **The eggs float in saturated salt solution.** About twice as many eggs are produced by *A. duodenale* than from *N. americanus*. Eggs are normally excreted in the faeces 4–7 weeks after infection.

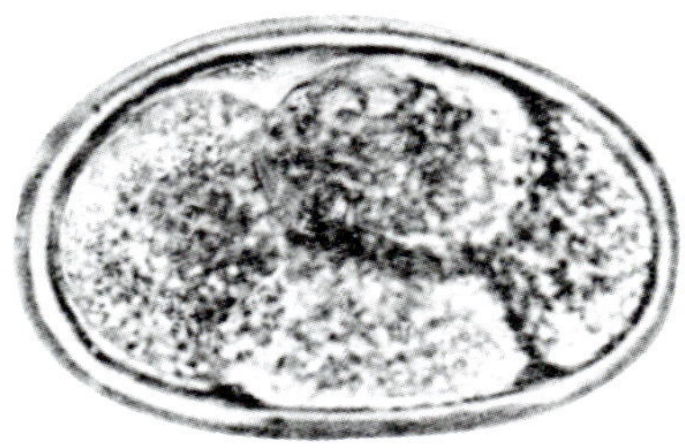

Fig. 11.7. Egg of *Ancylostoma duodenale* (saline wet mount, × 400).

Life cycle

Man is the only host (Figs. 11.5 and 11.8). No intermediate host is required. Adult worms inhabit the small

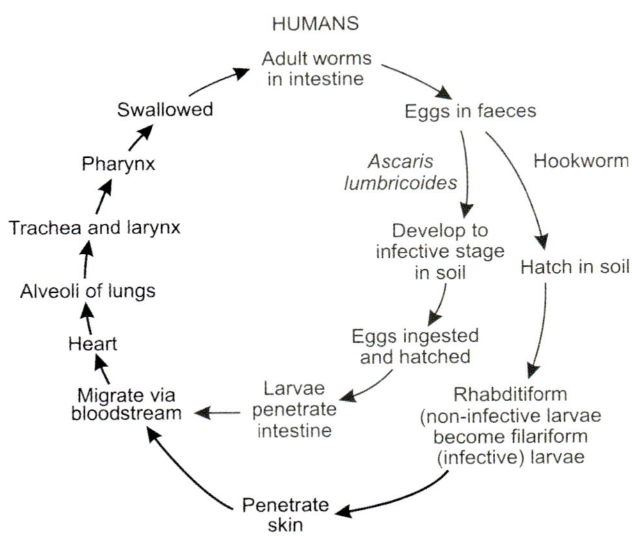

Fig. 11.8. Life cycle of hookworm and *Ascaris lumbricoides*.

Table 11.2. Differences between male and female *A. duodenale*		
	Male	**Female**
Size	5–11 mm × 0.4–0.5 mm	9–13 mm × 0.6 mm
Posterior end	Expanded in an umbrella-like fashion. This is known as copulatory bursa.	Tapering
Genital opening	Opens posteriorly with cloaca	Opens at the junction of the middle and posterior thirds of the body

intestine of man attaching themselves to the mucous membrane by means of their mouth parts. The eggs containing segmented ova are passed out in the faeces of infected person. In the warm and moist soil, **rhabditiform larvae** hatch out from the egg in 24–48 hours. These measure 250 µm in length and 17 µm in maximum diameter. These feed on bacteria and organic debris and moult twice on the third and fifth day and develop into **filariform larvae**, which no longer feed. These measure 500–700 µm in length and are the **infective stage of the parasite**. Depending on the temperature and moisture content of the soil, filariform larvae can remain infective for up to 6 weeks.

When a person walks barefoot on soil containing the filariform larvae they penetrate the skin, particularly the skin between the toes, the dorsum of the foot and the medial aspect of the sole. In farm workers the larvae may penetrate the skin of the hands. On reaching the subcutaneous tissue the larvae enter into the lymphatics or small venules. Through lymph-vascular system they enter into venous circulation and are carried via the right heart into the pulmonary capillaries. Here they breakthrough the capillary walls and enter into the alveolar spaces. From alveoli, the larvae migrate up the bronchi, trachea and larynx, crawl over the epiglottis to the pharynx and are swallowed.

During migration or on reaching oesophagus they undergo third moulting. Thereafter, they reach small intestine, undergo fourth moulting and develop into **adult worms**. They attach themselves to the mucous membrane of small intestine by means of their mouth parts. In about six weeks, from the time of infection, adult worms become sexually mature. Male fertilizes female and the latter lays eggs which are passed in faeces and the cycle is repeated.

Pathogenicity

Clinical disease in *A. duodenale* infection may be caused by the migrating larvae or adult worms.

Pathogenicity of migrating larvae

Migrating larvae of *A. duodenale* may cause two types of lesions:

1. Ancylostoma dermatitis or ground itch
2. Pulmonary lesions

Ancylostoma dermatitis or ground itch

When filariform larvae enter the skin they may lead to dermatitis. This causes intense itching and burning followed by erythema and oedema of the area which soon develops into papular and vesicular eruptions. This condition is more common with *N. americanus* than with *A. duodenale* infection. It disappears in 1–2 weeks.

Pulmonary lesions

When the filariform larvae breakthrough the pulmonary capillaries and enter the alveoli, they may lead to **bronchitis and bronchopneumonia**. A **marked eosinophilia** occurs at this stage.

Pathogenicity of adult worms

The disease caused by adult worms is responsible for the syndrome commonly referred to as **hookworm disease**. The maturing and adult worms attach themselves to the mucosa of small intestine by means of their mouth parts. Hookworms ingest blood. One adult worm each of ***A. duodenale* and *N. americanus* sucks 0.2 ml and 0.03 ml of blood daily, respectively**. They live for up to 5 years. In addition, the worms frequently leave one site and attach themselves to another site.

As the secretions of the worms contain anticoagulant activity, the bleeding from abandoned sites may continue for some time. These two facts are responsible for **microcytic, hypochromic type of iron deficiency anaemia**. Bleeding leads to anaemia, hypoproteinaemia, digestive disturbances and retarded development. The degree of anaemia depends on the number of worms, body iron store and dietary iron.

Patient develops epigastric pain, dyspepsia, vomiting and diarrhoea, the stool being reddish or black. Tongue, conjunctiva and skin become pale. Skin, in addition, becomes cold and dry. Hair become dry and lustreless and there is oedema of feet and ankle.

Laboratory diagnosis

Diagnosis of hookworm infection can be established by following methods:

Direct methods

- **Demonstration of characteristic eggs in the faeces** by direct microscopy or by concentration methods (Fig. 11.7). In heavy infections, a substantial amount of blood can be lost, and severe iron deficiency anaemia may develop in a short time. Therefore, faecal egg count may be indicated in assessing the severity (worm burden) in certain cases. Adult female hookworms produce about 2,500 to 5,000 eggs per day; thus, the faecal egg counts may reflect the number of adult hookworms and, in turn, indicate the severity of infection.

A number of more than 2,000 hookworm eggs per ml of faeces in women and children and more than 5,000 per ml in males is usually associated with anaemia. If the stool specimen is stored at room temperature (no preservative) for more than 24 hours, the eggs will continue to develop and larvae may hatch. These larvae may be confused with those of *Strongyloides stercoralis*.

- **Adult worms** may also be detected in the stool.
- Aspiration of duodenal contents by Ryle's tube may **reveal eggs or the adult worms**.

Indirect methods

- Blood examination may reveal microcytic, hypochromic anaemia and eosinophilia.
- In many cases of hookworm disease stool examination may show occult blood and Charcot-Leyden crystals.

NECATOR AMERICANUS

Necator americanus (the New World hookworm) adult worms are slightly smaller and thinner than those of *A. duodenale*. Differences between the adult worms of these two human hookworms are given in Table 11.3 and Fig. 11.6. The eggs of *N. americanus* are indistinguishable from those of *A. duodenale* and the life cycle, pathogenicity and diagnosis of the former is also similar to that of the latter.

Treatment

Albendazole is the drug of first choice and is considered far superior to mebendazole at removing adult hookworms from the gastrointestinal tract. If anaemia is present this should also be treated along with the specific anthelmintic drugs.

ANCYLOSTOMA BRAZILIENSE

Ancylostoma braziliense is a hookworm of dogs and cats in Brazil, India and Malaysia. The adult worms are much smaller than those of *A. duodenale*. The buccal capsule has a small orifice and the ventral dental plate contains one pair of large teeth. The bursa of the male is small and is supported by relatively short lateral rays. The eggs resemble those of *A. duodenale*. The filariform larvae are not able to penetrate below the level of stratum germinativum of human skin. Therefore, they are unable to negotiate their way into blood vessels and proceed to small intestine so the disease remains confined to the outer layers of the skin, and cause **cutaneous larva migrans** also called **ground itch** or **creeping eruption**.

ANCYLOSTOMA CEYLANICUM

Ancylostoma ceylanicum is one of the smaller species of the genus. It occurs in the intestine of cats and their wild relatives in Southeast Asia. To a lesser extent, it may cause intestinal infection in dogs and man. Human infection has been reported in the Philippines, Taiwan and India. Therefore, *A. ceylanicum* needs to be distinguished from *A. duodenale* and *N. americanus* which are more common human hookworms. It does not cause cutaneous larva migrans. The bursa of the male *A. ceylanicum* is broader, the lateral rays are more curved, the mediolateral and externolateral rays are more divergent and the externodorsal rays originate nearer to the stem of the dorsal ray.

ANCYLOSTOMA CANINUM

A. caninum is a dog hookworm. The adult male measures 10 mm by 0.4 mm and the female 14 mm by

Table 11.3. Differences between the adult worms of *A. duodenale* and *N. americanus*

	A. duodenale	***N. americanus***
Size	Larger and thicker	Smaller and thinner
Anterior end	Bends in the same direction as the body curvature	Bends in the opposite direction of the body curvature
Buccal capsule	Six teeth, four hook-like on ventral surface and two knob-like on dorsal surface	Four cutting plates, two each on ventral and dorsal surface
Copulatory bursa	Dorsal ray is single but partially divided at the tip and each division is tripartite; total number of rays is 13; two separate spicules	Dorsal ray is split from the base and each division is bipartite; total number of rays is 14; two spicules fused at the tip
Posterior end of female	A posterior spine is present	No posterior spine is present
Vulval opening	Situated behind the middle of the body	Situated in front of the middle of the body
Pathogenicity	More pathogenic	Less pathogenic

0.6 mm. It has a wide buccal capsule with three pairs of ventral teeth. Filariform larvae of *A. caninum*, like those of *A. braziliense*, cause creeping eruption in the skin of the infected humans.

Prophylaxis

Hookworms flourish under primitive conditions where people go barefoot, modern sanitary conditions do not exist and human faeces are deposited on ground. Therefore, for the prevention of hookworm infection, living conditions and sanitation should be improved and there should be sanitary disposal of human faeces. Wearing of shoes and gloves provides personal protection.

CUTANEOUS LARVA MIGRANS

Cutaneous larva migrans (CLM) is a parasitic skin infection caused by hookworm larvae that usually infect cats, dogs and other animals. Humans can be infected with the larvae by walking barefoot on moist soft soil that has been contaminated with animal faeces. It is also known as **creeping eruption** as once infected, the larvae migrate under the skin's surface and cause itchy red lines or tracks. Many types of hookworm can cause cutaneous larva migrans. It is caused by:

- *Ankylostoma braziliense*: hookworm of wild and domestic dogs and cats
- *Ankylostoma caninum*: dog hookworm found in Australia
- *Uncinaria stenocephala*: dog hookworm found in Europe
- *Bunostomum phlebotomum*: cattle hookworm
- *Gnathostoma* sp.

Occasionally *Ancylostoma duodenale*, *Necator americanus* and *Strongyloides stercoralis* may also cause cutaneous larva migrans.

People of all ages and races, and of both sexes can be affected if they have been exposed to the larvae. It is most commonly found in tropical and subtropical geographic locations. Groups at risk include those with occupations or hobbies that bring them into contact with warm, moist, sandy soil.

Parasite eggs are passed in the faeces of infected animals on warm, moist soil, where the larvae hatch. On contact with human skin, the larvae can penetrate through hair follicles, cracks or even intact skin to infect the human host. Between a few days and a few months after the initial infection, the larvae migrate beneath the skin.

In an animal host the larvae are able to penetrate the deeper layers of the skin (the dermis) and enter the blood and lymphatic system. Once in the intestine they mature sexually and lay eggs that are then excreted to start the cycle again. However, in a human host, the larvae are unable to penetrate below the level of stratum germinativum. So, the disease remains confined to the outer layers of the skin.

At the site of penetration a non-specific eruption occurs. There may be a tingling or prickling sensation within 30 minutes of the larvae penetrating. The larvae can then either lie dormant for weeks or months or immediately begin creeping activity that create 2–3 mm wide, snake-like tracks. These are slightly raised, flesh-coloured or pink and cause intense itching. Tracks advance a few millimetres to a few centimetres daily and if many larvae are involved a disorganised series of loops and tortuous tracks may form. Biopsy shows larvae with round cells, particularly eosinophil infiltration.

Sites most commonly affected are the feet, spaces between the toes, hands, knees and buttocks.

The disease is self-limiting. Humans are an accidental and "dead-end" host, so the larvae eventually die. The natural duration of the disease varies considerably depending on the species of larvae involved. In most cases, lesions will resolve without treatment within 4–8 weeks.

Treatment

Oral albendazole is the drug of choice for treating cutaneous larva migrans. Oral ivermectin or topical thiabendazole also can be used. Any secondary skin infections may require treatment with appropriate antibiotics.

ENTEROBIUS VERMICULARIS

Common names

Threadworm, pinworm, seatworm.

Leukart, 1865 was the first to describe the complete life cycle of this parasite. A second species, *Enterobius gregorii*, has been described and reported from Europe, Africa and Asia. For all practical purposes, the morphology, life cycle, clinical presentation, and treatment of *E. gregorii* is identical to that of *E. vermicularis*.

Geographical distribution

It has a cosmopolitan distribution. It is more common in temperate and cold climates than in warm climates because of less frequent bathing and infrequent changing of underclothing. It is the most common helminthic infection in North America. **Humans are considered to be the only hosts of *E. vermicularis*.**

Habitat

Adult worms inhabit the caecum, appendix (Fig. 11.9), and adjacent portions of the ascending colon, lying closely applied to the mucosal surface.

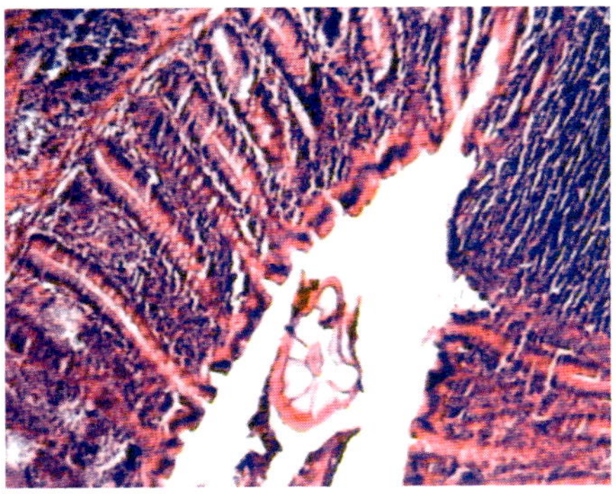

Fig. 11.9. *Enterobius vermicularis* in the lumen of the appendix (haematoxylin and eosin stain, × 100).

Morphology

Adult worms

These are small, white, spindle-shaped and resemble short pieces of thread (Fig. 11.10). At the anterior end, both male and female worms possess a pair of wing-like expansions, known as **cervical alae**. The male measures 2–4 mm in length and 0.1–0.2 mm in breadth. The posterior one-third of the body is curved. The female is longer, 8–12 mm in length and 0.3–0.5 mm in width. Its posterior extremity is straight and drawn out into a thin pointed pin-like tail. Males live for about 7 weeks and females live for 5–13 weeks.

Eggs

The eggs are **colourless, not bile-stained** and flattened on one side (planoconvex). They measure 60 µm in length and 30 µm in width. They are surrounded by a thin, smooth, transparent shell and usually contain fully developed larvae (Figs. 11.10 and 11.11). **They float in saturated solution of common salt.**

Life cycle

Of all the intestinal worms, it has the simplest life cycle (Fig. 11.10). **It is completed in a single host.** There is **no systemic migration** similar to that undertaken by *Ascaris lumbricoides*. The adult worms live in caecum, appendix, and adjacent portions of ascending colon. Male fertilizes female and dies, and is excreted in faeces. The gravid female migrates down the colon to the rectum. At night, when the host is in bed, it comes out of the anus. It then crawls on the perianal and perineal skin and deposits the eggs. As many as 20,000 eggs are deposited on the perianal and perineal skin. Crawling of the gravid female worm leads to intense pruritus and the patient scratches the affected part.

Such patients have eggs of *E. vermicularis* on the fingers and under the nails. These individuals may develop **autoinfection** by direct anus-to-mouth transfer by finger contamination. Persons handling night clothes and bedding of infected patients can also contract infection. Infection may also be acquired from contaminated objects like door knobs, table tops, etc. Eggs can become airborne when clothes, bedding or dust are disturbed. They may then contaminate food or the hands of people in the vicinity, but it has also been suggested that airborne eggs can be inhaled and then swallowed producing infection.

The larvae, from embryonated eggs, hatch out in the small intestine. They then migrate to the caecum and appendix and in 2–6 weeks develop into adult worms. Eggs laid on perianal skin may immediately hatch into infective-stage larvae and may ascend through anus to develop into adolescent worms in the caecum and appendix.

After laying eggs on the perianal skin the worm may retreat into the anal canal and come out again to lay more eggs. The worms may also wander into the vulva, vagina, uterus, fallopian tubes and peritoneum.

There is nine times higher incidence of *Dientamoeba fragilis* infection in patients with *E. vermicularis* infection. This, therefore, suggests that *E. vermicularis* eggs serve as the chief vector for the transmission of *D. fragilis* to humans.

Pathogenicity

Enterobiasis or **pinworm infection** is most frequent in school age children, but can occur in any age group. They are the commonest worm parasites in temperate, developed countries, where prevalence figure in young children may reach 80–90%, but infections are distributed globally. The itching associated with the movement of the female worms to the anal region leads to perianal and perineal pruritus. Infected children may show irritability, enuresis and weight loss. **Unlike the other intestinal nematodes, *Enterobius* infection is not associated with a pronounced eosinophilia or with elevated IgE.**

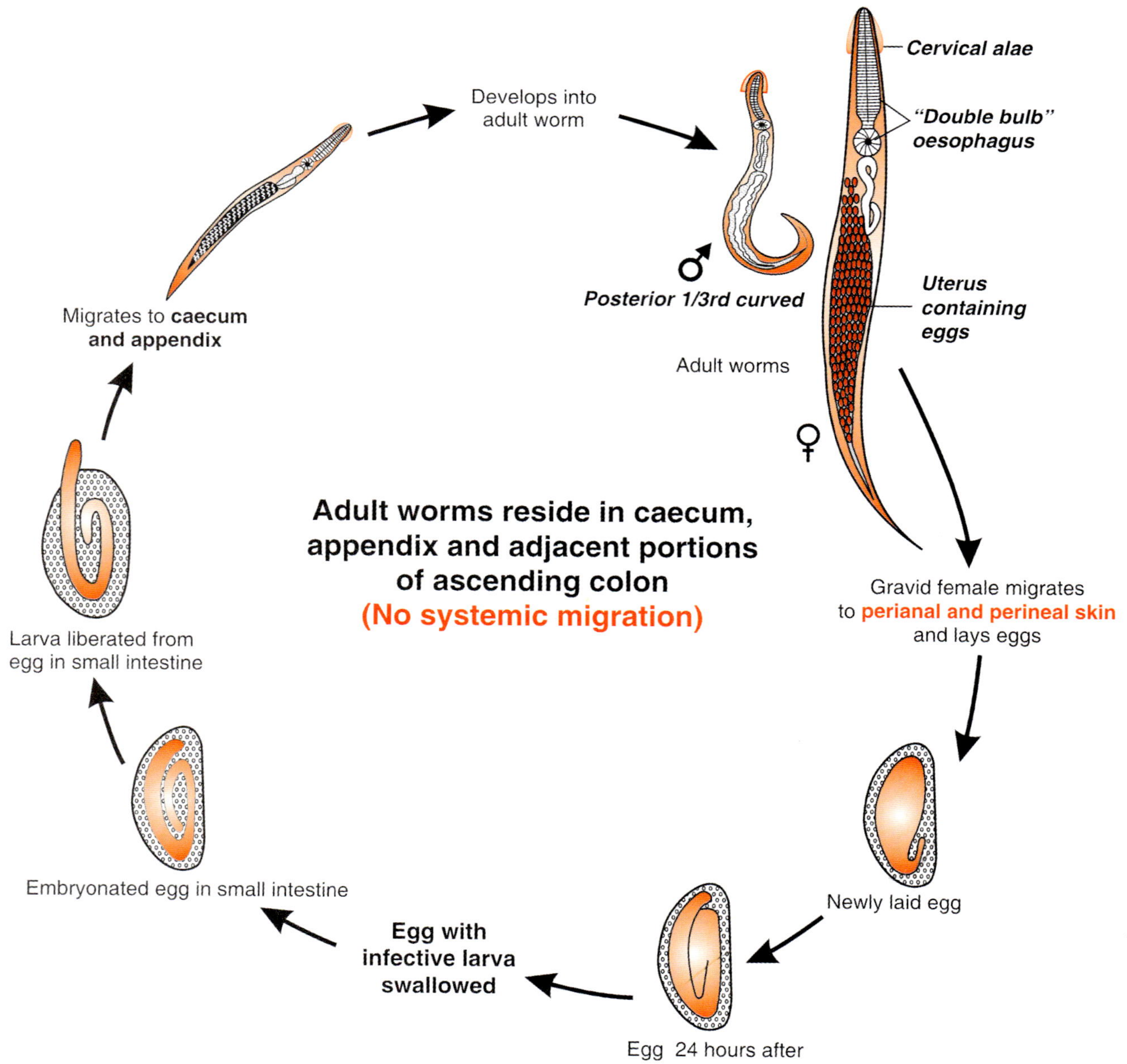

Fig. 11.10. Life cycle of *Enterobius vermicularis*.

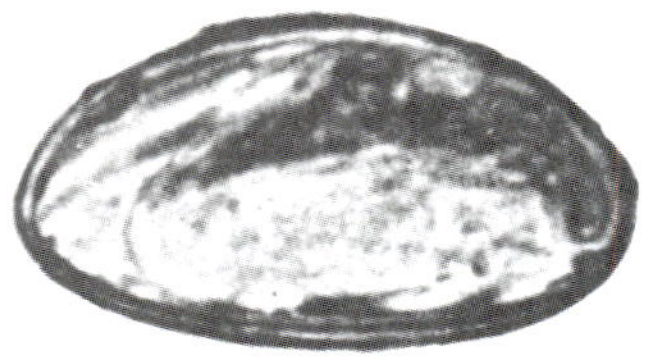

Fig. 11.11. Egg of *Enterobius vermicularis* (saline wet mount, × 400).

In girls the migrating female worms may enter into vagina and urethra leading to vaginitis and urethritis. These worms may cause appendicitis in 2.5–2.7% cases. If worms enter the peritoneum, either via intestinal perforation or following migration through the female reproductive tract, these may lead to more severe complications. Dead worms and eggs may be found in granulomata in vagina, cervix, fallopian tubes, omentum, peritoneum, liver, kidneys and lungs.

Laboratory diagnosis

1. Detection of adult worms

The adult worms may be detected in the perianal region or on the surface of the stool. These may also be detected in the appendix during appendicectomy (Fig. 11.9).

2. Demonstration of eggs

Since eggs are not discharged by the worm into faeces, therefore, faecal examination is not useful in the laboratory diagnosis of threadworm infection. However, in a small proportion of patients stool examination may show the presence of eggs of *E. vermicularis* (Fig. 11.11).

Eggs which are deposited in large numbers on the perianal and perineal skin at night can be demonstrated by scraping these areas with NIH (National Institute of Health) swab (Fig. 11.12) in the morning before the child goes to toilet and takes bath. NIH swab consists of a glass rod at one end of which a piece of transparent cellophane (with sticky surface out) is wrapped and held in place with a rubber band. The other end of the glass rod is fixed in a rubber stopper and kept in a test tube. The cellophane part is used for swabbing by rolling over the perianal and perineal area. Then the cellophane is detached, spread over glass slide and examined microscopically. This procedure should be repeated on three successive days (see also scotch cellophane tape method in Chapter 13).

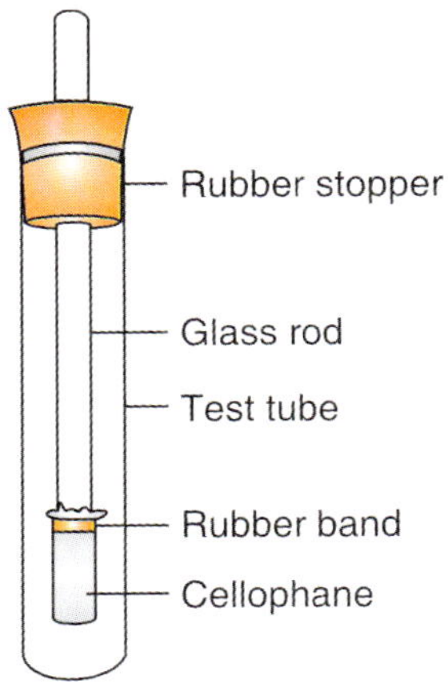

Fig. 11.12. NIH swab.

Eggs may also be recovered from under the fingernails and the washings from garments.

Treatment

Pyrantel pamoate, mebendazole, and albendazole are highly effective. Single oral doses of each should be repeated after 2 weeks. When their use is combined with rigid standards of hygiene, a very high proportion of cures can be obtained.

Prophylaxis

Enterobiasis can be prevented by:

- Personal hygiene, particularly hand washing, fingernail cleaning and regular bathing.
- Wearing of closed garments by the infected children during night.
- Frequent changing and washing of bed-linen and night clothes.
- Keeping the bedrooms clean and dust free.
- Treating the infected persons. If infection is confirmed in one individual in a household, other family members should be examined and treated.

ASCARIS LUMBRICOIDES

Common name

The common roundworm.

Geographical distribution

Ascaris lumbricoides is the most common intestinal nematode of the humans and is one of the major soil-transmitted helminths. It has worldwide distribution, being specially prevalent in the tropics, such as India, China and Southeast Asia. It is estimated that > 1.4 billion people worldwide are infected by this parasite. The highest prevalence is in areas where sanitation is poor and where human faeces is used as fertilizer. Areas with modern water and waste treatment have a low incidence of the infection with this parasite. No animal reservoir is known for *A. lumbricoides*. However, an almost identical species from pigs, *A. suum*, can infect humans.

Habitat

Adult worms reside in the small intestine, particularly the jejunum of man.

Morphology

A. lumbricoides is the largest nematode **parasitizing the human intestine**.

Adult worms

The body of *A. lumbricoides* is cylindrical, tapering gradually at the anterior end and somewhat less so at the posterior end (Fig. 11.13). White longitudinal streaks can usually be seen along the entire length of the pinkish cream body of the parasite. The mouth opens at the anterior end. It possesses three finely toothed lips, one dorsal and two ventral. The digestive

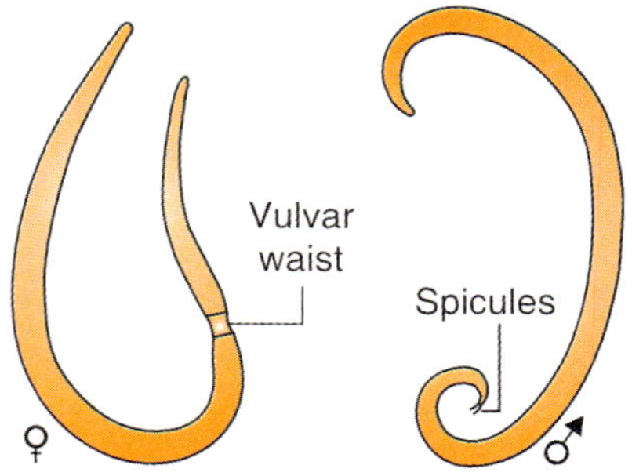

Fig. 11.13. Adult worms of *Ascaris lumbricoides*.

and respiratory organs of the worm float inside the body cavity possessing a toxic fluid known as **ascaron**. Allergic reactions seen in infected individuals are due to this toxin.

Male worm

It measures 15–30 cm in length and 3–4 mm in diameter. The posterior end is curved ventrally to form a hook. The ejaculatory duct along with the anus open into the cloaca from which arises a pair of copulatory spicules of equal size.

Female worm

It is longer and stouter than the male worm and measures 25–40 cm in length and 5 mm in diameter. The tail is straight and conical. The anus is subterminal and opens on the ventral surface in the form of a transverse slit. The vulva opens at the junction of the anterior and the middle-thirds of the body on the midventral aspect of the worm. This part of the worm is narrower and is known as **vulvar waist**. A mature female *A. lumbricoides* lays enormous number of eggs (nearly 200,000 eggs daily) which are passed in the faeces. Eggs are of two types:

Fertilized eggs

The fertilized eggs are round or oval in shape and measure 60–75 µm in length and 40–50 µm in breadth (Figs. 11.14 and 11.15). They are **bile-stained and brown in colour**. They are surrounded by a thick, transparent shell, consisting of a relatively nonpermeable innermost lipoidal vitelline membrane, a thick transparent middle layer and an outermost coarsely mammillated albuminoid layer. Outer mammillated coat is sometimes lost. Such eggs are called **decorticated eggs**. Each egg contains a large conspicuous unsegmented ovum with a clear crescentic area at each pole. **Fertilized eggs float in saturated solution of common salt.**

Unfertilized eggs

In the absence of a male worm, the female produces unfertilized (infertile) eggs. These are narrower and longer and measure 90 µm in length and 55 µm in breadth (Figs. 11.14 and 11.15). They are **bile-stained and brown in colour**. Each egg contains a small atrophied ovum and a thin shell within an irregular coating of albumin. The innermost lipoidal vitelline membrane of the shell is absent. The unfertilized eggs are heaviest of all the helminthic eggs, therefore, they **do not float in saturated solution of common salt**. The adult worms may live as long as 20 months, but usual life span is about 1 year.

Life cycle

The life cycle of *A. lumbricoides* is passed in **only one host, man** (Figs. 11.8 and 11.14). No intermediate host is required. Adult worms reside in the small intestine, particularly the jejunum of man. Fertilized eggs containing unsegmented ova are passed in the faeces. However, they are not immediately infective to man. **They have to undergo a period of incubation in soil before acquiring infectivity.** Depending on the temperature and humidity, a rhabditiform larva develops from the unsegmented ovum and undergoes **first moulting within the egg shell** in 10–40 days. The optimum temperature and humidity for the development of the larva within the egg shell is 22–30°C and more than 40%, respectively. **The embryonated eggs containing rhabditiform larvae are pathogenic to man.**

Man acquires infection by ingestion of food, water or raw vegetables contaminated with embryonated eggs. In the small intestine (duodenum), the ingested eggs hatch to liberate the larvae. These larvae then burrow their way through the mucous membrane of the small intestine and are carried by the portal circulation to the liver, where they reside for 3–4 days. They then pass via hepatic vein, inferior vena cava, right heart and pulmonary artery and reach the lungs. Here they grow in size and **moult twice** (first on 5th day and second on 10th day). The larvae then breakthrough the capillary wall and reach the lung alveoli.

From the alveoli, the larvae migrate up the bronchi, trachea and larynx, crawl over the epiglottis to the pharynx and are swallowed. They pass down the oesophagus and stomach and localize in the upper part of the small intestine, their normal abode. On twenty-fifth to twenty-ninth day of infection, the larvae undergo **another moulting** and transform into **adult worms**. In about 6–10 weeks, they become sexually

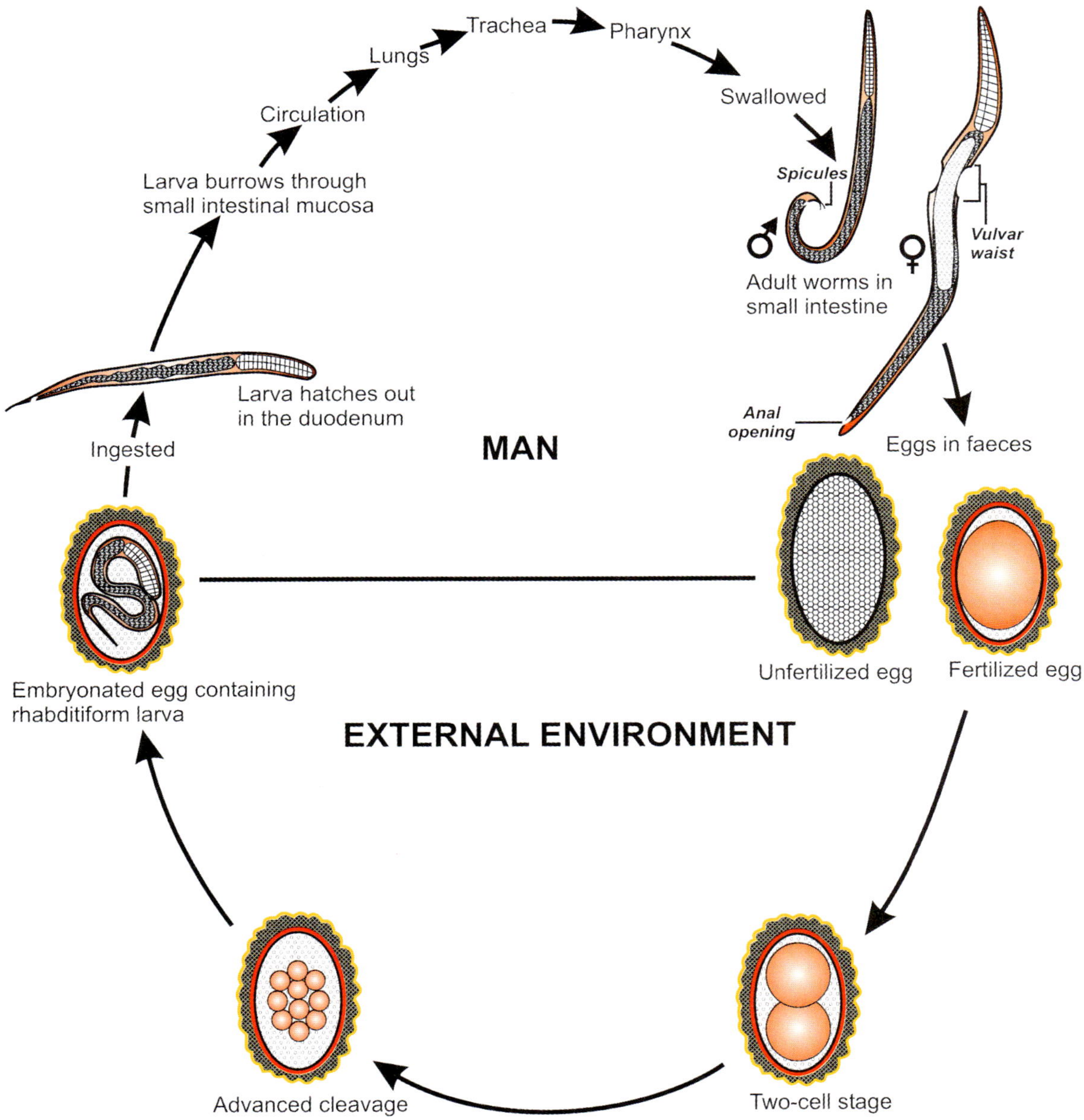

Fig. 11.14. Life cycle of *Ascaris lumbricoides*.

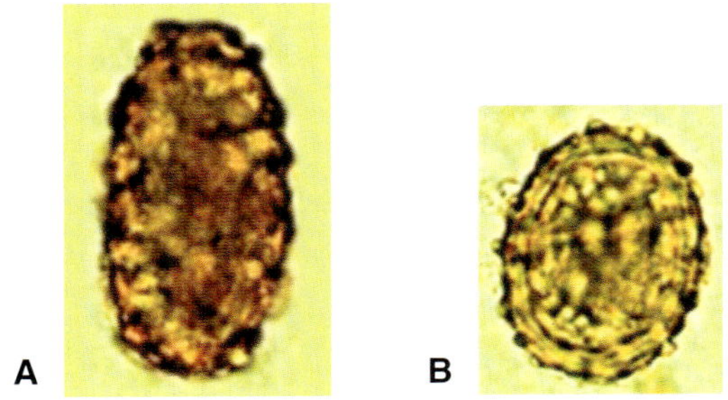

Fig. 11.15. Unfertilized (A) and fertilized (B) eggs of *Ascaris lumbricoides* (saline wet mount, × 400).

mature and by 12 weeks the gravid females begin to discharge eggs in the stool and the cycle is repeated.

Pathogenicity

Disease produced by *A. lumbricoides* is known as **ascariasis** and is caused by both adult worms and migrating larvae.

Pathogenicity of adult worm

- By robbing the host of its nutrition, the adult worms affect the nutritional status of the host leading to

malnutrition and night blindness due to vitamin A deficiency. The long-term effect of the malnutrition caused by ascariasis is **retardation of growth**.

- The presence of adult worms in the intestine may also lead to intermittent colicky cramps and loss of appetite. In heavy infection, adult worms may cause **obstruction of the intestinal tract**. Intestinal obstruction occurs in approximately 2 of every 1000 individuals infected.
- **The worms are restless wanderers.** They tend to probe and insinuate themselves into any aperture they find on the way. They may crawl out of mouth or may enter the nasal meatus via nasopharynx and pass out of a naris. From the oropharynx, the worm may enter a eustachian tube and penetrate to the middle ear and through the tympanic membrane to external auditory meatus. The worm may also enter into the trachea leading to **respiratory obstruction**. The worms may migrate downwards and lodge in appendix, bile duct and pancreatic duct leading to appendicitis, obstructive jaundice and acute haemorrhagic pancreatitis, respectively. They may perforate the intestinal wall (Fig. 11.16) weakened by ulcers or gangrene.
- Release of toxic body fluid (ascaron) of the adult worm in the body of the patient may lead to various **allergic manifestations** such as fever, urticaria, angioneurotic oedema, wheezing and conjunctivitis.

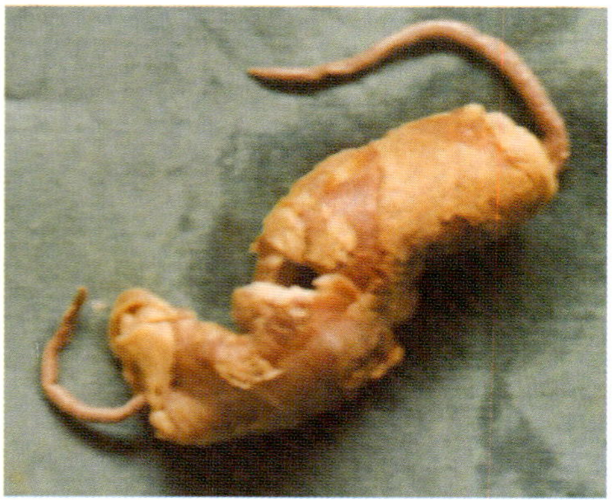

Fig. 11.16. *Ascaris lumbricoides* perforating the wall of small intestine.

Pathogenicity of migrating larvae

In persons repeatedly infected with *Ascaris* and sensitized to the parasite antigens, the migrating larvae may lead to inflammatory and hypersensitivity reactions in the lungs. There is formation of granuloma and eosinophilic infiltrates. It leads to fever, cough, dyspnoea, urticarial rash and eosinophilia. The sputum may be blood-tinged and may contain *Ascaris* larvae and Charcot-Leyden crystals. This condition is known as **Loeffler's syndrome**. Allergic inflammatory reaction to migrating larvae may involve other organs such as liver and kidneys.

If the *Ascaris* larvae pass beyond the pulmonary capillaries and reach the general circulation, they are filtered out to various organs, e.g., brain, spinal cord, heart and kidneys where they set up unusual clinical symptoms. Microorganisms may also be carried by the migrating larvae from the intestine to other tissues.

Larval and adult *A. lumbricoides* secrete allergens which elicit the production of IgE by the host leading to hypersensitivity and histamine release.

Laboratory diagnosis

1. Parasitic diagnosis

- **Demonstration of adult worms:** Worm may be passed through anus, mouth, nose and rarely through ear. Barium meal may occasionally reveal the presence of adult worms in the small intestine.
- **Demonstration of larvae:** *Ascaris* larvae and eosinophils may be detected in the sputum during the stage of migration.
- **Demonstration of both fertilized and unfertilized eggs:** These may be detected by direct microscopy or concentration of the faeces by salt floatation or formalin-ether sedimentation method. However, eggs may not be seen if only male worms are present.

2. Serodiagnosis

Ascaris antibody can be detected by indirect haemagglutination (IHA) and immunofluorescent antibody (IFA) test. These tests are useful for the diagnosis of extraintestinal ascariasis like Loeffler's syndrome.

3. Eosinophilia

It is seen in larval invasion stage.

Treatment

The preferred anthelmintics are mebendazole and albendazole, and the broad-spectrum drug pyrantel pamoate. Cure with any of these drugs can be achieved in nearly 100% of cases. Mebendazole and albendazole are preferred for therapy of asymptomatic to moderate ascariasis but should be used with caution to treat heavy *Ascaris* infections. Use of pyrantel for heavy *Ascaris* infections is recommended because this agent paralyzes the worms prior to their expulsion.

Prophylaxis

Ascariasis can be prevented by:

- Proper disposal of human faeces.
- Avoidance of eating raw vegetables and salads.
- Periodic treatment with an effective anthelmintic, in communities that lack sanitary facilities.

ASCARIS SUUM

Ascaris suum, also known as large roundworm of pigs, is an intestinal parasite of pig.

Geographical distribution

It has worldwide distribution.

Morphology

It is similar in morphology to that of *A. lumbricoides*. It has three prominent lips. Each lip contains a dentigerous ridge and no interlabia or alae.

Male worm

It measures 15–31 cm in length and 2–4 mm in diameter. The posterior end is curved toward the ventral side with pointed tail. It has simple spicules that measure 2.0–3.5 mm long.

Female worm

Female worm is larger than male worm. It measures 20–49 cm in length and 3–6 mm in diameter. Vulva occupies about one-third of the body length on the anterior end. It lays 200,000 eggs daily.

Fertilized eggs

The fertilized eggs are oval, 45–75 μm in length and 35–50 μm in breadth. The mammillated layer is thick, rough and **golden-brown (bile-stained) in colour**.

Unfertilized eggs

Before fertilization by male, female *A. suum* lays unfertilized eggs. These are narrower and longer than fertilized eggs, 88–94 μm in length and 44 μm in breadth.

Life cycle

Eggs laid by female worms pass to external environment in host faeces. Development to the infective stage takes place inside the egg with L2 larva inside the egg and undergoes first moulting within the egg shell. Pigs acquire infection by ingestion of embryonated eggs (eggs with L2 larvae). Rest of the cycle is similar to that of *A. lumbricoides* in man.

Human infection caused by *A. suum* is rare. The infection caused by accidental ingestion of eggs has been reported in the laboratory workers. A case of child infected with *A. suum* has been reported in Great Britain and a case of intestinal obstruction in Zimbabwe.

VISCERAL LARVA MIGRANS

Visceral larva migrans (VLM) is a syndrome caused by ingestion of embryonated eggs of nematodes of animals like *Toxocara canis* (dog roundworm) and *T. cati* (cat roundworm). These eggs are usually found in soil contaminated with dog or cat faeces. Larvae hatch in the small intestine and immediately penetrate the intestinal wall and migrate to liver. They may move onto the lungs or to other parts of the body or remain in the liver. Larva migrans caused by *Toxocara* spp. are widely recognized as zoonotic infections throughout the world. Several other roundworms are occasionally implicated in visceral larva migrans including:

- *Angiostrongylus cantonensis*,
- *Gnathostoma spinigerum*,
- *Anisakis simplex*, and
- *Baylisascaris procyonis*

Wherever the larvae settle, they are attacked by phagocytic cells, consisting mainly of eosinophils, histiocytes and occasionally giant cells leading to the formation of a granulomatous lesion and their progress is arrested. From lungs, like *A. lumbricoides*, they may even migrate through trachea and oesophagus and reach small intestine but, in the human body, they do not convert into adult worms.

Visceral larva migrans is characterized by hypereosinophilia (15–80%) together with hepatomegaly or pneumonitis or both, hypergammaglobulinaemia and fever. The larvae, usually of *T. canis*, may invade the eye (**ocular larva migrans**) producing an eosinophilic granulomatous reaction, usually in the retina, and lead to endophthalmitis.

Visceral larva migrans can be diagnosed by identification of larvae in autopsy or biopsy specimens, and by IHA and IFA test. However, biopsy specimens are usually not recommended.

BAYLISASCARIS PROCYONIS

Baylisascaris procyonis, an intestinal nematode of recoons, completes its life cycle in its host. Humans become accidentally infected when they ingest infective eggs from the environment; typically this occurs in young children playing in the dirt. After ingestion, the eggs hatch and larvae penetrate the gut wall and migrate to a wide variety of tissues (liver, heart, lungs, brain, eyes), and cause **visceral larva migrans** and **ocular larva migrans**, similar to toxocariasis. In contrast to *Toxocara* larvae, *Baylisascaris* larvae continue to grow in the human host.

Tissue damage and the signs and symptoms of baylisascariasis are often severe because of the size of *Baylisascaris* larvae, their tendency to wander widely, and the fact that they do not readily die. *B. procyonis* have a tendency to invade the spinal cord, brain and eye of humans, resulting in permanent neurologic damage, blindness, or death. Examination of tissue biopsies can be extremely helpful if a section of larva is contained. Serologic tests can also be extremely helpful.

FILARIAL NEMATODES

The filarial nematodes are a group of arthropod-borne worms that reside in the subcutaneous tissues, deep connective tissues, lymphatic system, or body cavities of humans. The adult worms measure 80–100 mm × 0.25–0.30 mm. The females are much longer than males. The worm has a simple lipless mouth, small buccal cavity, a cylindrical oesophagus without a bulb, and simple intestine which may be atrophied posteriorly.

The tail of the male worm has no caudal bursa, but carries perianal papillae and unequal spicules. The female worms are viviparous, giving birth to larvae known as **microfilariae** – embryos which develop within thin 'shells' that, in *Wuchereria bancrofti*, *Brugia* spp. and *Loa loa*, are retained as 'sheaths' after the microfilariae are released. Once released by the female worm, microfilariae can be detected in the peripheral blood or cutaneous tissues, depending on the species.

The life cycle of filarial nematodes is passed in two hosts – man and blood-sucking arthropods. The microfilariae complete their development in the arthropod host to produce the infective larval stages. These are then transmitted when the vectors next feed.

With the exception of *Loa loa*, adult filarial worms are rarely seen intact, sometimes only in histological sections (Fig. 11.17). On the other hand, the microfilariae, which appear in the blood, are easily seen and provide a good basis for the identification of the parasite. They measure 180–300 µm in length and 3–10 µm in diameter. They can be differentiated on the basis of size, the presence or absence of a sheath, the distribution of nuclei in the caudal region of the larvae and the periodicity of their appearance in the peripheral blood.

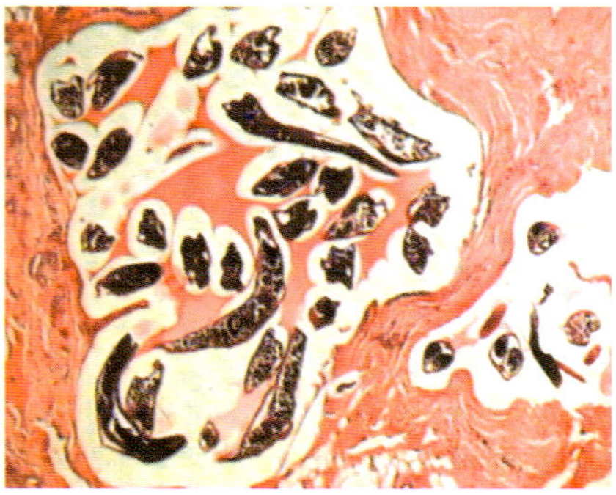

Fig. 11.17. *Wuchereria bancrofti* in lymph node (haematoxylin and eosin stain, × 400).

When largest number of microfilariae occurs in the blood at night, it is known as **nocturnal periodicity**. The microfilariae circulate in the peripheral circulation between 10 pm and 2 am. When largest number of microfilariae occurs in the blood during day, it is known as **diurnal periodicity**. Some species are **non-periodic**. In this case, the microfilariae circulate at somewhat constant levels during the day and night. **Subperiodic** or **nocturnally subperiodic** microfilariae are those that can be detected in the blood throughout the day but are detected at higher levels during the late afternoon or at night.

When not in the peripheral blood the microfilariae are found primarily in capillaries and blood vessels of lungs. The basis of filarial periodicity is unknown, however, it may be an adaptation to the biting habits of the relevant vector. Microfilarial periodicity may be altered by reversing the working and sleeping habits of the host. This reversal may take up to a week to complete. For species exhibiting nocturnal periodicity, it has been noted that the insect vector bites primarily at night, whereas in areas of non-periodic disease, the vector bites mainly during the day. Microfilariae of lymphatic filariasis may also appear in hydrocele fluid and urine.

Filarial nematodes belong to the phylum Nemathelminthes, class Secernentea, superfamily Filarioidea and family Onchocercidae (Table 1.6). Four species commonly cause disease in humans – *W. bancrofti*, *B. malayi*, *L. loa* and *Onchocerca volvulus*. The other four species *Mansonella ozzardi*, *M. perstans*, *M.*

streptocerca and *B. timori* are less important causes of human disease.

W. bancrofti, *B. malayi* and *B. timori* cause lymphatic filariasis. An estimated 300 million people, primarily in India, Southeast Asia, and sub-saharan Africa, live in areas where lymphatic filariasis is endemic, and at least 130 million people are probably currently infected. It is estimated that genital disease is present in 25 million infected men and that lymphoedema, or elephantiasis, of the leg is present in 15 million people, most of whom are women. Approximately 30 million people are exposed to onchocerciasis with probably at least 18 million being infected, 270,000 of whom are blind.

WUCHERERIA BANCROFTI

Common name

Bancroft's filarial worm.

Ancient Egyptian, Hindu, and Persian physicians (600 B.C.) were the first to note elephantiasis, which was probably due to *W. bancrofti*. The larval forms of *W. bancrofti* (microfilariae) were first demonstrated by Demarquay in 1863 in hydrocele fluid of a patient from Cuba and in 1866 Wucherer, in Brazil, first discovered their presence in chylous urine. In 1872 Lewis, in India, found the microfilariae in the peripheral blood. Adult female worms were first reported by Bancroft in Brisbane in 1876, and adult male worms by Sibthorpe in 1888.

Manson in 1878, first demonstrated that *Culex quinquefasciatus* was an intermediate host of *W. bancrofti*. **This was the first demonstration that arthropods could harbour an infective agent.** In 1881, Manson described nocturnal periodicity of *W. bancrofti,* the microfilariae circulating in the peripheral blood at night but then disappearing from the circulation and concentrating in the lungs during the day. The name *Filaria bancrofti* was proposed by Cobbold in 1877, and the generic name *Wuchereria* was given in 1878.

Geographical distribution

It occurs in Asia including India, Africa, Australia, Pacific and South America.

Habitat

Adult male and female worms reside in the lymph nodes and lymphatic vessels of man (Fig. 11.17). The microfilariae are found in blood (Fig. 11.18).

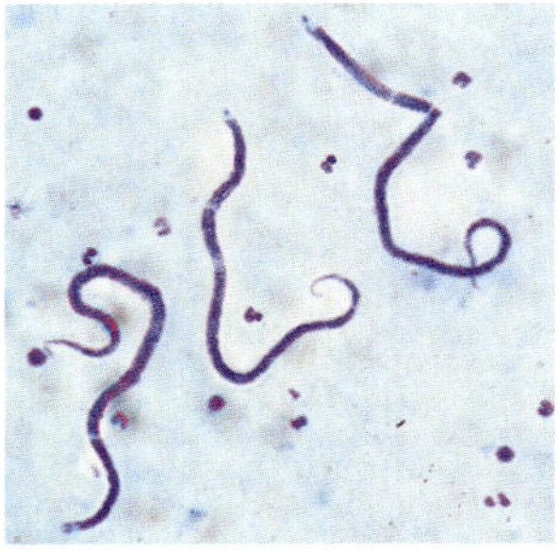

Fig. 11.18. *Microfilaria bancrofti* in peripheral blood (Giemsa stain, × 400).

Occasionally, microfilariae are also found in chylous urine or in hydrocele fluid. Humans are the only known reservoir hosts.

Morphology

Adult worms

Adult worms are transparent, creamy white, long, hair-like structures (Fig. 11.19). They are filiform in shape with both ends tapering. The male and female worms measure 2.5–4 cm × 0.1 mm and 8–10 cm × 0.2–0.3 mm respectively. The posterior end of the female worm is straight, while that of the male is curved ventrally and contains two spicules of unequal length. The spicules serve as organs of copulation. Both male and female worms remain coiled together and it is difficult to separate them. The female is viviparous and liberates sheathed embryos (microfilariae) into lymph from where they find their way into blood.

Microfilaria

It is transparent and colourless with blunt head and pointed tail. It measures 245–295 μm × 7.5–10 μm in size and is covered by a hyaline sheath which is much longer (359 μm) than the microfilaria. It can move forwards and backwards within the sheath. The somatic cells or nuclei appear as granules in the central axis of the microfilaria. At places, these granules are absent. These form the landmarks for recognition of various microfilariae. These are nerve ring, excretory pore and genital cells. At the anterior end there is space, devoid of granules, called the cephalic space. The tail-tip is free from nuclei (Table 11.4, and Figs. 11.18 and 11.20–11.22).

Life cycle

W. bancrofti passes its life cycle in two hosts (Fig. 11.19). Man is the definitive host and the female mosquitoes belonging to the genera *Culex*, *Aedes* and

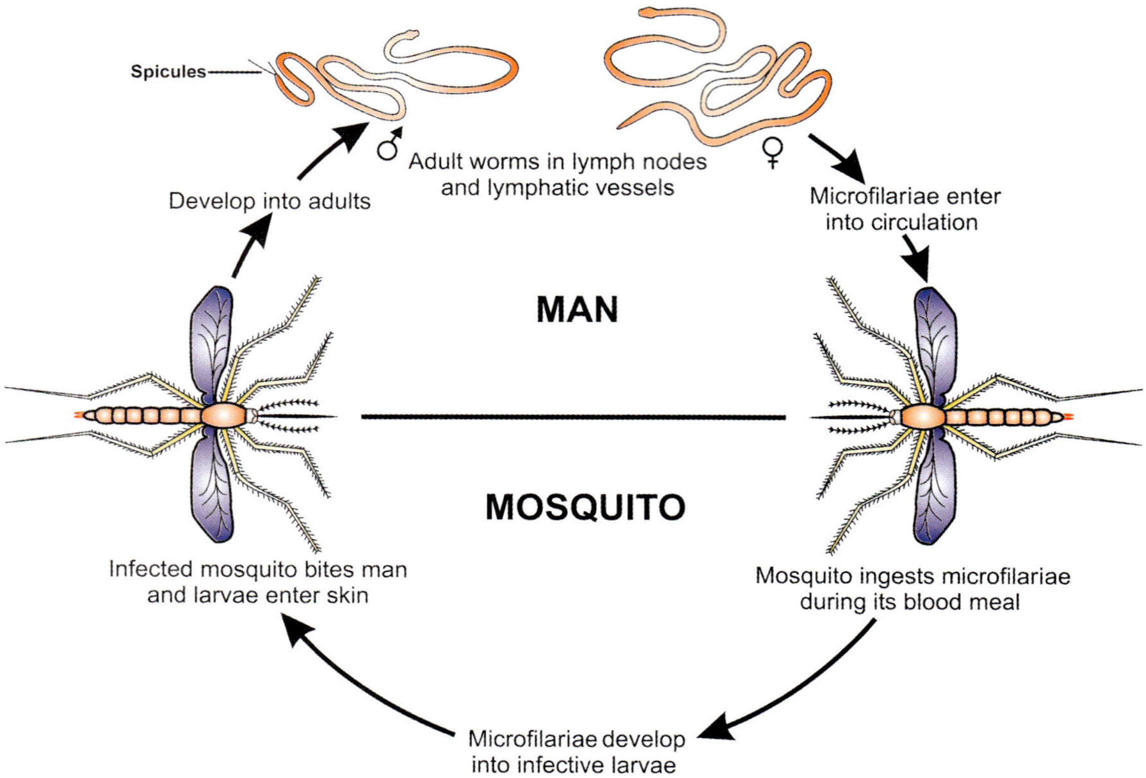

Fig. 11.19. Life cycle of *Wuchereria bancrofti*.

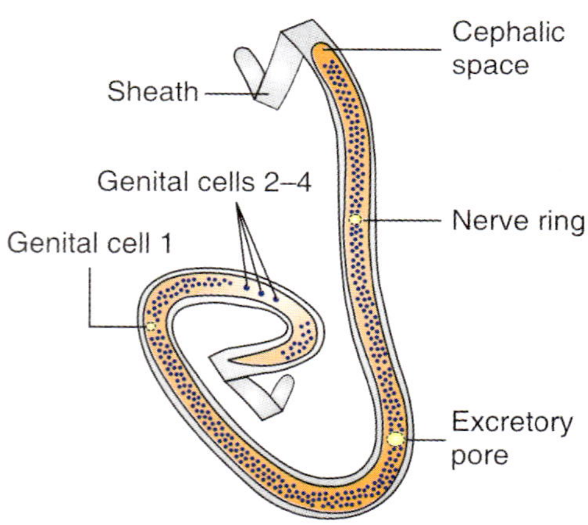

Fig. 11.20. *Microfilaria bancrofti*.

Anopheles act as intermediate hosts. *Culex quinquefasciatus* is the most important vector of *W. bancrofti* being responsible for more than 50% of cases of lymphatic filariasis. In rural areas, *Anopheles* species are the primary vectors often transmitting malaria as well.

Adult worms reside in lymph nodes and lymphatics (usually inguinal, scrotal and abdominal) of man. The lymph provides nutrition to the adult worms. The male fertilizes female and the gravid female gives birth to microfilariae. Through lymphatics, they find their way into general circulation. The appearance of microfilariae in the peripheral blood shows marked periodicity. The microfilariae appear for about 2 hours before and after midnight (10 pm–2 am) and then disappear more or less completely for the rest of the 24 hour period from the peripheral circulation and remain in pulmonary circulation. This correlates with the nocturnal biting habit of the insect vector. The periodicity may also be related to the sleeping habits of the hosts.

In Southeast Asia there are subperiodic forms of *W. bancrofti*, in which, although microfilariae are present throughout the 24 hour period, numbers in the blood are elevated at night. In Pacific areas like Polynesia and the Philippines a non-periodic or slightly diurnally periodic form is present in which microfilariae are present in the peripheral blood more or less constantly throughout much of the 24 hour period.

Sheathed microfilariae are ingested by the mosquito during its blood meal and reach the stomach of the mosquito. They cast off their sheaths in 2–6 hours, penetrate the stomach wall and in the course of 4–17

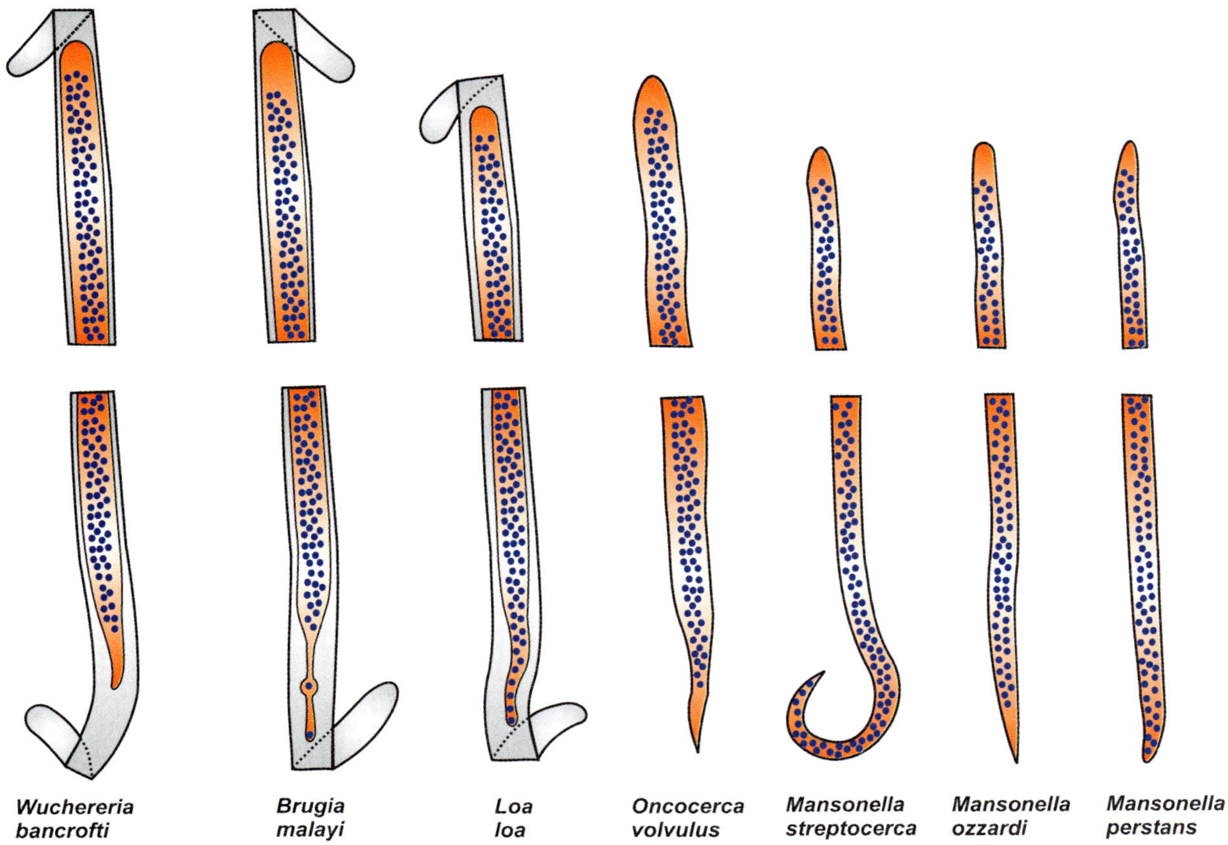

Fig. 11.21. Microfilariae.

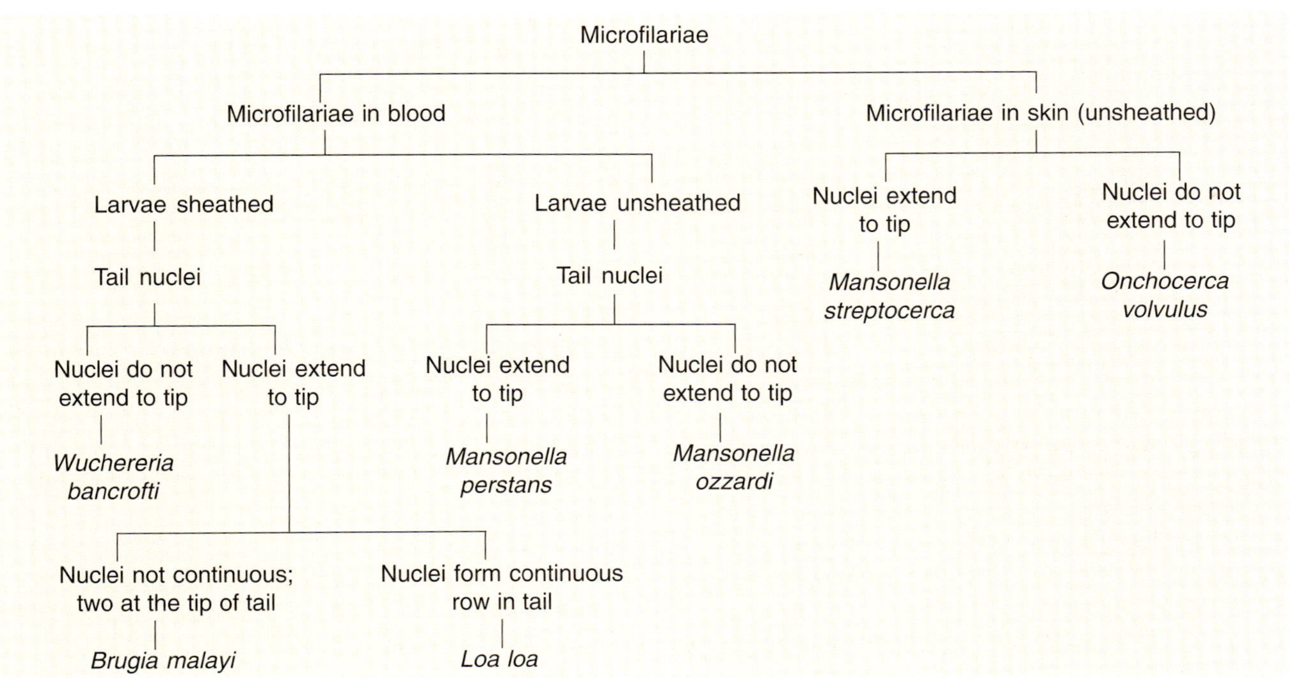

Fig. 11.22. Differential characters of microfilariae.

Table 11.4. Filarial nematodes infecting man

Parasite	Location in the body: Adult	Location in the body: Microfilaria	Periodicity of microfilaria	Characteristics of microfilaria	Vector
LYMPHATIC FILARIASIS					
Wuchereria bancrofti	Lymphatics	Blood	Nocturnal	Sheathed, the tail-tip is free from nuclei	*Culex, Anopheles, Aedes*
Brugia malayi	Lymphatics	Blood	Nocturnal	Sheathed, two discrete nuclei, one at the extreme tip of the tail and the other midway between the tip and the posterior column of nuclei	*Mansonia, Anopheles, Aedes*
Brugia timori	Lymphatics	Blood	Nocturnal	Sheathed, longer than that of *Microfilaria malayi*; the sheath of *Mf. timori* fails to take Giemsa stain	*Anopheles*
SUBCUTANEOUS FILARIASIS					
Loa loa	Subcutaneous connective tissue, subconjunctival tissue	Blood	Diurnal	Sheathed, nuclei up to the tail-tip	*Chrysops*
Onchocerca volvulus	Subcutaneous connective tissue	Skin	Non-periodic	Unsheathed, the tail-tip is free from nuclei	*Simulium*
Mansonella streptocerca	Dermis	Skin	Non-periodic	Unsheathed, the tail-end is bent in a crook-like curve and the column of nuclei extends to the tail-tip	*Culicoides*
SEROUS CAVITY FILARIASIS					
Mansonella ozzardi	Body cavities	Blood	Non-periodic	Unsheathed, the tail-end is sharply pointed and the column of nuclei does not extend to the tail-tip	*Culicoides*
Mansonella perstans	Body cavities	Blood	Non-periodic	Unsheathed, the tail-end is blunt and the nuclei extend to the tail-tip	*Culicoides*

hours reach thoracic muscles. In next 2 days they metamorphose into short, sausage-shaped organisms with a short spiky tail measuring 124–250 µm in length × 10–17 µm in diameter (the first-stage or L1 larvae).

In 3–7 days' time, they moult once or twice to become second-stage or L2 larvae measuring 225–300 µm in length × 15–30 µm in diameter. On the 10th or 11th day the metamorphosis become complete, the tail atrophies to a mere stump and the digestive system, body cavity and genital organs are fully developed. These are the third-stage or L3 larvae and are infective. They measure 1,400–2,000 µm in length × 18–23 µm in diameter and have three subterminal caudal papillae. These larvae then migrate from thoracic muscles to the proboscis sheath of the mosquito. In mosquitoes, microfilariae do not multiply to increase in numbers; instead give rise to infective larvae, each microfilaria developing into one infective third-stage or L3 larva.

When the infected mosquito bites a human being, the L3 larvae, in its proboscis, are deposited on the skin near the site of puncture. They then either enter through the puncture wound or penetrate through the skin on their own. Thereafter, they enter into lymphatics and settle down usually in inguinal, scrotal and abdominal lymph nodes, where they develop into adult worms. In one year or more they become sexually mature. Male fertilizes female, the gravid female gives birth to microfilariae and the cycle is repeated.

Pathogenicity

Infection caused by *W. bancrofti* is known as **wuchereriasis** or **bancroftian filariasis**. It is mainly due to the presence of adult worms in the lymph nodes and vessels. The lymph nodes become enlarged, firm and fibrotic. Microscopically, lymph nodes show the presence of many lymphocytes, plasma cells, polymorphs, eosinophils and there may be foci of necrosis. Sections of adult worms can be seen in the subcapsular sinuses or the lumen of the lymphatic vessels. In chronic disease the nodes and vessels may contain dead worms surrounded by fibrotic and eventually calcified tissues (Fig. 11.17).

Mechanical irritation caused by the movement of adult parasites inside the lymphatic system, liberation of metabolites by growing larvae, absorption of toxic products from dead worms and secondary bacterial infection leads to lymphangitis with swelling, redness, and pain. Because of the chronic inflammation, the lymph valves proximal to the worm become damaged and incompetent. Permeability of the walls of the lymphatics increases, which permits the leakage of fluid with high concentration of protein into the surrounding tissue. Lymphatic obstruction may result from mechanical blocking of the lumen by dead worms, obliterative endolymphangitis, obliterative excessive fibrosis of the lymphatic vessels and fibrosis of afferent lymph nodes draining particular area.

Repeated leakage of lymph into tissues results first in lymphoedema, then to **elephantiasis** of one or more limbs, breasts, penis, scrotum (Fig. 11.23) or vulva (Fig. 11.24) in which there is non-pitting oedema with growth of new adventitious tissue and thickened skin, often also with later verrucous growths and secondary bacterial and fungal infections.

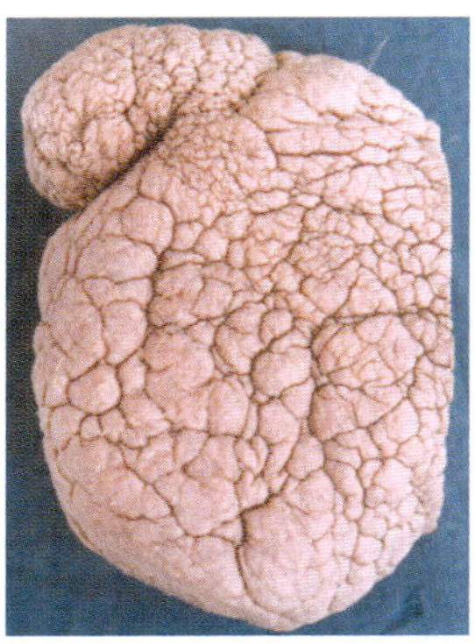

Fig. 11.23. Elephantiasis penis and scrotum.

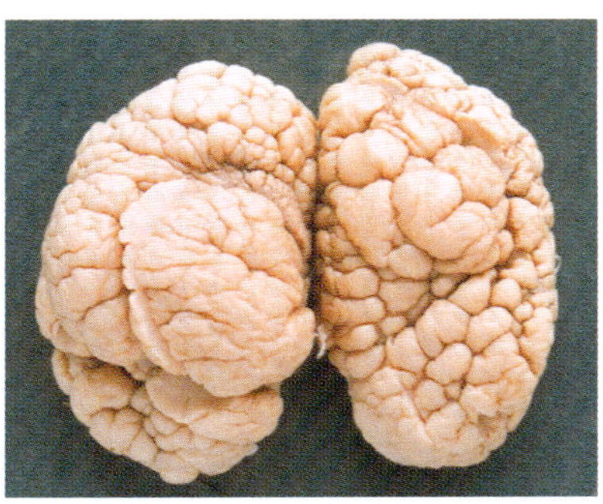

Fig. 11.24. Elephantiasis vulva.

In males, hydrocele, orchitis, funiculitis and epididymitis are common. The development of lymph scrotum results in chyluria, with lymph getting into the urine. In some parts of the world, hydrocele is very common. In East Africa, it occurs in up to 50% of infected males. Dilatation of lymph vessels (lymphangiovarices) commonly occurs in the inguinal, scrotal, testicular and abdominal sites. Rupture of lymph varices leads to the release of lymph or chyle. Depending on the site, it may lead to lymph scrotum, chyluria, chylous diarrhoea, chylous ascites and chylothorax.

The biological incubation or prepatent period in areas of endemic filariasis lasts 1 year or more. This is the period from the entry of the third-stage or L3 infective larvae into the skin until microfilariae first appear in peripheral blood. In many patients, acute attacks of 'filarial fever' ensue in a matter of a few months to many years after patency. Patient develops intermittent recurrent fever lasting 3–15 days, with headache, malaise, localized pain and tenderness with oedema and erythema above lymph vessels and glands, accompanied by acute lymphangitis and lymphadenitis of the groin or axilla. Examination of blood often shows high eosinophilia.

Occult filariasis

This is a **hypersensitivity reaction to microfilarial antigens**. Patient develops massive eosinophilia (30–80%; absolute count more than 3,000/μl), generalized lymph node enlargement, hepatosplenomegaly and pulmonary symptoms. The adult worm produces the microfilariae continuously but they do not reach the peripheral blood because they are destroyed in the tissues. In the affected organs, eosinophil granulomas develop in which a large number of eosinophils aggregate around a microfilaria or its remnants.

Tropical pulmonary eosinophilia (TPE)

This is a manifestation of occult filariasis characterized by malaise, fever, weight loss and respiratory symptoms such as dry nocturnal cough, dyspnoea and asthmatic wheezing with a marked increase in blood eosinophil counts of over 3,000/μl. Chest radiography shows increased bronchovascular markings or diffuse miliary "mottling" in the lung fields. It occurs in children and adults in areas of endemic filariasis including the Indian subcontinent, Southeast Asia, and South Pacific Islands, but imported cases in temperate climates are being recognized with increasing frequency.

TPE is associated with marked increase in total serum IgE and antibodies to filaria are of high titre. The disease is a hypersensitivity reaction to microfilariae. It is associated with *W. bancrofti* and *Brugia malayi* infections, and the disease responds to treatment with diethylcarbamazine that acts on microfilariae. Microfilariae are not usually detectable in blood, but lung biopsies have shown microfilariae in some cases.

Laboratory diagnosis

Bancroftian filariasis can be diagnosed by:

Detection of microfilariae

Microfilariae of *W. bancrofti* circulate in the peripheral blood with a regular nocturnal periodicity. Therefore, to diagnose bancroftian filariasis, blood must be taken during night, optimally between 10 pm and 2 am. In adults blood should be obtained from the ear or finger and in infants from the heels.

Microscopy of stained blood film

Thin and thick smears are prepared. The thick smear is dehaemoglobinized and both the smears are stained with Leishman or Giemsa stain. The smears are then examined under microscope for the presence of characteristic microfilariae (Fig. 11.18).

W. bancrofti, as well as *B. malayi* and *Loa loa*, demonstrate a sheath on their microfilariae. This is the first step in identifying the specific types of filariasis. Further identification is based on study of head and tail structures (Table 11.4 and Figs. 11.21 and 11.22). Clinically, an exact species identification is not critical, because treatment for all the filarial infections, except that caused by *O. volovulus*, is identical.

Direct wet mount

- Microfilariae can also be seen in microscopic mounts of anticoagulated blood by their undulating motion, displacing the red blood cells from side to side as they move.
- Acridine orange-microhaematocrit tube technique can also be used for the detection of microfilariae. A microhaematocrit tube incorporating heparin, EDTA, and acridine orange serves the basis for this test. After centrifugation, parasites become concentrated in the buffy coat and can be visualized through the clear glass wall of the tube. The acridine orange stains the DNA of the parasites, and the morphologic characteristics, including the nuclear patterns in the tail sections, can be examined by fluorescence microscopy in making a species identification.

Concentration methods

- **Knott concentration method:** 2 ml of blood is thoroughly mixed with 10 ml of 2% solution of formalin and allowed to stand for 10 minutes or longer. It is then centrifuged at 200 *g* for 2 minutes and the sediment is examined microscopically for microfilariae.
- **Membrane filtration method:** The presence of small numbers of microfilariae in blood can be detected by a membrane-filtration technique in which anticoagulated blood is mixed with saline, and forced through a 5-µm membrane filter. After several washes with saline or distilled water, the filter is examined microscopically for living microfilariae, or it is dried, fixed, and stained with Leishman or Giemsa stain and examined microscopically for microfilariae.

Diethylcarbamazine provocation test

In areas where microfilaraemia is nocturnal or is present throughout the day but at low levels, microfilariae may be induced to appear in the blood during the day by giving diethylcarbamazine in a single dose of 2 mg per kg body weight. Usually, peak numbers are reported to occur 15–20 minutes after administration of the drug.

Urine, exudate of lymph varix and hydrocele fluid microscopy

Microfilariae may also be demonstrated in the centrifuged deposits of chylous urine, exudate of lymph varix and in the hydrocele fluid.

Detection of adult worms

Adult worms can be seen in the biopsied lymph node (Fig. 11.17) and the calcified worm may be seen on X-ray examination.

Immunodiagnosis

- Filarial antigen may be detected in the patient serum by enzyme immunoassays using monoclonal antibodies against microfilarial larval surface antigens. However, because antigen shedding may be irregular, particularly during times when circulating microfilariae may not be detected, detection of antibody to larval antigens may be more appropriate.
- Antibodies may be detected by indirect haemagglutination assay, indirect fluorescent antibody test, enzyme-linked immunosorbent assay and radioimmunoassay.

Molecular diagnosis

Polymerase chain reaction is available for *W. bancrofti* and *B. malayi*. This may be used for the diagnosis of infection caused by these parasites.

Treatment

Diethylcarbamazine (DEC) is the drug of choice for the treatment of bancroftian filariasis. It is given orally in a dose of 6 mg/kg body weight daily in divided doses for 12 days. It kills microfilariae but its action on adult worms is much less dramatic.

Prophylaxis

- Bancroftian filariasis can be prevented by control of vectors by spraying residual insecticides such as DDT, malathion, etc. onto common resting sites. A difficulty in this approach has been that many vector species have become resistant to the available insecticides. Insecticides can be effectively used against larval stages.
- A film of oil may be sprayed over water surfaces.
- Larvivorous fish may be added to the ponds.
- Open drains, septic tanks, soakage pits and flood pit laterines should be adequately maintained.
- All at-risk individuals should be treated once yearly with an oral 2-drug combination. For most countries, the WHO recommends DEC for its micro- and macrofilarial effect in combination with albendazole to enhance macrofilaricidal activity.

BRUGIA MALAYI

Common name

Malayan filaria.

Brugia malayi was first observed by Lichtenstein in its microfilaria stage in blood films of natives of northern Sumatra. Brug (1927) described it as a new species. Adult males and females were first described by Rao and Maplestone (1940) from human material from India.

Geographical distribution

B. malayi is prevalent in India, the Far East and Southeast Asia. In India it has been chiefly reported from Kerala, Assam, Orissa, West Bengal and Madhya Pradesh. *W. bancrofti* and *B. malayi* may co-exist at one place.

Habitat

As in case of *W. bancrofti*, adult male and female *B. malayi* reside in the lymph nodes and lymphatic vessels, and the microfilariae in the blood of man.

Morphology

Adult worms

The adult worms of *B. malayi* bear a general resemblance to those of *W. bancrofti*, though smaller in size. Mature females vary from 43–55 mm in length and 130–170 μm in breadth. Mature males vary from 13–23 mm in length and 70–80 μm in breadth.

Microfilariae

Microfilaria malayi is enveloped. Like *Mf. bancrofti* the sheath extends beyond the anterior and posterior ends of the larvae. As compared to *Mf. bancrofti*, it is smaller in size measuring 177–230 μm in length and 6 μm in diameter. It possesses secondary kinks, its cephalic space is longer, it carries double stylets at the anterior end, and its nuclear column appears blurred in Giemsa stained films.

Tail-tip of *Mf. malayi* is not free from nuclei. There are two discrete nuclei, one at the extreme tip of the tail and the other midway between the tip and the posterior column of nuclei (Table 11.4 and Figs. 11.21 and 11.22). Microfilariae of *B. malayi*, like those of *W. bancrofti*, are also released into the blood stream with nocturnal periodicity. Subperiodic forms also exist in *B. malayi*.

Life cycle

The life cycle of *B. malayi* is similar to that of *W. bancrofti*, however, the intermediate hosts of *B. malayi* are mosquitoes of the genera *Mansonia*, *Anopheles* and *Aedes*. The intermediate hosts in India are *M. annulifera*, *M. indiana*, *M. uniformis* and *Anopheles barbirostris*. Larval development of *B. malayi*, in the mosquito, is completed in 6–8 days and adult mature females develop in lymph vessels of man in about 7 months.

Pathogenicity

B. malayi causes brugian filariasis. The course of brugian filariasis is similar to that of bancroftian filariasis but elephantiasis, when it occurs, is usually restricted to the legs and there is no chyluria and involvement of male genitalia. Like *W. bancrofti*, it may also cause tropical pulmonary eosinophilia.

Laboratory diagnosis

As in case of bancroftian filariasis, the diagnosis of brugian filariasis can be made by the demonstration of microfilariae and adult worms of *B. malayi*. DNA probes and PCR for *B. malayi* have also been developed.

Treatment

Same as that of bancroftian filariasis.

Prophylaxis

Preventive measures of brugian filariasis are similar to those of bancroftian filariasis. Larval *Mansonia* vectors obtain oxygen from the roots of underwater aquatic plants, such as water lettuce (*Pistia stratioides*). In Sri Lanka and southern India, where *M. annulifera* is the chief vector of *B. malayi*, the transmission of this parasite has been effectively reduced by removal of these water plants. Herbicides have also been employed successfully to kill aquatic plants.

BRUGIA TIMORI

Common name

The Timor filaria.

Brugia timori was first recognized as distinct from *B. malayi* by David and Edeson (1965) from island of Timor at the eastern end of the Indonesian Archipelago. The adult worms were obtained from experimentally infected Mongolian jirds and described by Partono and associates in 1977.

Morphology

Adult worms

The adult worms inhabit the lymphatics of man. The adult male measures 2 cm in length and 70 µm in breadth. The females are longer and measure 3 cm in length and 100 µm in breadth. The anterior end of both male and female worms is expanded into a bulb-like head. The tail is long, tapered, and smoothly rounded.

Microfilariae

The microfilariae of *B. timori* like those of *W. bancrofti* and *B. malayi* show nocturnal periodicity and are ensheathed. The sheath in the microfilariae of all these parasites extends beyond the anterior and posterior ends of the larvae. The microfilariae of *B. timori* can be differentiated from those of *B. malayi* by:

- failure of the sheath to stain with Giemsa,
- the long cephalic space,
- longer in size (average size 310 µm × 6 µm), and
- greater number (5–8) of contiguous nuclei in the tail and smaller nuclei in the distal portion of the tail.

Life cycle

Man is the only definitive host and the intermediate host is *Anopheles barbirostris*, which breeds in rice fields and feeds at night. *B. timori* is limited in its distribution to the Lesser Sunda Islands in the Indonesian Archipelago extending from Wallaces line on the west to Weber's line beyond Timor on the east.

Pathogenicity

The lesions caused by *B. timori* are few and mild. It causes lymphadenitis, lymphangitis and elephantiasis which is confined to oedema of the legs below the knee. The laboratory diagnosis, treatment and preventive measures for the prophylaxis of *B. timori* infection are similar to those for *B. malayi* infection.

LOA LOA

Common name

The eye worm

Loa loa was first noted in the eye of a Negro girl in West Indies in 1770. In 1895, Argyll–Robertson described the adult worms that he extracted from the eye of a woman who had resided at Old Calabar in West Africa.

Geographical distribution

This worm is restricted in distribution to central and western parts of tropical Africa. Sporadic cases have been reported from other parts of the world including India.

Habitat

The adult worms live in subcutaneous connective tissues of man. They may also occur in the subconjunctival tissue though a few cases have been reported from India with worm in the anterior chamber of the eye. For this reason, *L. loa* is known as the **eye worm**. The sheathed microfilariae are found in the blood.

Morphology

Adult worms

Adult worms are thin, whitish and taper somewhat towards the cephalic end. Male measures 30–34 mm × 0.35–0.43 mm and female, 40–70 mm × 0.5 mm. The caudal end of the male is curved ventrally and is provided with narrow alae. The vulva in female opens in the cervical region.

Microfilariae

Microfilariae of *L. loa* resemble those of *W. bancrofti*, *B. malayi* and *B. timori* except that the column of nuclei extends completely to the tip of the tail (Table 11.4 and Figs. 11.21 and 11.22). The sheath in the microfilariae of all these parasites extends beyond the anterior and posterior ends of the larvae. *Mf. loa* measures 250–300 μm in length and 6–8 μm in breadth. Because the sheath stains poorly in ordinary blood films, it may be overlooked. It has a diurnal periodicity, number of microfilariae peaking at about midday. On the other hand *Mf. bancrofti*, *Mf. malayi* and *Mf. timori* show nocturnal periodicity.

Life cycle

L. loa passes its life cycle in two hosts – man and day-biting female mango fly (*Chrysops dimidiata*, *C. silacea* and other species). Man acquires infection by the bite of infected female *Chrysops*. The infective larvae enter in large numbers through the punctured wound on the skin made by the vector during the blood meal. The larvae enter the subcutaneous tissue, moult and develop to mature adult worms. Development into adult worms takes about 6–12 months and they can survive up to 17 years. Female worms produce microfilariae which circulate in the peripheral blood during the day time and are also found in the subcutaneous tissue. The optimum site for the microfilariae during their non-circulation phase is the lungs.

Sheathed microfilariae are ingested by female *Chrysops* during its blood meal. They cast off their sheaths, penetrate the stomach wall and reach thoracic muscles where they develop into the infective larvae. Development in *Chrysops* is completed in about 10 days. The mature infective larvae then migrate to the mouth parts of *Chrysops* for transmission to human hosts during their next blood meal.

Pathogenicity

L. loa produces the disease in man called **loiasis**. The adult worms live in subcutaneous connective tissues and wander round the body causing, usually painless, oedematous swellings known as **fugitive** or **Calabar swellings**. The swellings measure 5–10 cm in diameter and last for a few hours to a few days and reappear elsewhere. They may occur anywhere on the body but are most common on the back of the hand or arm. These are hypersensitivity reactions, probably to excretory products of the adults or perhaps to the microfilariae, and sometimes are accompanied by itching, erythema, fever and generalized pruritus. There is usually also a very high eosinophilia.

Sometimes adult worms may **wander slowly across the conjunctiva**, causing some discomfort and oedema of the eyelid. In addition, it may cause **granulomata in the bulbar conjunctiva**, and proptosis. The conjunctival granulomata present as solitary or multiple small yellow nodules about 2 mm in diameter. They are in the deep layers of the conjunctiva close to the episcleral tissue.

Laboratory diagnosis

Loiasis may be suggested by the presence of fugitive swellings in association with high eosinophilia. However, the specific diagnosis is made by identification of the microfilariae in peripheral blood during the day. Microfilariae are inconsistently shed by the females; therefore, multiple samples over a period of days may need to be tested.

Microfilariae exhibit diurnal periodicity; therefore, blood samples should be collected during daytime, preferably between 10 am and 2 pm. Demonstration of the sheathed microfilariae with nuclei extending to the tip of the tail is sufficient for the diagnosis.

The infection can also be diagnosed by detection or removal of adults from the eye or Calabar swellings.

Treatment

Loiasis can be treated by surgical removal of the adult worms. The most favourable time is when the worms are migrating through the bridge of the nose or through conjunctiva. Diethylcarbamazine is the drug of choice. It kills both microfilariae and adults of *L. loa* when given at 2–6 mg/kg body weight daily for 2–4 weeks. Glucocorticoids may be administered to ameliorate post-treatment acute reactions.

Prophylaxis

Loiasis can be prevented by:

- Protection from *Chrysops* bites in endemic areas by application of repellents to exposed skin.
- Destructive campaigns against *Chrysops*.
- Detection and treatment of infected individuals with diethylcarbamazine.

ONCHOCERCA VOLVULUS

Common name: The convoluted filaria.

Onchocerca volvulus microfilariae were first found by O'Neal in 1875, and the adult worms were described by Leuckart in 1893 in nodules removed from the scalp and chest of a West African native. **It is the leading cause of blindness in the world.**

Geographical distribution

This filarial worm is common in parts of tropical Africa and Central America.

Habitat

Adult worms are located in nodules in the subcutaneous tissue of man.

Morphology

Adult worms

Adult worms are white, opalescent and transparent with transverse striations on the cuticula. Male measures 1.9–4.2 cm in length × 0.13–0.21 mm in diameter and has a coiled tail. The female is much longer, measuring 33.5–50 cm in length × 0.27–0.40 mm in diameter.

Microfilariae

Microfilariae are unsheathed, non-periodic and measure 220–360 μm in length by 5–9 μm in diameter. The column of nuclei does not extend to the tail-tip (Table 11.4 and Figs. 11.21 and 11.22). Microfilariae are normally found in dermis and rarely in the blood, sputum, or urine.

Life cycle

O. volvulus completes its life cycle in two hosts. Man is the definitive host and day-biting female blackfly of the genus *Simulium* is the intermediate host. The fly has its main habitat in the underbrush lining the banks of fast-moving streams. Humans become infected by the bite of blackfly, which possesses in its mouth parts the infective third-stage larvae. The larvae enter the skin through the punctured wound and migrate to the subcutaneous tissue in which they moult twice and develop into male and female adult worms. The adult worms become encased in fibrous subcutaneous nodules within which they may remain viable for as long as 15 years. The female worm, after fertilization by the male, begins producing as many as 2000 actively motile, unsheathed microfilariae each day. The microfilariae exit out of the nodule and migrate to the skin, the eye, and other body tissues.

When a blackfly again bites a diseased human at one of the infected sites, the microfilariae are taken up with the blood meal. They migrate from the gut of the vector into the thoracic muscles. Here they moult twice and develop into infective larvae over a period of 6–8 days. These larvae then migrate to the mouth parts of the blackfly where they may be transmitted to humans at the next blood meal. The cycle is thus repeated.

Pathogenicity

O. volvulus produces **onchocerciasis** in man. The disease is also known as **river blindness** because invasion of the eye can lead to loss of vision. It is a major health and socioeconomic problem, especially in endemic areas in Africa. Adult worms develop in the subcutaneous tissue often encapsulated in dense fibrous nodules ranging from 5 to 25 mm in diameter. These nodules tend to occur over anatomic sites where the bone is superficial, such as knees, hips, iliac crests, trochanters, sacrum, ribs, scapulae, elbows and scalp. The nodules are fully movable, but they may be attached to the periosteum, deep fascia or skin. The microfilariae live in the superficial layers of the skin causing itching and, in heavy, chronic infections, gross thickening of skin.

Although the microfilariae may remain localized to the site of infection, they may wander through the adjacent skin and reach other tissues, including the eye, which may cause corneal and retinal lesions that lead to blindness. Ocular lesions are a result of the host immune response to the microfilariae. Circulating antibodies to retinal antigens have been found in patients with onchocercal retinopathy. Because of the association of the vector with rivers, the condition is known as river blindness.

Laboratory diagnosis

The diagnosis of onchocerciasis can be made by:

1. Demonstration of adult worms

These can be demonstrated inside the excised nodule. At times, the nodules may be inhabited only by females or males or by dead worms. In such cases no microfilariae can be demonstrated.

2. Demonstration of microfilariae

These can be demonstrated in skin snips. Two to six skin snips are taken from iliac crests, buttocks, calves and shoulders. The skin is cleaned with spirit and allowed to dry before a piece of skin 2–3 mm in diameter and 0.5–1 mm deep is taken. The skin is raised with a needle and the tip sliced off with a razor blade. Biopsy specimens are placed in normal saline or distilled water on a slide or in the well of a microtitre plate for 60 minutes and are examined for microfilariae that migrate from the tissue. If no microfilariae are seen, the preparation should be left overnight and re-examined for the microfilariae. Live microfilariae can be seen moving vigorously in the medium by direct microscopy. They can be distinguished from other species of microfilariae after staining with Giemsa or Mayer's haemalum.

Slit lamp examination

In patients with ocular manifestations, live microfilariae may be demonstrated in the substantia propria of the cornea and in the anterior chamber of the eye by slit lamp examination. Rarely, the microfilariae may be found in the peripheral blood.

Diethylcarbamazine provocation test

A provocative test (**Mazzotti test**) can also be done. A single oral dose of 50 mg diethylcarbamazine is given to the patient. The development of pruritus and rash within 24 hours suggests the presence of cutaneous microfilariae.

3. Serological tests

Serological diagnosis can be made by the detection of circulating antigen or by the detection of specific antibodies to the parasites. Tests based on the detection of circulating antigen are more desirable as they define the current infection status of an individual. ELISA detects antibodies against onchocercal microfilarial antigens. However, main limitations of the test is that it cannot distinguish past and current infections.

4. Polymerase chain reaction

Parasitic genome of *O. volvulus* can be detected by polymerase chain reaction (PCR) in skin snip specimens. In comparison to skin snip tests PCR is more sensitive in patients with low-level infections.

Treatment

Treatment consists of surgical removal of detectable nodules (nodulectomy). It is simple, easy to perform and produces immediate results. Ivermectin is the drug of choice for control and treatment of onchocerciasis. DEC is no longer recommended because ivermectin produces far milder systemic reactions and few, if any, ocular complications. Although suramin kills adult *O. volvulus* worms, treatment with this relatively toxic agent is generally not advised.

Prophylaxis

Onchocerciasis can be prevented by application of insecticides to the streams where the vector *Simulium* is breeding. Mass chemotherapy as a control measure is not recommended because the available drugs produce severe side effects.

MANSONELLA STREPTOCERCA

Mansonella streptocerca occurs primarily in Africa, especially in the Congo basin.

Habitat

The adult worms live in the dermis, usually less than 1 mm below the skin surface.

Morphology

Adult worms

The adult male measures 17–18 mm × 0.4 mm and the adult female measures 25–27 mm × 0.6–0.8 mm.

Microfilariae

The microfilariae measure 180–240 μm × 5 μm and are unsheathed. The tail-end is bent in a crook-like curve and the column of nuclei extends to the tail-tip (Table 11.4 and Figs. 11.21 and 11.22). They are non-periodic. The microfilariae are found in the skin, where they can be ingested by *Culicoides* spp. (midges), the insect vectors.

Life cycle

During a blood meal, an infected midge (*Culicoides* spp.) deposits third-stage filarial larvae onto the skin of the human host, where they penetrate into the bite wound. They develop into adults in the dermis most commonly less than 1 mm from the skin surface. Adult females produce unsheathed non-periodic microfilariae which reside in the skin but can also reach the peripheral blood.

A midge ingests the microfilariae during a blood meal. After ingestion, the microfilariae migrate from the midge's midgut through the hemocoel to the thoracic muscles. There the microfilariae develop into first-stage larvae and subsequently into third-stage larvae. The third-stage larvae migrate to the midge's proboscis and can infect another human when the midge takes another blood meal.

Pathogenicity

Microfilariae of *M. streptocerca* which are found in the skin cause **streptocerciasis**. It is characterized by oedema and thickening of the skin, hypopigmented macules, pruritus and papules mimicking mild onchocerciasis or leprosy. Hypopigmented macules do not tend to occur in onchocerciasis, whereas iridocyclitis and subcutaneous nodules seen in onchocerciasis are not features of streptocerciasis.

Laboratory diagnosis

Diagnosis of the condition is made by demonstration and identification of characteristic microfilariae in the skin snips. These should be differentiated from those of *O. volvulus*.

Treatment

Diethylcarbamazine administered as in treatment of bancroftian filariasis is effective in streptocerciasis.

MANSONELLA OZZARDI

Mansonella ozzardi occurs in West Indies, and Central and South America.

The infection was first noted by Ozzard in an Indian in South America and was described by Manson in 1897. Humans are the only known natural definitive hosts. The **adult female** measures 65–81 mm × 0.21–0.25 mm. **Adult male** measures about half the size of female. It has a smooth surface with a coiled tail. The tail contains single spicule. **Microfilariae** are small (150–200 µm × 4.5 µm), unsheathed and non-periodic. The tail-end is sharply pointed and the column of nuclei does not extend to the tail-tip (Table 11.4 and Figs. 11.21 and 11.22).

Adult male and female worms live in the subcutaneous and connective tissues, and the microfilariae are found in the blood, where they can be ingested by *Culicoides* spp. (midges) or *Simulium* spp. (blackflies), the insect vectors.

M. ozzardi infections have been associated with cutaneous itching, pruritus, articular pains, subcutaneous inflammation, enlarged inguinal lymph nodes and vague abdominal symptoms, accompanied by high eosinophilia.

Diagnosis is made by demonstration of unsheathed, non-periodic microfilariae in the blood and also in skin snips.

MANSONELLA PERSTANS

Mansonella perstans occurs in tropical Africa, and Central and South America.

Adult worms reside in body cavities, most commonly in the peritoneal cavity next in pleural cavity, and rarely in the pericardium. The adult male measures about 45 mm × 60 µm and the female, 70–80 mm × 120 µm. The microfilariae are found in the blood. They are unsheathed, non-periodic and measure 200 µm × 4.5 µm. The tail-end is blunt and the nuclei extend to the tail-tip (Table 11.4 and Figs. 11.21 and 11.22). The insect vector is *Culicoides* spp. (midges). Humans acquire infection by the bite of these mosquitoes.

Live adults appear to produce little or no host reaction; however, eosinophilia is common. Pruritus, abdominal pain, urticaria and Calabar-like swellings on the arms, shoulders, and face have been described.

Recovery of the characteristic microfilariae from peripheral blood provides a diagnosis.

DIROFILARIA

Genus *Dirofilaria* includes *D. immitis*, *D. repens*, *D. tenuis* and *D. ursi*. These are common parasites of dog, cat and raccoon. They can cause occasional zoonotic infections in man.

DIROFILARIA IMMITIS

D. immitis (dog heartworm) is a common parasite of dogs in the tropical, subtropical and warm temperate regions of the world. Human cases have been reported from the USA, Japan, Australia, Brazil and New Zealand.

The adult worms inhabit the right heart and large blood vessels joining it, in dog. The female measures 25–30 cm in length and about 1 mm in width. The male is smaller and measures 12–18 cm in length. Microfilariae are unsheathed, 300–325 µm in length and about 7 µm in width. They are found in the blood, where they are ingested by mosquitoes.

Dog is the definitive host and the mosquitoes are the intermediate hosts. The infective larval forms, from the proboscis of the mosquito, are injected into the subcutaneous tissue of the dog by the bite of the mosquito. The larvae enter into the circulation and ultimately find their way to the heart, where they develop into adults. The diagnosis in dogs may be made by observing circulating microfilariae in the peripheral blood.

When humans, as accidental hosts, are bitten by infected mosquitoes the larvae are incapable of completing their life cycle because they are in the wrong host. They lodge and obstruct pulmonary arterioles and develop into local granulomatous nodules. Occasionally, they may reach sufficient size to be diagnosed as "**coin lesions**" radiologically. Microfilariae do not circulate in human blood.

The diagnosis is made by histologic observation of larvae of *D. immitis* within the pulmonary granulomatous nodules. Blood examination reveals eosinophilia.

OTHER DIROFILARIA SPECIES

Occasional human infections by other species of *Dirofilaria* have been reported. *D. repens*, *D. tenuis* and *D. ursi* are the subcutaneous parasites of dog and cat, raccoon and bear respectively. However, these may also cause subcutaneous dirofilariasis in man.

Zoonotic filariasis occurs when humans are accidentally infected by filariae normally found in animals. *Dirofilaria* spp. being one among them. Transmission occurs through mosquito bite. In human infection, parasite development is impaired and microfilariae are not produced. Dirofilariasis is a common zoonotic infection in Sri Lanka. Subconjunctival dirofilariasis caused by *D. repens* and subcutaneous dirofilariasis of the medial aspect of the left upper lid caused by *D. repens* has been reported from Karnataka. The first author has also reported subconjunctival dirofilariasis caused by *D. repens* from Haryana.

OTHER NEMATODES

DRACUNCULUS MEDINENSIS

Common names

The guinea worm, serpent worm, dragon worm, medina worm.

Dracunculiasis, caused by the nematode *Dracunculus medinensis*, is the only parasitic infection of which a good description is given in the Bible. It is not a filarial worm but a tissue-invading nematode of medical importance.

Geographical distribution

Guinea worm infection (dracunculiasis) is the subject of a global eradication campaign, initiated in 1980. In India, the last reported case was in July 1996. **On completion of three years of zero incidence, India was declared free of guinea worm disease.** At present it occurs in many parts of Asia and equatorial Africa infecting an estimated 10 million people.

Habitat

The adult females inhabit the subcutaneous tissue, especially of the legs, arms and back of man.

Morphology

Adult worms

Female

The mature female of *D. medinensis* is a slender, long worm, measuring 50–80 cm × 1.0–2.0 mm. It resembles a piece of long twine thread. The body is cylindrical, smooth and milk-white in colour. The anterior end is bluntly rounded and the posterior extremity is tapering and is bent to form a hook. The worm is viviparous and discharges embryos in successive batches for a period of 3 weeks until the gravid female completely empties its uterine contents. The body fluid is toxic and causes a blister if it escapes into the tissues.

Male

Males recovered from experimental infections in animals measure 15–40 mm × 0.4 mm. The posterior end of the male is coiled on itself one or more times.

The life span of the female is about 1 year and that of male is not more than 6 months.

Embryos

These are coiled bodies with rounded heads and long slender tapering tails. They measure 500–750 μm in length by 15–25 μm in the greatest diameter. The embryos are set free only at the time of parturition when the affected part is submerged in water (Fig. 11.25).

Life cycle

D. medinensis passes its life cycle in two hosts. Man is the definitive host and *Cyclops* is the intermediate host. In human body each female worm takes about one year to mature and the cephalic end of the worm approaches the skin liable to come in contact with water, such as the backs of water-carriers, arms and legs of washermen, and legs of those who fill water in containers in "step wells" and ponds. It provokes a blister which bursts and leaves an ulcer through which about 5 cm of the worm is extruded, particularly after immersion of the affected part in water (Fig. 11.25). The anterior end of the worm and its uterus are ruptured, releasing many thousands of motile first-stage

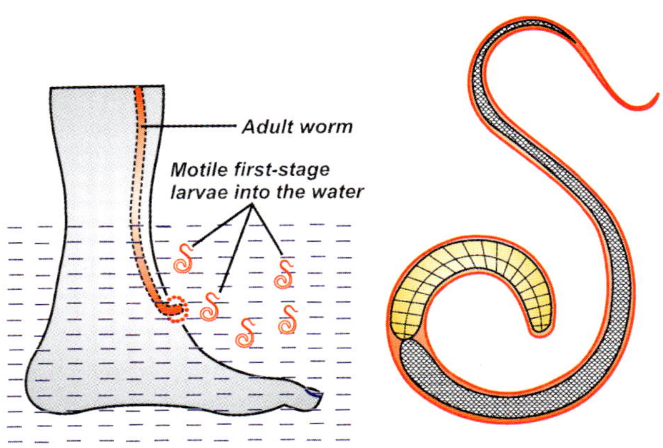

Fig. 11.25. First-stage larvae of *Dracunculus medinensis*. On right side is the magnified view of the larva.

larvae into the water. This may happen several times until all the larvae are discharged.

The larvae move about with a stiff motion, briskly coiling and uncoiling the body. In the water they can live for only a few days. For further development they have to be ingested by an appropriate species of *Cyclops*. On reaching the midintestine of the *Cyclops*, they break through the soft wall, come to lie in the coelomic cavity, moult twice and are infective in about 2 weeks.

Humans become infected by drinking water containing infected *Cyclops*. On reaching the stomach the *Cyclops* are digested by the gastric juice and the larvae are liberated. These larvae penetrate the wall of the digestive tract and migrate to the retroperitoneal space, where they mature into male and female adult worms in about 6 months time after entering into man. Male fertilizes the female and dies. In another 6 months, the fertilized female migrates to subcutaneous tissue of those parts of the body which are likely to come in contact with water and discharges the embryos in water. The cycle is thus repeated.

Pathogenicity

D. medinensis causes **dracunculiasis**. It is typically a disease of rural communities which obtain their drinking water from ponds or from large "step wells" where *Cyclops* can breed. Migrating worm in the subcutaneous regions may cause some tenderness, but the presence of the parasite may not be apparent until the gravid female worm has reached the skin, has produced a blister at the outer end of the tunnel, and the blister has burst in contact with water. Thereafter, because of the discharge of the worm's metabolites together with motile larvae, symptoms may decrease. Incubation period is about 1 year.

A few hours preceding the development of the local cutaneous lesion there may be pronounced systemic symptoms including erythema and urticarial rash, with intense pruritus, nausea, vomiting, diarrhoea, giddiness, and syncope. In a few hours the local lesion develops. It is a reddish papule with a vesicular centre and an indurated margin measuring 2–7 cm in diameter. It may be painful and may cause considerable inflammation. Lesion may be single or multiple. These lesions are most common between the metatarsal bones of the soles of the feet or on the ankles, but may be found on the hands or arms, trunk, buttocks, scrotum, knee joint, calf, thigh, shoulder, or even the angle of the jaw. The fluid in the blister is bacteriologically sterile and yellow in colour. It contains many mononuclear, eosinophilic, and polymorphonuclear leucocytes.

On rupture of the blister about 5 cm of the worm is extruded and many thousands of motile first-stage larvae are discharged. Secondary infection along the track of the worm in tissues is very common, often with spreading cellulitis. Tetanus is not an uncommon complication.

Laboratory diagnosis

Diagnosis of dracunculiasis can be made by:

1. Detection of adult worm

This is possible when the gravid female worm appears at the surface of the skin. Worms in deeper tissues after death may become calcified. These can be detected by X-ray examination.

2. Detection of embryos

Cold water is placed on the ulcer. On contact with water a large number of motile larvae are discharged which can be examined under microscope.

3. Immunological tests

Antibodies to *D. medinensis* may be detected in patient serum by ELISA, Western blot and fluorescent antibody test using deep frozen first-stage larvae.

4. Intradermal test

Injection of *Dracunculus* antigen intradermally in patients suffering from dracunculiasis causes a wheal to appear in the course of 24 hours.

5. Blood examination

It reveals eosinophilia.

Treatment

As soon as the female worm shows herself, the end is tied with a fine silk to a match stick, it is then wound out daily with gentle traction, combined with sterile dressing and acriflavine cream until the whole parasite is extracted. This takes about 15–20 days. There is no effective anthelmintic for treatment of *D. medinensis* infection. Metronidazole 250 mg given three times a day for 10 days may provide symptomatic relief.

Prevention

Dracunculiasis can be prevented by:

- Filtering or boiling drinking water.

- Individuals with open blisters and ulcers, and infected persons with an emerging worm should not be permitted to come in contact with any source of drinking water.
- Treating water sources. The insecticide temephos added to ponds at a concentration of 1 ppm will kill *Cyclops*.

ANGIOSTRONGYLUS

The genus *Angiostrongylus* (the rat lungworm) belongs to the order Strongylida and the superfamily Metastrongyloidea. It includes 20 species infective to small mammals, of which two are pathogenic to humans. *A. cantonensis* is neurotropic causing eosinophilic meningoencephalitis and *A. costaricensis* causes abdominal angiostrongyliasis. In addition, *A. mackerrase* and *A. malaysiensis* have been reported to cause eosinophilic meningitis in Australia and eosinophilic meningoencephalitis in Southeast Asia.

ANGIOSTRONGYLUS CANTONENSIS

Human infection with *A. cantonensis* was first described in 1945 in a 15-year-old Taiwanese boy with suspected meningitis. It is prevalent in Pacific islands and Southeast Asia. Three human cases have been reported from Greater Mumbai (India).

Morphology

Adult males measure 20–25 mm × 0.32–0.42 mm and adult females measure 22–34 mm × 0.34–0.56 mm.

Life cycle

A. cantonensis passes its life cycle in rat (definitive host) and molluscs (intermediate host). The adult worms inhabit mainly in branches of the pulmonary artery, but sometimes in the right ventricle of rat. The gravid female worm lays eggs into the blood stream. These are carried to the lung capillaries where they form emboli. After about one week they embryonate and hatch. First-stage (L1) larvae enter alveoli, then migrate up the trachea and larynx. They are subsequently swallowed and passed out with faeces.

These larvae are ingested by molluscs (terrestrial and aquatic snails and slugs) and undergo two moults to the second (L2) and third (L3) stage, after 7–9 and 12–16 days respectively. The L3 larvae are 460–510 μm long and, in molluscan intermediate host, remain enclosed in the L1 and L2 sheaths. When the mollusc is ingested by a rat, L3 larvae exsheathe and penetrate into the intestinal wall and reach the heart via the portal system and the inferior vena cava. Larvae then reach the left ventricle through the pulmonary circulation. From here some larvae migrate to the brain directly, whereas others migrate first through other organs or tissues. In either case, L3 larvae reach the CNS within 2–3 days, after which they migrate within the brain and grow. The larvae moult twice to become young adults that migrate through brain tissue to the subarachnoid space. After about 26–29 days of infection, the worms penetrate cerebral veins and return to pulmonary arteries via the heart. The worms further grow and females lay eggs and the cycle is thus repeated.

Pathogenicity

Humans are infected by ingestion of L3 larvae in raw or undercooked intermediate hosts. Animals that acquire L3 larvae by eating infected molluscs may act as **paratenic (transport) host** and may transmit *A. cantonensis* to humans. Known paratenic hosts are toads, frogs, freshwater prawns, land planarians and land crabs. Infection may also be acquired by ingestion of water or vegetables contaminated with L3 larvae and oral contact with larvae released from molluscs.

L3 larvae after entering the alimentary canal of man follow the same route, as in the rat, to reach the brain. Here they moult twice and develop into young adults. They probably do not develop to sexual maturity and die in the brain without returning to the heart and lungs and cause **eosinophilic meningoencephalitis**.

Patient develops severe headache, nausea, vomiting, fever, neck stiffness, paraesthesia, weakness of extremities, muscle twitching, diplopia, strabismus and facial paralysis with peripheral eosinophilia. The worms are mostly found in the medulla, pons and cerebellum and in the adjacent leptomeninges.

L3 larvae may migrate to the base of the brain, move anteriorly into the orbit and finally penetrate the eye via the cribriform plate. The worms may be found in the anterior chamber, retina and other sites. This condition is known as **ocular angiostrongyliasis**. This form is rarely accompanied by meningoencephalitis.

Laboratory diagnosis

A. cantonensis infection can be diagnosed by:

- A history of eating raw or undercooked molluscs.
- Peripheral eosinophilia.
- Spinal fluid eosinophilia.

- Demonstration of larvae and young adults in CSF.
- IgM and IgE serum antibodies by ELISA and immunoblot analyses.

Treatment

Mebendazole 100 mg BD for 5 days is the drug of choice.

Prevention

For prevention of the disease, ingestion of infected hosts and water or vegetables contaminated with L3 larvae must be avoided. Larvae can be killed by boiling for 2–3 minutes or by freezing at –15°C for more than 12 hours.

ANGIOSTRONGYLUS COSTARICENSIS

A. costaricensis was discovered in the mesenteric arteries of patients in Costa Rica by Morera and Céspedes (1971) who established it as the cause of abdominal angiostrongyliasis. It has subsequently been reported from Latin America, USA, and more recently from Africa.

Morphology

Adult males measure 17.4–22.2 × 0.28–0.31 mm and adult females measure 28.2–42.0 × 0.322–0.35 mm. The eggs are oval and about 90 µm long, have a thin shell, and are unembryonated (they may be embryonated in humans, with some larvae being released from the egg).

Life cycle

A. costaricensis inhabits the ileo-caecocolic branches of the anterior mesenteric artery of cotton rat and other rodents. Coatimundi, marmosets and dogs can also serve as definitive hosts. L1 larvae from the definitive hosts enter slugs (intermediate hosts), develop to L3 stage. When the slug is eaten by a cotton rat and the larvae are digested free, they migrate through the intestinal tissues to the lymphatics. Here they moult twice on the fourth and fifth days, respectively. On about the tenth day, they migrate to the mesenteric arteries and reach maturity and release eggs by eighteenth day. Eggs deposited in the intestinal wall develop and hatch, the L1 larvae appearing in faeces 24 days after infection.

Pathogenicity

Human infection with *A. costaricensis* is acquired by ingestion of infected slugs, either intentionally or by the accidental ingestion of slugs hidden on vegetables. Human infections have been reported from California to Argentina. Incidence is particularly high in Costa Rica. In Brazil, the incidence of infection is still increasing.

A. costaricensis causes **abdominal angiostrongyliasis**. Pathogenesis is attributed either to adult worms in the mesenteric arteries or eggs in the intestinal wall. Eggs cause a granulomatous inflammatory reaction, with oedema and marked thickening of the intestinal wall and a narrow lumen. There is also a dense eosinophilic infiltration of the vessels occupied by the worms, with marked thickening of the walls. Frequently, the vessel is partially occluded. Rarely, the worms may be located in the liver, causing conditions suggestive of **visceral larva migrans**.

Most patients complain of pain and tenderness and a palpable tumour-like mass in the right iliac fossa and right flank, fever, anorexia, vomiting and diarrhoea. Clinical findings, in general, resemble those of appendicitis.

Laboratory diagnosis

L1 larvae are not discharged in stools of man as they are in the rat, although larvae in eggs may be seen in sections of the involved area, usually the caecum, appendix, and adjacent parts of the colon and ileum. Sections may show adult worms in functional or occluded vessels. In most cases there is leucocytosis with eosinophilia ranging up to 60%. Serological tests have been employed, including ELISA and latex agglutination. Radiological examination shows a mass in the right lower quadrant, thickening of the intestinal wall at the ileo-caecal region and a narrowed intestinal lumen.

Treatment

Abdominal angiostrongyliasis may be treated with:

1. thiabendazole in combination with diethylcarbamazine,
2. thiabendazole alone, or
3. high dose mebendazole.

However, for definitive cure surgical treatments are generally required.

GNATHOSTOMA

The genus *Gnathostoma* contains 12 distinct species, four of which are zoonotic in Southeast Asia and the

Far East. These include *G. spinigerum*, *G. hispidum*, *G. doloresi* and *G. nipponicum*.

GNATHOSTOMA SPINIGERUM

G. spinigerum was first described in 1836 by Richard Owen in a stomach nodule of a tiger. It causes **gnathostomiasis**, a less frequent zoonotic infection in man. The first human infection was reported by Levinsen in 1890 in a breast abscess of a woman living in Siam. Human cases have been reported from Thailand, Japan, Malaysia, China, India, Java, Israel, Vietnam, and the Philippines. In recent years, however, gnathostomiasis has become an increasing problem in Central and South America, most notably in Mexico. As the scope of international travel expands, an increasing number of travellers are coming into contact with helminthic parasites rarely seen outside the tropics. As a result, the occurrence of *Gnathostoma spinigerum* infection leading to the clinical syndrome gnathostomiasis is increasing. In areas where *Gnathostoma* is not endemic, few clinicians are familiar with this disease.

Morphology

Adult worms

The adult worms may be curved ventrally at one or both ends. The male measures 12–30 mm in length and 2 mm in breadth. The female is relatively larger and measures 15–33 mm in length and 3 mm in breadth. The cephalic end bears 8–11 rows of cuticular hooklets.

Eggs

The eggs are oval, brownish and unsegmented. They measure 65–70 μm × 38–40 μm and possess a transparent knob-like thickening at one pole (Fig. 11.26).

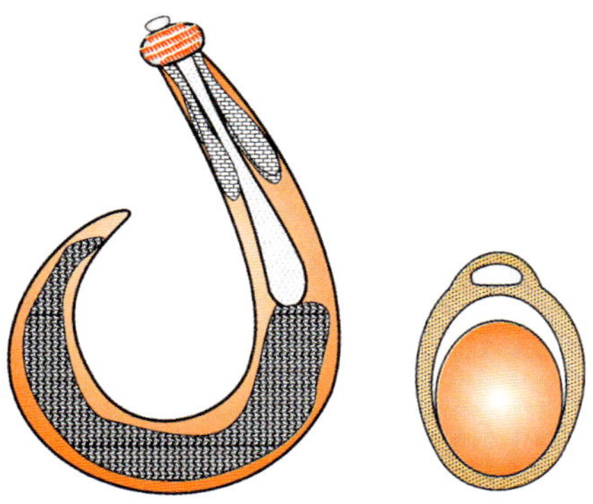

Fig. 11.26. Third-stage larva and egg of *Gnathostoma spinigerum*.

Third stage larva resembles the adult worm in morphology, having 4–8 rows of sharp hooklets.

Life cycle

Adult *G. spinigerum* resides in the tumours or granulomatous lesions of the stomach wall of cat, dog and many other carnivores (definitive hosts). Eggs are laid in these tumours. They pass into gastric lumen through a small aperture and are discharged in faeces into water. L1 larvae develop in the eggs and moult to the L2 stage after which the eggs hatch. L2 larvae are ingested by *Cyclops* (first intermediate host) after which they develop in the haemocoel and moult into the early L3 stage in 6–10 days (Fig. 11.27).

When the infected *Cyclops* are eaten by freshwater fish, frog or snake (second intermediate host), early L3 larvae develop into the advanced L3 larvae in the flesh of these animals. Other hosts that are not suited to be a definitive host (reptiles, birds or mammals), may ingest the vertebrate host containing advanced L3 larvae and become infected. Since the larva undergoes no further development, such a host is **paratenic**.

When the suitable definitive host eats either the infected second intermediate host or the paratenic host, the L3 larvae penetrate the gastric wall to the peritoneal cavity to reach the liver. Subsequently, they migrate through the host and, 4 weeks later, they return to the stomach, penetrating the stomach wall from the outside to form a tumour that connects with the stomach lumen through a small aperture. The adult worm develops within six months after infection, completing the cycle.

Pathogenicity

Humans acquire infection by ingestion of second intermediate or paratenic hosts or, possibly, by drinking water containing *Cyclops* or free L3 larvae. Advanced L3 larvae can also penetrate the intact skin. In humans, the larvae penetrate the gastric wall and migrate throughout the tissues. Although, adult stage can develop in humans, the worms cannot return to the stomach. Clinical symptoms of gnathostomiasis occur because of the inflammatory reaction provoked by these migrating larvae. Traditionally the disease has been divided into cutaneous and visceral forms depending on the site of larval migration and subsequent symptoms.

Deep cutaneous or subcutaneous tunnels in which the larvae migrate may develop, causing **larva migrans** or **creeping eruption**. The lesions of cutaneous larva migrans of gnathostomiasis differ from those of hook-

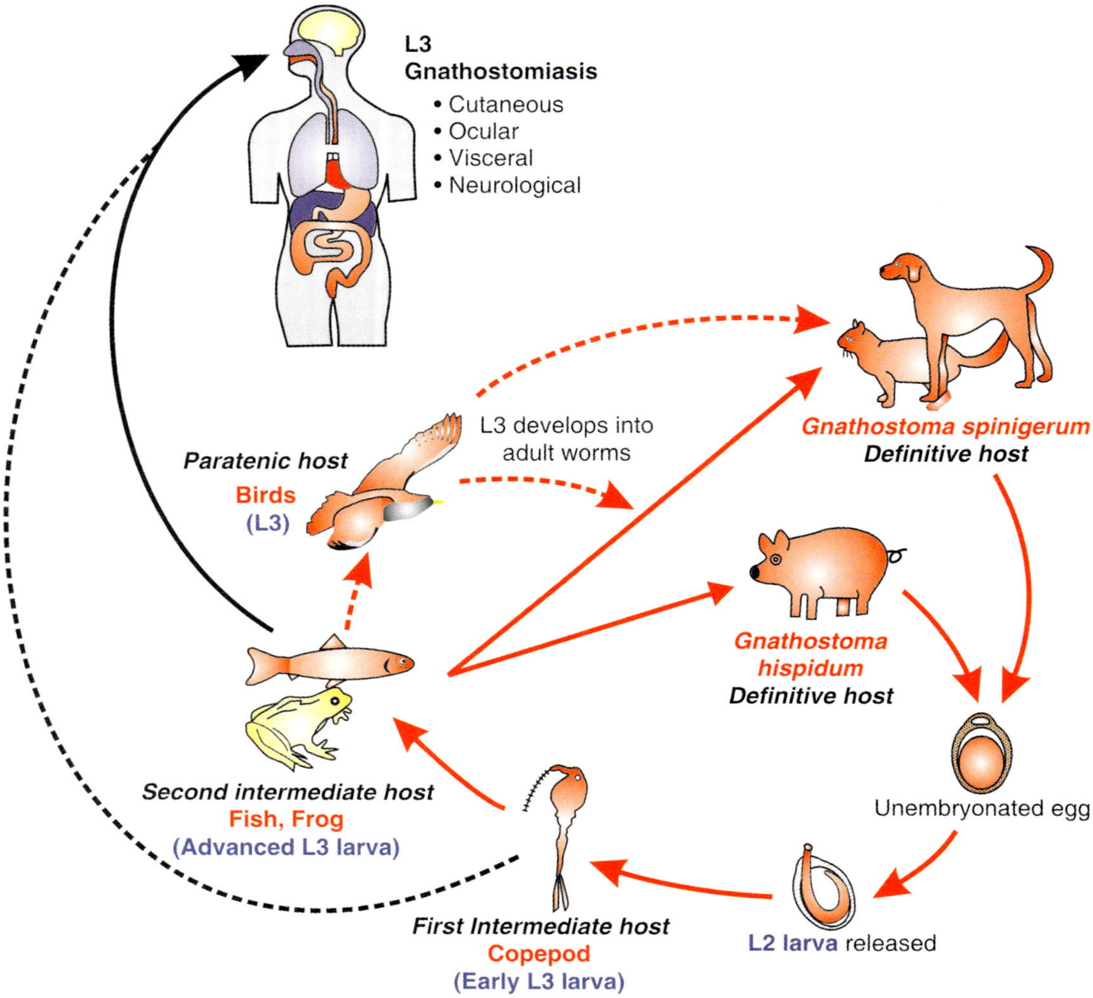

Fig. 11.27. Life cycle of *Gnathostoma* spp.

worm in that they are usually deeper, i.e., subcutaneous or even more frequently in the muscles. They appear as migratory swellings that frequently appear first in the abdominal area, after which the lesions migrate at random. The swellings are rather hard, normally painless, up to several centimeters in diameter and mostly erythematous. Swellings last 1–2 weeks, and then disappear, another swelling appearing elsewhere. Migratory swellings may recur intermittently for up to 10–12 years. Worms migrating near the body surface may also cause cutaneous abscesses or cutaneous nodules in which the worms can be demonstrated.

Migrating worms in deeper tissues produce **visceral gnathostomiasis** or **visceral larva migrans**. Signs and symptoms depend on the organs and tissues affected. They may invade central nervous system, eye, lung, urinary bladder, gastrointestinal tract, ear, nose and throat. An acute or chronic inflammatory reaction occurs around invading larvae and local haemorrhage, necrosis, oedema, fibrosis and tumour formation may occur. Entry to the central nervous system appears to be by migration along a peripheral nerve into the spinal cord, thence to the brain. It leads to **encephalomyelitis**. As in case of eosinophilic meningoencephalitis caused by *Angiostrongylus cantonensis*, eosinophils are found in the cerebrospinal fluid. However, encephalomyelitis caused by *G. spinigerum* is more severe. It has frequently fatal course with paralysis or coma and bloody cerebrospinal fluid.

Laboratory diagnosis

The diagnosis of gnathostomiasis can be established by:

- Demonstration and identification of the larvae in the surgical specimens.

- Demonstration of IgE or IgG antibody by ELISA test using crude extracts of advanced L3 larvae as antigen.
- Intradermal test employing, an antigen prepared from larval or adult *G. spinigerum,* read in 15 minutes.

Treatment

The only available treatment is incision of the lesion and removal of larva. Reported efficacy of albendazole in the treatment of gnathostomiasis is > 90%, and similar success has been reported for ivermectin.

Prevention

Preventive measures include avoidance of ingestion of raw or inadequately cooked second intermediate or paratenic hosts that may contain L3 larvae, and avoidance of drinking water that may contain infected *Cyclops*.

GNATHOSTOMA HISPIDUM

G. hispidum is a relatively common parasite in the stomach wall of wild and domestic pigs in Europe, Asia and Australia.

Morphology

Adult males and females are 20 mm and 25 mm long, respectively. The head end bears 9–12 rows of cephalic hooklets and the entire body surface is covered with cuticular spines. Eggs resemble those of *G. spinigerum* but are slightly larger (72 × 40 µm).

Life cycle

Domestic and wild pigs are the definitive hosts of *G. hispidum*. Adult worms live in the stomach wall without producing a tumour. The first and second intermediate hosts, the paratenic hosts, the life cycle and the mode of acquisition of infection by humans with *G. hispidum* are similar to those of *G. spinigerum* (Fig. 11.27). Unlike *G. spinigerum*, *G. hispidum* cannot mature in humans.

Pathogenicity

G. hispidum causes creeping eruption with erythema and itch (**cutaneous gnathostomiasis**) and peripheral eosinophilia. It normally occurs on the trunk or extremities. A few cases of human infection have been reported from India and Japan.

Laboratory diagnosis

The diagnosis of *G. hispidum* infection can be established by:

- demonstration and identification of the worms in the surgical specimens,
- peripheral eosinophilia, and
- detection of antibodies in patient serum by ELISA test.

Crude *G. spinigerum* antigens are commonly used, because *G. hispidum* antigens are not available.

GNATHOSTOMA DOLORESI

Morphology

Adult *G. doloresi* males and females are 20 mm and 34 mm long, respectively. They occur in the gastric walls of domestic pigs or wild boars, inserting the anterior body into the thickened gastric wall. Eggs measure 61.3 µm × 30.9 µm on average, with transparent knob-like bulges at both ends.

Life cycle and pathogenicity

Life cycle and transmission of infection to humans are similar to those of *G. hispidum*. *G. doloresi* causes creeping eruption with local pain and itch on the skin particularly the trunk, and migratory swellings sometime develop. Creeping eruption may be preceded by fever, vomiting, abdominal pain, weakness and malaise.

Laboratory diagnosis

Diagnosis can be established by:

- demonstration and identification of worms in the surgical specimen, and
- detection of antibodies by various serological tests which employ *G. doloresi* crude extract as an antigen.

GNATHOSTOMA NIPPONICUM

Morphology

Adult *G. nipponicum* males and females are 20–23 mm and 29–34 mm long, respectively. They reside in hard tumours in the oesophageal wall of the weasel. The anterior body is embedded and the posterior lies free in the lumen. Eggs measure 72.3 µm × 42.1 µm on average, with a transparent knob-like bulge at one end.

Life cycle and pathogenicity

Life cycle and transmission of infection to humans are similar to those of *G. hispidum* and *G. doloresi*. *G. nipponicum* causes creeping eruption on the abdomen, waist and hip areas with peripheral eosinophilia.

Laboratory diagnosis

Diagnosis can be established by demonstration and identification of worms in the surgical specimens.

TERNIDENS DEMINUTUS

T. deminutus belongs to the order Strongylida, and the superfamily Strongyloidea. It is a relatively common parasite of the large intestine of several species of simian hosts in Africa, India and Indonesia. It has also been reported in man from southern Africa, Comoros and Mauritius.

Morphology

Adult males and females are 6–13 mm and 9–17 mm long, respectively. Superficially *T. deminutus* resembles hookworm, but it can be readily distinguished by the anteriorly directed buccal capsule, which has a double crown of 22 stout bristles. Males have cup-shaped copulatory bursa, two spicules and a gubernaculum. Females have protuberant vulva slightly anterior to the anus. The eggs are ovoid, transparent and closely resemble those of human hookworms. However, they are larger (85 × 50 μm) in size (Fig. 11.28).

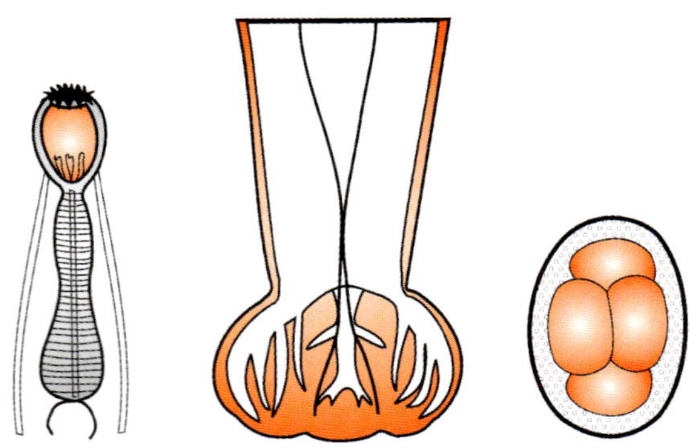

Fig. 11.28. Anterior end (A), copulatory bursa (B) and egg (C) of *Ternidens deminutus*.

Life cycle

Eggs discharged in the faeces develop in the soil. They hatch into L1 larvae in 2–3 days. Subsequently, they moult to L2 larvae and L3 filariform larvae in 2–3 days and 8–10 days respectively.

Pathogenicity

Infection is acquired by ingestion of L3 filariform larvae. They penetrate the mucosa of large intestine and moult to L4 larvae. These larvae produce nodules or ulcerations. Finally, L4 larvae moult to the adult stage. *T. deminutus* does not suck blood, but if worm loads are heavy, anaemia might result.

Laboratory diagnosis

Diagnosis can be established by demonstration and identification of adult worms and eggs.

Treatment

Thiabendazole and albendazole can be used for the treatment.

CAPILLARIA PHILIPPINENSIS

This parasite was first discovered in 1963, in a male patient from Ilocos Norte, the Philippine, who died 3 days after admission to the Philippine General Hospital with a diagnosis of malabsorption syndrome. *Capillaria philippinensis* is prevalent in the Philippines and Thailand. Infection with *C. philippinensis* has also been reported from Japan, Indonesia, India, Iran, Egypt and South America.

Morphology

Fish-eating birds are the natural definitive hosts of *C. philippinensis*. In man, it lives burrowed into the mucosa of the small intestine, predominantly the jejunum. Adult males measure 1.5–3.9 mm in length and females measure 2.3–5.3 mm in length. Females produce ova which are barrel-shaped and bear a superficial resemblance to those of *T. trichiura*. They are, however, smaller (36–45 μm × 20 μm), more cylindrical in shape, have thin shell and the plugs (one at each end of the egg) are smaller and do not protrude like those of *T. trichiura*.

Eggs in faeces of infected persons and birds embryonate in water in 5–10 days and develop further if swallowed by small freshwater and brackish water fish. Upon ingestion the eggs hatch, giving rise to larvae that penetrate the intestine and migrate to tissues.

Pathogenicity

Man acquires infection by ingestion of raw, undercooked, or pickled fish containing larvae of *C. philippinensis*. They develop into adult worms in the lumen of the small intestine, where they burrow in the mucosa. The females deposit unembryonated eggs. Some of these become embryonated in the intestine, and release larvae that can cause autoinfection. ***C. philippinensis* and *Strongyloides stercoralis* are the**

two major nematodes that can undergo auto-infection and hyperinfection in the human host.

C. philippinensis causes intestinal capillariasis. It invades the small intestine, predominantly the jejunum and causes severe enteropathy, which is manifested by derangement of intestinal function with malabsorption and loss of fluid, electrolytes, and plasma proteins into the intestinal tract. Patient complains of diarrhoea, abdominal pain, vomiting, and anorexia. Infections lasting 2–3 months result in a severe protein losing enteropathy characterized by cachexia, dehydration and anasarca, and unless treated, death is often the outcome.

Laboratory diagnosis

The diagnosis of intestinal capillariasis can be made by detection of characteristic eggs in the stool. Larvae and adult worms may also be detected.

Treatment

Albendazole 200 mg twice daily for 10 days or mebendazole 200 mg daily for 20 days can be used for the treatment of intestinal capillariasis.

Prevention

The disease can be prevented by sanitary disposal of faeces and thoroughly cooking the fish before eating.

CAPILLARIA HEPATICA

Capillaria hepatica is a relatively common parasite of rat and other rodent species. It has been reported from the muskrat, opossum, and rarely humans. It lives in the liver, and the eggs are laid in the surrounding parenchyma.

Morphology

Adult female measures about 20 mm long by about 100 μm wide and the male is about half as long. The eggs resemble those of *Trichuris trichiura*, but the poles are less tapered and measure 51–68 μm × 30–35 μm.

Life cycle

The female worm lays eggs in the liver. When the eggs contained within the infected liver are eaten by another animal during cannibalism, the eggs are released by digestion, excreted in the faeces of the second animal, and develop into the infective-stage larvae in damp soil. Alternatively, the eggs can be released following the death and decomposition of the first animal and mature in the soil.

Pathogenicity

When the infective eggs are ingested by humans with contaminated food or drink, they hatch in the small intestine and produce larvae that migrate through the portal system to the liver. They mature in about one month and the female worms lay eggs. *C. hepatica* causes acute or subacute hepatitis with hypereosinophilia.

Laboratory diagnosis

A definitive diagnosis can be made by demonstrating the eggs or adults of *C. hepatica* in liver biopsy specimens.

CAPILLARIA AEROPHILA

Capillaria aerophila is a worldwide parasite of cats, dogs, foxes and other carnivores where it lives beneath the mucosa of upper and lower respiratory tree.

Morphology

Males measure up to 18 mm × 70 μm and females up to 20 mm × 105 μm. Female worm lays eggs that measure 59–80 μm × 39–40 μm with characteristic polar plugs.

Life cycle

The adult worms live beneath the mucosa of the upper and lower respiratory tree where they produce eggs that are coughed and swallowed. Eggs passing out with the faeces embryonate in moist soil. In summer temperatures it takes about 6 weeks. Embryonated eggs enter a new host via contaminated food or water. The larvae hatch in the intestines and migrate to the lungs. They mature into adults in about 40 days after infection and lay eggs in the lungs, and cycle is repeated.

Pathogenicity

Human infections with *C. aerophila* have been reported from Russia, Morocco and Iran. It causes tracheobronchitis usually with asthma and productive cough.

Laboratory diagnosis

Diagnosis may be made by demonstration of eggs in the sputum or faeces or both, and the adult worm in the lung biopsy.

ANISAKIS SIMPLEX

Anisakis simplex was first discovered as cause of **larva migrans** by van Thiel, Kuiper and Roskam in 1960.

They noted a nematode larva in the intestinal wall of a patient suffering from acute abdominal pain after eating raw herrings. Many cases of gastric anisakiasis have been reported in Japan. These have been linked to eating raw fish (sashimi or sushi). Anisakiasis has also been reported from the Netherlands, where infections are acquired from eating raw herrings. Cases have also been reported from the USA and Europe. No case has been reported from India.

Life cycle

Adult worms reside in clusters, with their anterior ends embedded in the gastric wall of marine mammals such as whales, porpoises and dolphins. The eggs (40×50 μm) of these worms, passed in the host's faeces, embryonate and hatch free in the water as microscopic second-stage larvae. These are free-swimming and able to survive for 2–3 months. When ingested by small marine crustacea (krill), they develop into third-stage larvae. When infected krill are eaten by squids or marine teleosts, e.g., salmon, cod, herring and mackerel, the larvae encyst in the viscera or muscles but do not develop further. When these **paratenic hosts** are eaten by marine mammals, the larvae moult twice in the stomach and develop into adult worms. These lay eggs which are discharged in the host's faeces and the cycle is thus repeated. Humans are not suitable hosts; third-stage larvae are found but never adult worms.

Pathogenicity

Man acquires infection by consuming raw, freshly salted or smoked marine fish containing *Anisakis* larvae. These larvae penetrate the gastric or intestinal mucosa in the same manner as they do in their natural final host. In the stomach and intestine these are usually found embedded in a dense eosinophilic granuloma in the wall below the mucosa. These larvae measure 1–3 cm long or more by 1 mm wide. In the stomach, a portion of the larvae can be seen in the lumen.

Occasionally, the site of attachment and partial penetration by *A. simplex*, is the throat. *A. simplex* larvae readily penetrate the gastrointestinal wall and invade the abdominal cavity, provoking peritonitis and intruding into various organs and tissues.

The disease is also classified into gastric, intestinal and extra-gastrointestinal (ectopic) anisakiasis. The last form is caused by larvae that penetrate into the abdominal or pleural cavity, entering organs or tissues (e.g. omentum, mesentery, peritoneum, liver, pancreas, ovary, oviduct, utero-cervix, lymph node, lung, and even the subcutaneous tissue), and provoking inflammatory foci.

Acute gastric anisakiasis occurs approximately 6 hours after ingestion of raw seafood. Larvae normally parasitize the fundus of the stomach (rarely tongue, tonsil, uvula, and oesophagus). Intestinal anisakiasis usually develops within 2 days after infection and occurs in any region between the duodenum and the rectum, most frequently in the ileal region.

The patients develop moderate leucocytosis and, in some cases, eosinophilia (4–41%). They may complain of abdominal pain, nausea, vomiting and diarrhoea. The symptoms last for 1–5 days.

Laboratory diagnosis

- Diagnosis of gastric anisakiasis and sometimes duodenal anisakiasis can be made by **endoscopy**. The site of larval penetration shows oedema, hyperaemia, erosion and bleeding. The penetrating larvae can be easily removed endoscopically with biopsy forceps.
- An **immunoblot assay**, using antigens of *A. simplex* larvae can be used for detection of IgA and IgE antibodies in the patient serum.

Treatment and prevention

Supportive treatment is recommended until the larvae die and are absorbed. Anisakiasis can be prevented by thorough cooking or freezing at –20°C for 3–5 days of seafood. These processes kill the larvae of *A. simplex* in the seafood.

OESOPHAGOSTOMUM SPECIES

Genus *Oesophagostomum* belongs to the order Strongylida and the superfamily Strongyloidea. Species of this genus are common parasites of large intestines of monkeys and apes in Africa, Asia and South America. Certain species are also common in swine and sheep. Human oesophagostomiasis occurs predominantly in Africa with some cases reported in Indonesia, China and South America. Five species are known in humans of which, *O. bifurcum* is most common in Africa and Asia and *O. aculeatum* occurs in Southeast Asia.

Morphology

They resemble hookworms in size but differ in the character of the buccal capsule which, as in *Ternidens*, is cylindrical and opens forward with a crown of bristles around the mouth. Eggs are indistinguishable from those of hookworms but are passed in the faeces in an advanced stage of development.

Life cycle

Life cycle of *Oesophagostomum* is similar to that of *Ternidens*. Humans acquire infection by ingestion of L3 larvae which produce nodules in the large intestine wall. When development is complete, the worms emerge, attach to the mucosa, mate and produce eggs which are discharged in the faeces. The cycle is thus repeated.

Pathogenicity

In human infection, L3 larvae penetrate the intestinal wall and produce a solitary, tumour-like inflammatory mass or abscess (**helminthoma**) measuring 1–2 cm in diameter, usually in the ileo-caecal region. Other levels of large and small intestines are affected less commonly and the masses or nodules may be multiple. Symptoms include abdominal pain, with localized tenderness (usually right lower quadrant). There may be gradual onset of pain, with a low grade fever and no diarrhoea, vomiting, or anorexia. Careful examination of the patient may reveal a mass in the abdominal cavity adherent to the abdominal wall. L3 larvae of *oesophagostomum* occasionally produce subcutaneous nodules by direct skin penetration or by vascular dissemination of larvae from the bowel.

Laboratory diagnosis

Clinically oesophagostomiasis may be misdiagnosed as carcinoma, amoeboma, ileo-caecal tuberculosis and appendicitis. However, diagnosis can be established by demonstration and identification of worms in the nodules. Worm-specific IgG antibody can be detected in patient serum by ELISA test.

Treatment

Albendazole and pyrantel pamoate can be used for the treatment of oesophagostomiasis. It may occasionally require surgical intervention to relieve mechanical problems.

TRICHOSTRONGYLUS SPECIES

Genus *Trichostrongylus* belongs to the order Strongylida and superfamily Trichostrongyloidea. Various species of this genus are commonly parasitic in the digestive tract of herbivorous animals throughout the world. At least 10 *Trichostrongylus* species are capable of parasitizing humans of which *T. colubriformis* and *T. orientalis* are important.

Trichostrongylus infections have been reported from parts of Africa, Egypt, Indonesia, Iran, Iraq, Southeast Asia, India, Japan and Chile. These are more prevalent in Iran.

Morphology

These worms are small and slender, measuring 4–8 mm long. The head is unarmed and lacks a distinct buccal capsule. The males have a copulatory bursa with long lateral and poorly developed dorsal rays. Eggs resemble those of hookworms, but are longer and narrower (measuring 75–91 μm × 39–47 μm), with one end more pointed than the other. They are usually discharged at 16–32 cell stage.

Life cycle

Adult worms live embedded in the mucosa of the small intestine. Eggs are discharged in the faeces and develop in the soil. Under favourable conditions of moisture and temperature, they hatch into L1 larvae in 1–2 days. L1 larvae moult to L2 larvae in 2–3 days and to the ensheathed filariform L3 larvae in 7–8 days. Humans acquire infection by ingestion of vegetables or drinking water contaminated with L3 larvae. On reaching the small intestine the larvae develop in the intestinal mucosa, moult twice and develop to sexual maturity in about 3–4 weeks **without requiring migration through the lungs. However, percutaneous infection may also occur.**

Pathogenicity

Trichostrongylus penetrates into intestinal mucosa, producing erythema, erosion and local bleeding. Patient complains of epigastric pain, diarrhoea, anorexia, nausea and malaise. If the worms enter into biliary tract then they may provoke cholecystitis. If worm loads are light patients may be asymptomatic, but heavy worm loads are associated with anaemia.

Laboratory diagnosis

Diagnosis can be established by the demonstration of characteristic eggs in the faeces, or by culturing faeces and recovering typical larvae.

Treatment

Several anthelmintic agents are available, including pyrentel pamoate, mebendazole, and albendazole, some of which are also used for other nematode infections.

Prophylaxis

Infection can be prevented by avoiding ingestion of raw vegetables contaminated with L3 larvae. These should be properly cooked.

THELAZIA CALLIPAEDA

T. callipaeda is a parasite of dog, rabbit and occasionally man. It occurs in India, Burma, China, Russia, Thailand, Japan and Korea.

Morphology

The adult worms are thread-like, creamy-white. Male worm measures 4.5–13 mm × 0.25–0.75 mm and female 6.2–17 mm × 0.3–0.85 mm. Eggs are oval, thin-shelled and fully embryonated when laid. They measure 54–60 μm × 34–37 μm.

Life cycle

T. callipaeda occurs in the orbit, conjunctival sac or lacrimal glands. First-stage larvae occur in eye secretions. When these larvae are ingested by a fly, they moult twice in its tissues, migrate to the mouth parts and are transmitted to dog, rabbit and occasionally man, when the fly feeds upon eye secretions. Two more moults occur in the eye.

Pathogenicity

The presence of *T. callipaeda* in the conjunctival sac provokes excessive lacrimation, itching, or pain with the sensation of a foreign body in the eye.

Laboratory diagnosis

The diagnosis can be established by demonstration of thread-like, creamy-white worms in the conjunctival sac or migrating over the cornea. After application of topical anaesthetic to the eye, worms can be easily removed with forceps and identified by microscopic examination. If all worms are removed, the symptoms subside. If not, re-examine and remove the remaining worms.

DIOCTOPHYMA RENALE

D. renale was first reported by Goeze in 1782 in the kidney of a dog. Since then the parasite has been isolated from a large number of mammals including man. It has been widely reported from the Americas and China.

Morphology

The adult worm is cylindrical in shape and has a blood-red colour. Male measures 14–20 cm in length × 4–6 mm in diameter. At the posterior extremity, it has a bursa that is not supported by rays. Female is much larger and measures 20–100 cm in length × 5–12 mm in diameter. The eggs are ellipsoidal, yellowish-brown in colour and measure 60–80 μm × 39–46 μm (Fig. 11.29).

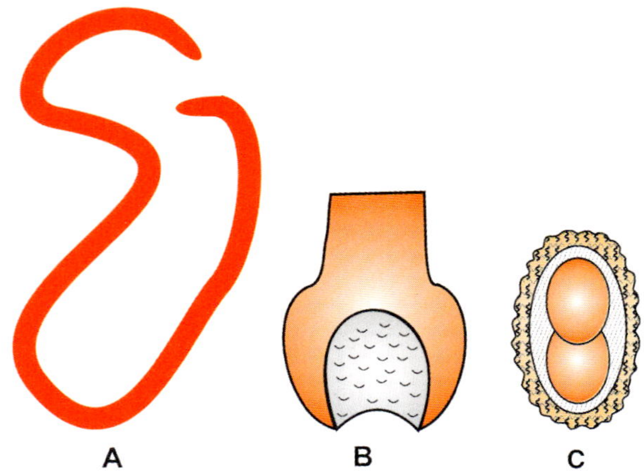

Fig. 11.29. *Dioctophyma renale*: (A) Adult male worm, (B) Bursa, and (C) Egg.

Life cycle

Adult worms inhabit the pelvis of the kidney, usually the right kidney, of many mammals including man. Female worm produces eggs which are excreted in the urine. They develop in water to first-stage larvae in 4 weeks. On ingestion by aquatic oligochaetes, the larvae hatch out of eggs in the intestine and after 2 months they metamorphose to the infective larvae. Dog acquires infection by ingesting these infected oligochaetes wherein larvae penetrate intestinal lining and migrate to liver. After maturing for about 50 days the larvae then migrate to kidneys (typically the right kidney), develop into adult worms and excrete eggs in urine. Infective larvae may be taken up by tadpoles or frogs or fish, which serve as **paratenic** or **transport hosts**. Man acquires infection by ingestion of raw or inadequately cooked fish or frog containing infective larvae.

Pathogenicity, laboratory diagnosis and prevention

In man, *D. renale* causes **dioctophymiasis**. It is a rare zoonotic infection. The presence of the parasite in the kidney causes renal colic and haematuria. The presence of characteristic eggs in the urine provides specific diagnosis. Dioctophymiasis can be prevented by thorough cooking of fish and frogs.

Further Reading

1. Barua, P., Barua, N., et al. 2005. *Loa loa* in the anterior chamber of the eye: a case report. *Indian J. Med. Microbiol.*, **23**: 59–60.
2. Cairncross, S., Muller, R. and Zagaria, N. 2002. Dracunculiasis (Guinea Worm Disease) and the eradication initiative. *Clin. Microbiol. Rev.*, **15**: 223–46.
3. Cook, J.A., Steel, C. and Ottesen, E.A. 2001. Towards a vaccine for onchocerciasis. *Trends Parasitol.*, **17**: 555–7.
4. Crompton, D.W.T. 2001. *Ascaris* and ascariasis. *Adv. Parasitol.*, **48**: 286–375.
5. Despommier, D.D. 2003. Toxocariasis: clinical aspects, epidemiology, medical ecology, and molecular aspects. *Clin. Microbiol. Rev.*, **16**: 265–72.
6. Diaz-Camacho, S.P., Wilms, K., et al. 2002. Morphology of *Gnathostoma* spp. isolated from natural hosts in Sinaloa, Mexico. *Parasitol. Res.*, **88**: 639–45.
7. Dreyer, G., Noroes, J., et al. 2000. Pathogenesis of lymphatic disease in bancroftian filariasis: clinical perspective. *Parasitol. Today*, **16**: 544–8.
8. Figueredo-Silva, J., Noroes, J., et al. 2002. The histopathology of bancroftian filariasis revised: the role of the adult worm in the lymphatic-vessel disease. *Ann. Trop. Med. Parasitol.*, **96**: 531–41.
9. Gautam, V., Rastagi, I.M., Singh, S., Arora, D.R. 2002. Subconjunctival infection with *Dirofilaria repens*. *Japanese J. Infect. Dis.*, **55**: 47–48.
10. Hoerauf, A., Büttner, D., et al. 2003. Onchocerciasis. *Br. Med. J.*, **326**: 207–10.
11. Intapan, P.M., Maleewong, W., et al. 2003. Evaluation of human IgG subclass antibodies in the sero–diagnosis of angiostrongyliasis. *Parasitol. Res.*, **89**: 425–9.
12. Juncker-Voss, M., Prosl, H., et al. 2000. Serological detection of *Capillaria hepatica* by indirect immunofluorescence assay. *J. Clin. Microbiol.*, **38**: 431–3.
13. Liu, M. and Boireau, P. 2002. Trichinellosis in China: epidemiology and control. *Trends Parasitol.*, **18**: 553–6.
14. Loutfy, M.R., Wilson, M., et al. 2002. Serology and eosinophil count in the diagnosis and management of strongyloidiasis in a non-endemic area. *Am. J. Trop. Med. Hyg.*, **66**: 749–52.
15. Machado, E.R., Ueta, M.T., et al. 2001. Diagnosis of human strongyloidiasis using particulate antigen of two strains of *Strongyloides venezuelensis* in indirect immunofluorescence antibody test. *Exp. Parasitol.*, **99**: 52–5.
16. Maraha, B., Buiting, A.G.M., et al. 2001. The risk of *Strongyloides stercoralis* transmission from patients with disseminated strongyloidiasis to the medical staff. *J. Hosp. Infect.*, **49**: 222–4.
17. Ottesen, E.A. 2000. The global programme to eliminate lymphatic filariasis. *Trop. Med. Int. Health*, **5**: 591–4.
18. Quinnell, R.J., Griffin, J., et al. 2001. Predisposition to hookworm infection in Papua New Guinea. *Trans. R. Soc. Trop. Med. Hyg.*, **95**: 139–42.
19. Satyanarayana, S., Nema, S., et al. 2005. Disseminated *Strongyloides stercoralis* in AIDS: a report from India. *Indian J. Pathol. Microbiol.*, **48**: 472–74.
20. Satyavani, M. and Chinnaya Rao, K.N. 1993. Live adult male *Loa loa* in the anterior chamber of the eye: a case report. *Indian J. Pathol. Microbiol.*, **36**: 154–157.
21. Slom, T.J., Cortese, M.M., et al. 2002. An outbreak of eosinophilic meningitis caused by *Angiostrongylus cantonensis* in travellers returning from the Caribbean. *N. Engl. J. Med.*, **346**: 668–75.
22. Taylor, M.R. 2001. The epidemiology of ocular toxocariasis. *J. Helminthol.*, **75**: 109–18.

Important Questions

1. Classify nematodes.
2. Classify filarial nematodes.
3. Discuss geographical distribution, habitat, morphology, life cycle, pathogenicity and laboratory diagnosis of:
   (a) *Trichinella spiralis*.
   (b) *Trichuris trichiura*.
   (c) *Strongyloides stercoralis*.
   (d) *Ancylostoma duodenale*.
   (e) *Enterobius vermicularis*.
   (f) *Ascaris lumbricoides*.
   (g) *Wuchereria bancrofti*.
   (h) *Brugia malayi*.
   (i) *Loa loa*.
   (j) *Onchocerca volvulus*.
   (k) *Dracunculus medinensis*.
4. Write short notes on:
   (a) General characters of nematodes
   (b) Cutaneous larva migrans
   (c) Visceral larva migrans
   (d) *Anisakis simplex*
   (e) Tropical eosinophilia
   (f) Occult filariasis
   (g) *Brugia timori*
   (h) *Mansonella streptocerca*
   (i) *Mansonella ozzardi*
   (j) *Mansonella perstans*
   (k) *Dirofilaria immitis*
   (l) *Angiostrongylus cantonensis*
   (m) *Angiostrongylus costaricensis*

(n) *Gnathostoma spinigerum*
(o) *Gnathostoma hispidum*
(p) *Gnathostoma doloresi*
(q) *Capillaria philippinensis*
(r) *Capillaria hepatica*
(s) *Capillaria aerophila*
(t) *Ternidens deminutus*
(u) *Oesophagostomum* spp.
(v) *Trichostrongylus* spp.
(w) *Thelazia callipaeda*
(x) *Dioctophyma renale*

5. Tabulate differences between *Ancylostoma duodenale* and *Necator americanus*

Multiple Choice Questions

1. Largest nematode parasite known to cause infection in man is:
   (a) *Ascaris lumbricoides*.
   (b) *Strongyloides stercoralis*.
   (c) *Ancylostoma duodenale*.
   (d) *Dracunculus medinensis*.
2. Which of the following nematodes is ovo-viviparous?
   (a) *Ascaris lumbricoides*.
   (b) *Dracunculus medinensis*.
   (c) *Strongyloides stercoralis*.
   (d) *Trichinella spiralis*.
3. Which of the following nematodes lays unsegmented eggs?
   (a) *Necator americanus*.
   (b) *Trichuris trichiura*.
   (c) *Strongyloides stercoralis*.
   (d) *Trichinella spiralis*.
4. Which of the following nematodes lays eggs containing larvae?
   (a) *Trichinella spiralis*.
   (b) *Enterobius vermicularis*.
   (c) *Brugia malayi*.
   (d) *Ascaris lumbricoides*.
5. Best site for taking biopsy for diagnosis of trichinellosis is:
   (a) deltoid muscle.
   (b) diaphragm.
   (c) pectoralis major.
   (d) liver.
6. Bachman's test is done to diagnose infection with:
   (a) *Schistosoma japonicum*.
   (b) *Trichinella spiralis*.
   (c) *Trichuris trichiura*.
   (d) *Ancylostoma duodenale*.
7. Rectal prolapse is seen in infection with:
   (a) *Enterobius vermicularis*.
   (b) *Trichuris trichiura*.
   (c) *Ascaris lumbricoides*.
   (d) *Ancylostoma duodenale*.
8. Disseminated systemic infection in AIDS patients is seen with:
   (a) *Ancylostoma duodenale*.
   (b) *Dracunculus medinensis*.
   (c) *Strongyloides stercoralis*.
   (d) *Trichinella spiralis*.
9. "Larva currens" is the name given to the migrating larvae of:
   (a) *Ancylostoma braziliense*.
   (b) *Strongyloides stercoralis*.
   (c) *Ancylostoma caninum*.
   (d) *Wuchereria bancrofti*.
10. Which of the following nematodes **does not** pass through lungs during its life cycle?
    (a) *Ancylostoma duodenale*.
    (b) *Necator americanus*.
    (c) *Ascaris lumbricoides*.
    (d) *Trichuris trichiura*.
11. Cutaneous larva migrans is the name given to migrating larvae of:
    (a) *Ancylostoma braziliense*.
    (b) *Enterobius vermicularis*.
    (c) *Wuchereria bancrofti*.
    (d) *Trichuris trichiura*.
12. All of the following parasites may cause iron deficiency anaemia **except**:
    (a) *Ancylostoma duodenale*.
    (b) *Diphyllobothrium latum*.
    (c) *Trichuris trichiura*.
    (d) *Necator americanus*.
13. Which of the following stages of *Ancylostoma duodenale* is infective to human beings?
    (a) Rhabditiform larva.
    (b) Filariform larva.
    (c) Eggs.
    (d) Adult worm.

14. Which of the following characteristics possessed by fertilized eggs of *Ascaris lumbricoides* differentiates them from unfertilized?
    (a) Do not float in the concentrated salt solution.
    (b) Larger in size.
    (c) Always non-mammilated.
    (d) Possess a clear crescentic space at each pole.
15. Visceral larva migrans is caused by the migrating larvae of which of the following worms?
    (a) *Ancylostoma caninum*.
    (b) *Ancylostoma braziliense*.
    (c) *Toxocara canis*.
    (d) *Enterobius vermicularis*.
16. Life cycle of larvae of *W. bancrofti* in mosquito is:
    (a) cyclo-developmental.
    (b) cyclo-propagative.
    (c) propagative.
    (d) cyclo-propagative and propagative.
17. Diurnal periodicity is shown by larvae of:
    (a) *Wuchereria bancrofti*.
    (b) *Brugia malayi*.
    (c) *Loa loa*.
    (d) *Mansonella perstans*.
18. Tail-tip contains 2 nuclei in case of microfilariae of:
    (a) *Wuchereria bancrofti*.
    (b) *Brugia malayi*.
    (c) *Loa loa*.
    (d) *Onchocerca volvulus*.
19. Diethylcarbamazine provocation test is done to:
    (a) test sensitivity of microfilariae to the drug.
    (b) test hypersensitivity reaction to the drug.
    (c) make a peripheral blood film for diagnosis.
    (d) to induce production of antibodies for serology.
20. Dose of diethylcarbamazine for the treatment of bancroftian filariasis is:
    (a) 6 mg/kg body weight daily for 12 days.
    (b) 9 mg/kg body weight daily for 12 days.
    (c) 12 mg/kg body weight daily for 12 days.
    (d) 15 mg/kg body weight daily for 12 days.
21. Which of the following microfilariae is unsheathed?
    (a) *Mf. perstans*.
    (b) *Mf. bancrofti*.
    (c) *Mf. malayi*.
    (d) *Mf. loa*.
22. Microfilariae can be diagnosed in peripheral blood film examination in all of the following **except**:
    (a) *Mf. malayi*.
    (b) *Mf. loa*.
    (c) *Mf. perstans*.
    (d) *Mf. streptocerca*.
23. Microfilaria of *B. malayi* differs from that of *W. bancrofti* in that the latter:
    (a) is smaller in size.
    (b) possesses secondary kinks.
    (c) has longer cephalic space.
    (d) has tail-tip free from nuclei.
24. River blindness is the name given to disease caused by:
    (a) *Loa loa*.
    (b) *Onchocerca volvulus*.
    (c) *Toxoplasma gondii*.
    (d) *Acanthamoeba culbertsoni*.
25. Fugitive or Calabar swellings are seen in infection with:
    (a) *Onchocerca volvulus*.
    (b) *Loa loa*.
    (c) *Wuchereria bancrofti*.
    (d) *Brugia timori*.
26. Mazzotti test is the name given to:
    (a) complement fixation test for *Loa loa*.
    (b) serological test for *Onchocerca volvulus*.
    (c) provocation test for *Onchocerca volvulus*.
    (d) intradermal skin test for *Loa loa*.
27. Which stage of *Gnathostoma spinigerum* is infective to man?
    (a) Adult worm.
    (b) L1 larvae.
    (c) L2 larvae.
    (d) L3 larvae.
28. Dog heartworm is the common name for:
    (a) *Toxocara canis*.
    (b) *Dirofilaria immitis*.
    (c) *Mansonella streptocerca*.
    (d) *Toxoplasma gondii*.
29. The blister formed by *Dracunculus medinensis* contains:
    (a) many polymorphs and bacteria.
    (b) haemorrhagic fluid.
    (c) sterile fluid and inflammatory infiltrate.
    (d) dead larvae.

30. The parasite which has been eradicated from India is:
    (a) *Leishmania donovani*.
    (b) *Dracunculus medinensis*.
    (c) *Babesia microti*.
    (d) *Toxoplasma gondii*.
31. Eosinophilic meningoencephalitis is caused by:
    (a) *Naegleria fowleri*.
    (b) *Angiostrongylus cantonensis*.
    (c) *Angiostrongylus costaricensis*.
    (d) *Toxoplasma gondii*.
32. Rat lungworm is the common name of:
    (a) *Paragonimus westermani*.
    (b) *Toxocara canis*.
    (c) *Angiostrongylus cantonensis*.
    (d) *Mansonella streptocerca*.
33. Lesions produced by which of the following worms mimic those of leprosy?
    (a) *Ancylostoma caninum*.
    (b) *Mansonella streptocerca*.
    (c) *Angiostrongylus cantonensis*.
    (d) *Schistosoma haematobium*.
34. Adult worms of which of the following parasites reside in human body cavity?
    (a) *Mansonella streptocerca*.
    (b) *Wuchereria bancrofti*.
    (c) *Brugia malayi*.
    (d) *Mansonella perstans*.
35. Dracunculiasis was a health problem in which state of India?
    (a) Rajasthan.
    (b) Haryana.
    (c) Bihar.
    (d) Kerala.
36. Paratenic host for *Angiostrongylus cantonensis* is:
    (a) man.
    (b) rat.
    (c) frog.
    (d) sheep.
37. In *Angiostrongylus costaricensis*, species name is given after:
    (a) name of the scientist who discovered it.
    (b) name of the patient in which it was first seen.
    (c) name of the place where incidence is high.
    (d) name of the university where it was first reported.
38. Clinical illness caused by which worm resembles appendicitis?
    (a) *Ancylostoma duodenale*.
    (b) *Dracunculus medinensis*.
    (c) *Angiostrongylus costaricensis*.
    (d) *Trichuris trichiura*.
39. All of the following parasites inhabit ocular tissues **except**:
    (a) *Thelazia callipaeda*.
    (b) *Onchocerca volvulus*.
    (c) *Loa loa*.
    (d) *Mansonella streptocerca*.
40. Which of the following parasitic eggs can be demonstrated in urine of infected patient?
    (a) *Dioctophyma renale*.
    (b) *Schistosoma japonicum*.
    (c) *Ascaris lumbricoides*.
    (d) *Trichuris trichiura*.
41. A 50-year-old patient reported in surgery outpatient department with multiple subcutaneous nodules over the right iliac crest. They measured 5–15 mm in diameter and were fully movable. Adult worms and microfilariae could be detected inside the excised nodules and skin snips taken from the vicinity of the lesions respectively. Which of the following nematodes is most likely to be the causative agent?
    (a) *Onchocerca volvulus*.
    (b) *Wuchereria bancrofti*.
    (c) *Brugia malayi*.
    (d) *Brugia timori*.
42. Loeffler's syndrome may be seen in infection with:
    (a) *Ancylostoma duodenale*.
    (b) *Ascaris lumbricoides*.
    (c) *Trichinella spiralis*.
    (d) *Trichuris trichiura*.
43. NIH swab is used for the detection of eggs of:
    (a) *Ascaris lumbricoides*.
    (b) *Necator americanus*.
    (c) *Enterobius vermicularis*.
    (d) *Ancylostoma duodenale*.
44. Which of the following parasites is **not** transmitted by ingestion of eggs?
    (a) *Ancylostoma duodenale*.
    (b) *Ascaris lumbricoides*.
    (c) *Enterobius vermicularis*.
    (d) *Trichuris trichiura*.

45. Which of the following adult worms resides in the subcutaneous nodules?
 (a) *Onchocerca volvulus.*
 (b) *Gnathostoma spinigerum.*
 (c) *Wuchereria bancrofti.*
 (d) *Brugia malayi.*

46. Which of the following adult worms resides in lymphatics and lymph nodes?
 (a) *Dracunculus medinensis.*
 (b) *Loa loa.*
 (c) *Brugia malayi.*
 (d) *Gnathostoma spinigerum.*

47. Infection with which of the following parasites may cause enuresis?
 (a) *Ascaris lumbricoides.*
 (b) *Enterobius vermicularis.*
 (c) *Trichuris trichiura.*
 (d) *Wuchereria bancrofti.*

48. Humans acquire infection with *Dracunculus medinensis* by:
 (a) penetration of the skin by the larva.
 (b) drinking water containing infected *Cyclops*.
 (c) bite of female *Aedes* mosquito.
 (d) bite of female sand fly.

49. Which of the following parasites **does not** penetrate human skin?
 (a) *Ascaris lumbricoides.*
 (b) *Ancylostoma duodenale.*
 (c) *Strongyloides stercoralis.*
 (d) *Schistosoma haematobium.*

50. Which of the following nematodes is oviparous?
 (a) *Wuchereria bancrofti*
 (b) *Strongyloides stercoralis.*
 (c) *Ancylostoma duodenale.*
 (d) *Trichinella spiralis.*

51. Which of the following filarial worms produces sheated microfilariae?
 (a) *Mansonella oozardi.*
 (b) *Mansonella perstans.*
 (c) *Onchocerca volvulus.*
 (d) *Loa loa.*

52. Autoinfection is seen with following parasites **except**:
 (a) *Strongyloides stercoralis.*
 (b) *Ascaris lumbricoides.*
 (c) *Enterobius vemicularis.*
 (d) *Taenia solium.*

53. Which of the following filarial worms resides in the subconjunctival tissue of the eye?
 (a) *Loa loa.*
 (b) *Brugia malayi.*
 (c) *Wuchereria bancrofti.*
 (d) *Onchocerca volvulus.*

54. Fish is **not** the source of infection with:
 (a) *Diphyllobothrium latum.*
 (b) *Clonorchis sinensis.*
 (c) *Heterophyes heterophyes.*
 (d) *Trichinella spiralis.*

55. Microfilariae of which of the following filarial worms are found in skin?
 (a) *Onchocerca volvulus.*
 (b) *Brugia malayi.*
 (c) *Wuchereria bancrofti.*
 (d) *Mansonella oozardi.*

56. *Dracunculus medinensis* resides in:
 (a) subcutaneous tissue.
 (b) small intestine.
 (c) liver.
 (d) lung.

57. Smallest nematode known to cause infection in man is:
 (a) *Trichinella spiralis.*
 (b) *Ancylostoma duodenale.*
 (c) *Strongyloides stercoralis.*
 (d) *Trichuris trichiura.*

58. Which of the following nematodes **does not** occur in the intestine?
 (a) *Trichuris trichiura.*
 (b) *Enterobius vermicularis.*
 (c) *Ascaris lumbricoides.*
 (d) *Wuchereria bancrofti.*

59. Infection with *Dracunculus medinensis* is acquired through ingestion of infective larvae harboured in which of the intermediate hosts listed below?
 (a) Snails.
 (b) Coppods (Cyclops).
 (c) Fish.
 (d) None of the above.

60. Which of the following helminth genera **does not** need an intermediate host in its life cycle?
 (a) *Schistosoma haematobium.*
 (b) *Strongyloides stercoralis.*
 (c) *Dracunculus medinensis.*
 (d) *Anisakis simplex.*

61. Which of the following stages of the specific parasites could be found in a human muscle squash preparation?
    (a) Metacercariae of *Paragonimus*.
    (b) Encysted larvae of *Trichinella spiralis*.
    (c) Metacercariae of *Fasciolopsis buski*.
    (d) Metacercariae of *Clonorchis sinensis*.
62. In *Trichinella spiralis* infection encysted, coiled larvae can be seen in:
    (a) stool.
    (b) cerebrospinal fluid.
    (c) sputum.
    (d) muscle tissue.
63. Man acquires infection by ingestion of eggs of:
    (a) *Ancylostoma duodenale*.
    (b) *Schistosoma haematobium*.
    (c) *Enterobius vermicularis*.
    (d) *Strongyloides stercoralis*.
64. Which of the following parasites lays eggs with mucoid polar plugs?
    (a) *Ascaris lumbricoides*.
    (b) *Ancylostoma duodenale*.
    (c) *Trichuris trichiura*.
    (d) *Enterobius vermicularis*.
65. Which of the following parasites can cause dysentery in heavy infection?
    (a) *Trichuris trichiura*.
    (b) *Necator americanus*.
    (c) *Giardia lamblia*.
    (d) *Cryptosporidium parvum*.
66. Eye worm is the common name of which of the following nematodes?
    (a) *Onchocerca volvulus*.
    (b) *Loa loa*.
    (c) *Mansonella oozardi*.
    (d) *Dirofilaria bancrofti*.

ANSWERS TO MCQs

1 (d), 2 (c), 3 (b), 4 (b), 5 (a), 6 (b), 7 (b), 8 (c), 9 (b), 10 (d), 11 (a), 12 (b), 13 (b), 14 (d), 15 (c), 16 (a), 17 (c), 18 (b), 19 (c), 20 (a), 21 (a), 22 (d), 23 (d), 24 (b), 25 (b), 26 (c), 27 (d), 28 (b), 29 (c), 30 (b), 31 (b), 32 (c), 33 (b), 34 (d), 35 (a), 36 (c), 37 (c), 38 (c), 39 (d), 40 (a), 41 (a), 42 (b), 43 (c), 44 (a), 45 (a), 46 (c), 47 (b), 48 (b), 49 (a), 50 (c), 51 (d), 52 (b), 53 (a), 54 (d), 55 (a), 56 (a), 57 (c), 58 (d), 59 (b), 60 (b), 61 (b), 62 (d), 63 (c), 64 (c), 65 (a), 66 (b).

SECTION 4

Applied Parasitology, Diagnostic Procedures and Overview

12

Parasitic Opportunistic Infections in AIDS Cases and Nosocomial Parasitic Infections

Toxoplasma gondii
Cryptosporidium parvum
Isospora belli
Microsporidia
Entamoeba histolytica
Giardia lamblia
Cyclospora cayetanensis
Leishmania spp.
Strongyloides stercoralis
Free-living protozoa
Nosocomial parasitic infections

PARASITIC OPPORTUNISTIC INFECTIONS IN AIDS CASES

Patients with HIV disease, sometimes during the course of their illness, become a microbial zoo. Most of the patients with HIV disease die of infections other than HIV. Because of a progressive decline in their immunological responses, patients with HIV infection are extremely susceptible to a variety of common as well as opportunistic infections.

Opportunistic parasitic infections can cause severe morbidity and mortality. Since many of these infections are treatable, an early and accurate diagnosis is important. This can be accomplished by a variety of methods such as direct demonstration of the parasite and by serological tests to detect antigen and/or specific antibodies. *Antibody response may be poor in AIDS patients, therefore, immunodiagnostic tests have to be interpreted with caution.* Parasitic opportunistic infections in AIDS cases are given in Table 12.1.

Table 12.1. Parasites causing opportunistic infections in AIDS cases

• *Toxoplasma gondii*	• *Cryptosporidium parvum*
• *Isospora belli*	• Microsporidia
• *Entamoeba histolytica*	• *Giardia lamblia*
• *Cyclospora cayetanensis*	• *Leishmania* spp.
• *Strongyloides stercoralis*	• Free-living protozoa

TOXOPLASMA GONDII

Toxoplasma gondii is an obligate intracellular protozoan. It is the most common cause of secondary CNS infection in patients with AIDS accounting for 38% of all such patients. It is also the common cause of intracerebral mass lesions in patients with HIV infection (accounting for 50–60%). Overall, toxoplasmosis is seen in approximately 15% of patients with AIDS. It is generally a late complication of HIV infection and usually occurs in patients with CD4+ T cell count less than 100/µl.

Toxoplasmosis is thought to represent a reactivation syndrome and is 10 times more common in patients with antibodies to the organisms, an indicator of prior infection, than in patients who are seronegative. Approximately 30% of AIDS patients with antibodies to *T. gondii* go on to develop CNS infection at sometime during the course of their disease. However, owing to abnormalities of B cell functions seen in patients with HIV infection, serologic testing cannot be used to rule out a diagnosis of toxoplasmosis, and approximately 5% of cases occur in HIV-infected patients who are seronegative for *T. gondii*.

The most common clinical presentation in patients with HIV infection is one of fever, headache, and focal neurologic deficits, with the latter occurring in approximately 90% of patients. Patients may present with seizure, hemiparesis or aphasia as a manifestation of focal neurologic defects or with a picture more related to accompanying cerebral oedema and consisting of confusion, dementia, lethargy, and progression to coma. In addition to the CNS involvement, *T. gondii* has been reported to cause a variety of other clinical problems in HIV-infected patients. These include chorioretinitis, pneumonia, peritonitis with ascites, gastrointestinal involvement, cystitis and orchitis. Patients can minimize their risk of developing toxoplasmosis by avoiding the consumption of undercooked meat and careful hand washing after contact with soil.

CRYPTOSPORIDIUM PARVUM

Cryptosporidium parvum produces mild and self-limited (1–2 weeks) diarrhoea in immunocompetent persons. It is spread through faecal-oral contact, and nosocomial outbreaks have been reported. In HIV-infected individuals, cryptosporidial infection may present in a variety of ways, ranging from a self-limited or intermittent diarrhoeal illness in patients in the early stages of HIV disease to a severe life-threatening diarrhoea in severely immunodeficient individuals. The diarrhoea is profuse and watery; it may contain mucus but rarely blood and leucocytes, and it is often associated with weight loss. Fluid loss in AIDS patients with cryptosporidiosis is often excessive; 3–6 litres of watery stool per day. In 75% cases, diarrhoea is accompanied by crampy abdominal pain, approximately 25% of patients have nausea and/or vomiting.

C. parvum is not always confined to gastrointestinal tract, additional symptoms (respiratory cryptosporidiosis, cholecystitis, hepatitis and pancreatitis) have been associated with extraintestinal lesions.

The characteristic finding is the presence of oocysts, in the faeces, that can be stained by modified acid-fast staining. On electron microscopy of small bowel biopsy specimens, organisms can be seen adhering to the brush border of the intestinal epithelium. Therapy is purely symptomatic. Patients can minimize their risk of developing cryptosporidiosis by avoiding contact with human and animal faeces and by not drinking faecally contaminated water from lakes or rivers.

ISOSPORA BELLI

Isospora belli is a coccidian parasite most commonly found as a cause of diarrhoea in patients from the Caribbean and Africa. Currently, it is being seen in increasing frequency as one of the causes of the diarrhoeal syndrome in AIDS patients. Fever, headache, steatorrhoea, and weight loss may occur in protracted cases. Deaths due to water loss and electrolyte imbalance have been reported in overwhelming infections. In patients with AIDS, this infection may disseminate beyond the intestinal wall, e.g., mesenteric and tracheobronchial lymph nodes, gall bladder, liver and spleen. Diagnosis can be established by demonstration of characteristic oocysts in the faeces. This infection can be treated with trimethoprim/sulphamethoxazole.

MICROSPORIDIA

Microsporidia are small, unicellular, obligate intracellular parasites that reside in the cytoplasm of enteric cells. With the spread of HIV infection and AIDS, microsporidia are becoming increasingly recognized as important causes of opportunistic disease in infected individuals. Microsporidian species most frequently reported in association with AIDS are *Enterocytozoon bieneusi*, *Encephalitozoon intestinalis* and *Encephalitozoon hellem*.

Intestinal microsporidiosis is the commonest infection, caused mainly by *E. bieneusi*. It produces persistent diarrhoea with wasting. *E. intestinalis* infects the intestine, gall bladder, liver and kidney. *E. hellem* is associated with infection of the cornea and conjunctiva, causing keratoconjunctivitis. Other species have been reported as causing hepatitis and disseminated infections. Infection is probably by spores being ingested, inhaled or inoculated (eye). Spores are highly resistant in the environment.

ENTAMOEBA HISTOLYTICA

Entamoeba histolytica, although not strictly opportunistic pathogen in that it can also cause disease in immunocompetent individuals, is more common in patients with HIV infection. It should be carefully looked in any patient with HIV infection and persistent diarrhoea.

It appears that invasive amoebiasis is becoming more important as one of the opportunistic parasitic infections in patients with HIV infection in areas of endemicity for amoebiasis.

GIARDIA LAMBLIA

Although patients with HIV infection have also been found to have giardiasis, the infection does not appear to be more severe among this group, regardless of the CD4+ T cell count. With giardiasis, symptoms may range from none to the malabsorption syndrome, characterized by gas, bloating, frothy green foul-smelling stools, and abdominal pain.

CYCLOSPORA CAYETANENSIS

In normal host it causes self-limiting infection with abdominal pain and diarrhoea lasting for 3–4 days. In AIDS patients diarrhoea may persist for 12 weeks or more. Biliary disease has also been reported in AIDS patients.

LEISHMANIA spp.

Leishmaniasis is emerging as third most frequent opportunistic infection in AIDS patients in various parts of the world particularly in *Leishmania* endemic countries where in 25–70% of adult cases of visceral leishmaniasis are found to be HIV co-infected. Both HIV and *Leishmania* spp. are obligate intracellular parasites. It is reported that like HIV, leishmanial infection also causes depletion of helper T cells. HIV related immunosuppression increases the risk of reactivating leishmaniasis by 100–1000 times in endemic areas and enhances the chances of drug-resistant leishmaniasis.

In AIDS patient *Leishmania* spp. lead to more serious manifestations of visceral leishmaniasis. The presentation of visceral leishmaniasis is very atypical. Some cutaneous species manifest visceral disease. HIV may either activate subclinical leishmaniasis or make the patient susceptible to a new infection. *L. infantum* causes visceral leishmaniasis classically restricted to children, especially those below 2 years. However, it may also cause infection in HIV-infected adults.

The results of different serological tests need to be interpreted with care as up to 42% of co-infected patients have been found to have a negative antibody response.

STRONGYLOIDES STERCORALIS

In normal host, *Strongyloides stercoralis* causes asymptomatic to mild abdominal symptoms. Infection may remain latent for many years owing to low-level infection maintained by internal autoinfective life cycle. In AIDS patients, it may result in disseminated disease (hyperinfection syndrome due to autoinfective nature of life cycle). During hyperinfection, filariform larvae may enter arterial circulation and lodge in various organs, e.g., lymph nodes, endocardium, pancreas, liver, kidneys and brain.

Patient may present with abdominal pain, pneumonitis and there may be repeated episodes of unexplained bacteraemia or meningitis with enteric bacteria. This occurs when the larvae penetrate the bowel and reinitiate the cycle. In doing so, they carry members of the bowel flora with them. The other consistent finding in these patients is an unexplained eosinophilia, which may range from 10–50%.

FREE-LIVING PROTOZOA

Infections caused by free-living protozoa are being recognized clinically as important parasitic pathogens, particularly in immunocompromised patients. Primary amoebic meningoencephalitis caused by *Naegleria fowleri* and granulomatous amoebic encephalitis caused by *Acanthamoeba* spp. and *Balamuthia mandrillaris* (including cases in patients with AIDS) are now well recognized.

NOSOCOMIAL PARASITIC INFECTIONS

Nosocomial (*nosocomion* means hospital) infection, healthcare-associated or hospital-acquired infection is defined as infection developing in a patient after admission to the hospital, which was neither present nor in its incubation period when the subject entered the hospital. Such an infection may manifest during the stay in the hospital or some time after the patient is discharged. Parasites causing nosocomial infections are given in Table 12.2.

Table 12.2. Nosocomial parasitic infections

Nosocomial gastrointestinal infections	
• *Cryptosporidium parvum*	• *Giardia lamblia*
• *Entamoeba histolytica*	• Microsporidia
• *Hymenolepis nana*	• *Taenia solium*
• *Strongyloides stercoralis*	
Nosocomial blood and tissue infections	
• *Plasmodium* spp.	• *Babesia* spp.
• *Trypanosoma brucei gambiense*	• *Trypanosoma brucei rhodesiense*
• *Trypanosoma cruzi*	• *Leishmania donovani*
• *Toxoplasma gondii*	
Nosocomial infection in the paediatric patient	
• *Cryptosporidium parvum*	• *Giardia lamblia*

Nosocomial gastrointestinal infections

Patients at highest risk for gastrointestinal infections include neonates, the elderly patients with achlorhydria, and those who are immunosuppressed. The transmission of the organism is generally via the faecal-oral route. Parasites that have been implicated in parasitic nosocomial gastrointestinal infections include *C. parvum*, *G. lamblia*, *E. histolytica*, microsporidia, *H. nana*, *T. solium* (cysticercosis) and *Strongyloides stercoralis*.

Nosocomial blood and tissue infections

Plasmodium spp., *Babesia* spp., *T. brucei gambiense*, *T. brucei rhodesiense*, *T. cruzi* and *L. donovani* may be transmitted by blood transfusion. Nosocomial infection with *T. gondii*, primarily in cardiac or renal transplant patients, has been documented.

Nosocomial infections in the paediatric patients

Specific infections that can be acquired in the paediatric patients include those caused by *C. parvum* & *G. lamblia*.

Further Reading

1. Benator, D.A., French, A.L. et al. 1994. *Isospora belli* infection associated with acalculous cholecystitis in a patient with AIDS. *Ann. Intern. Med.*, **121**: 663–4.
2. Boothe, C.C., Salvin, C. et al. 1980. Immunodeficiency and cryptosporidiosis demonstration at the Royal College of Physicians of London. *Br. Med. J.*, **281**: 1123–7.
3. Centres for Disease Control. 1982. Cryptosporidiosis: an assessment of chemotherapy of males with acquired immunodeficiency syndrome (AIDS). *Morbid Mortal Weekly Rep.*, **31**: 589–92.
4. Friedberg, D.N., Stenson, S.M. et al. 1990. Microsporidial keratoconjunctivitis in acquired immunodeficiency syndrome. *Arch. Ophthalmol.*, **108**: 504–8.
5. Lowder, C.Y., Meisler, D.M. et al. 1990. Microsporidia infection of the cornea in a man seropositive for human immunodeficiency virus. *Am. J. Ophthalmol.*, **109**: 242–4.
6. Luft, B.J., Hafner, R. et al. 1993. Toxoplasmic encephalitis in patients with the acquired immunodeficiency syndrome. *N. Engl. J. Med.*, **329**: 995–1000.
7. Luft, B.J. and Remington, J.S. 1992. Toxoplasmic encephalitis in AIDS. *Clin. Infect. Dis.*, **15**: 211–22.
8. Machtinger, L., Telford, S.R. III et al. 1993. Treatment of babesiosis by red blood cell exchange in an HIV positive splenectomised patient. *J. Clin. Apheresis*, **8**: 78–81.
9. Michiels, J.F., Hofman, P. et al. 1994. Intestinal and extraintestinal *Isospora belli* infection in an AIDS patient. A second case report. *Pathol. Res. Pract.*, **190**: 1089–93.
10. Modigliani, R., Boris, C. et al. 1985. Diarrhoea and malabsorption in acquired immunodeficiency syndrome: a study of four cases with special emphasis on opportunistic protozoan infestations. *Gut*, **26**: 179–87.
11. Raband, C., May, T. et al. 1994. Extracerebral toxoplasmosis in patients infected with HIV. A French National Survey. *Medicine*, **73**: 306–14.
12. Restrepo, C., Macher, A.M. and Radany, E.H. 1987. Disseminated extraintestinal isosporiasis in a patient with acquired immunodeficiency syndrome. *Am. J. Clin. Pathol.*, **87**: 536–42.
13. Shanker, S.K., Satishchandra, P., et al. 2003. Low prevalence of progressive multifocal leucoencephalopathy in India and Africa. *J. Neurovirol.*, **9** (Suppl. 1): 59–67.
14. Singh, S. 2002. Human strongyloidiasis in AIDS era: its zoonotic importance. *J. Assoc. Physicians India*, **50**: 415–22.
15. Smith, P.D., Lane, H.C. et al. 1988. Intestinal infection in patients with acquired immunodeficiency syndrome (AIDS). *Ann. Intern. Med.*, **108**: 328–33.
16. Yee, R.W., Tio, F.O. et al. 1991. Resolution of microsporidial epithelial keratopathy in a patient with AIDS. *Ophthalmology*, **98**: 196–201.

Important Questions

1. Name and discuss briefly parasitic opportunistic infections in AIDS cases.
2. Name and discuss briefly nosocomial parasitic infections.

Multiple Choice Questions

1. The most common clinical presentation of toxoplasmosis in patients with HIV infection is:
   (a) chorioretinitis.
   (b) pneumonia.
   (c) CNS involvement.
   (d) peritonitis with ascites.
2. In AIDS cases, *Isospora belli* may disseminate beyond the intestinal wall to:
   (a) mesenteric and tracheobronchial lymph nodes.
   (b) gall bladder.
   (c) liver and spleen.
   (d) All of the above.
3. Most important microsporidia causing opportunistic infection in AIDS cases is:
   (a) *Enterocytozoon bieneusi.*
   (b) *Microsporidium ceylonensis.*
   (c) *Encephalitozoon cuniculi.*
   (d) *Nosema connori.*
4. Diarrhoea in AIDS patients may be caused by:
   (a) *Cryptosporidium parvum.*
   (b) microsporidia.
   (c) *Isospora belli.*
   (d) All of the above.

ANSWERS TO MCQs

1 (c), 2 (d), 3 (a), 4 (d).

13

Diagnostic Procedures

Laboratory diagnosis of a parasitic infection can be carried out by detection and identification of the parasite or a stage in the life cycle of the parasite (trophozoite, cyst, egg, or larva) in various specimens (faeces, blood, bone marrow, urine, and biopsy material from spleen, liver, lymph nodes, etc.), cultivation of parasites, immunoassays, DNA probes and polymerase chain reaction.

EXAMINATION OF FAECES

COLLECTION OF THE SPECIMEN

Specimens should be collected in a wide-mouthed, clean, leak-proof container without contamination with urine, water or disinfectants because water may contain free-living organisms that can be mistaken for human parasites, and urine and disinfectants may destroy motile organisms. Faecal specimens, like other specimens received in the laboratory, must be handled with care to avoid acquiring infection from infectious parasites, bacteria, or viruses. Faeces may contain:

- **Infective forms of parasites** such as *Strongyloides stercoralis*, *Enterobius vermicularis*, *Taenia solium*, *Entamoeba histolytica*, *Giardia lamblia*, *Balantidium coli* and *Cryptosporidium parvum*.
- **Bacteria** such as *Shigella*, *Salmonella* and *Vibrio cholerae*.
- **Viruses** such as hepatitis A virus, hepatitis E virus and rotavirus.

Optimum time of specimen collection should ideally be as close to the onset of symptoms as possible, before initiation of antiparasitic therapy and first morning sample. Normally passed stool is preferable. Specimens obtained by purgation are generally less satisfactory. The specimen should be free of oil and other nonfaecal substances such as barium or bismuth. Patients who have received a barium enema may not excrete organisms in their stools for at least 1 week following barium enema, therefore, stool examination must be delayed for at least 1 week following the enema.

The amount of faeces required may range from the whole stool, or series of stools over a specified period, to milligram amounts scraped from the gloved finger after rectal examination. The collection of three faecal specimens usually suffices to make the diagnosis of intestinal parasitic diseases, two obtained on successive days during normal bowel movement and a third after magnesium sulphate purge.

A total of six specimens, collected on successive days, may be required if intestinal amoebiasis or giardiasis is suspected. For obtaining scrapings of the ulcers in the rectum or the sigmoid colon, a proctoscope or a sigmoidoscope should be used. Every specimen should be identified with the following minimal information – patient's name and identification number, physician's name, and the date and time specimen was collected. The specimen should also be accompanied by a request form indicating which laboratory procedures are to be performed.

Because trophozoites disintegrate rapidly after defecation and do not encyst, liquid stool specimens should be examined within 30 minutes after collection (not 30 minutes after receipt in the laboratory) or semi-formed stools within 60 minutes, to detect motile trophozoites, particularly in suspected infections with *Entamoeba histolytica* and *Giardia lamblia*. Formed stools, in which trophozoites are not expected, may be examined up to 24 hours after passage.

Preservation of stool

If there is delay from the time of collection of specimen and transport until examination in the laboratory, the use of stool preservatives should be considered. Several preservatives are available for permanent fixation of stool specimens that may be sent to reference laboratory for analysis. Preservation of stool helps in maintaining morphology of protozoan parasites and preventing further development of some helminthic eggs and larvae. Intestinal parasites which can be detected in faeces are given in Table 13.1.

Commonly used preservatives

Following are the commonly used preservatives:

Formalin solution

Faecal sample can be preserved in 10% formalin saline (100 ml formaldehyde in 900 ml 0.85% sodium chloride). Three parts of formalin preservative solution is thoroughly mixed with one part of stool specimen.

Table 13.1. Intestinal parasites found in faeces

• *Entamoeba histolytica*	• *Giardia lamblia*
• *Dientamoeba fragilis*	• *Cryptosporidium parvum*
• *Isospora belli*	• *Cyclospora cayetanensis*
• *Balantidium coli*	• *Encephalitozoon intestinalis*
• *Enterocytozoon bieneusi*	• *Diphyllobothrium latum*
• *Taenia* species	• *Hymenolepis nana*
• *Hymenolepis diminuta*	• *Dipylidium caninum*
• *Schistosoma mansoni*	• *Schistosoma japonicum*
• *Fasciola hepatica*	• *Fasciolopsis buski*
• *Clonorchis sinensis*	• *Opisthorchis* species
• *Heterophyes heterophyes*	• *Metagonimus yokogawai*
• *Ascaris lumbricoides*	• *Ancylostoma duodenale*
• *Necator americanus*	• *Enterobius vermicularis*
• *Strongyloides stercoralis*	• *Trichuris trichiura*
• *Capillaria* species	

Advantages

- It is readily available, is easy to prepare, and serves as an all-purpose fixative.
- The prepared reagent has long shelf life.
- The morphology of helminth eggs, larvae, protozoan cysts, and coccidial forms are well preserved.
- Formalin preserved specimens are suitable for concentration procedures.

Disadvantages

- Formalin preserved specimens are not suitable for the preparation of trichrome-stained smears.
- Preservation is inadequate to maintain the morphology of protozoan trophozoites.
- Since the preservatives kill the parasites, therefore, characteristic motility of trophozoites cannot be seen.

Polyvinyl alcohol (PVA)

It preserves intestinal protozoa especially trophozoite stage. It is prepared by mixing 62.5 ml of 95% ethyl alcohol, 125 ml of saturated aqueous solution of mercuric chloride, 10 ml of glacial acetic acid, and 3 ml of glycerine in a 500 ml beaker. Then 10 gram of PVA powder is added, without stirring. The beaker is then covered and allowed to soak overnight. It is then heated slowly to 75°C. When this temperature is reached, the mixture is removed from heat and it is stirred until a homogenous, slightly milky solution is obtained. For the preservation of stool, three parts of PVA is mixed with one part of the specimen.

Advantages

- The morphology of protozoan trophozoites and cysts is well preserved.
- Preserved samples remain stable for several months.
- Permanent slides can be prepared from PVA preserved stool specimens.

Disadvantages

- The morphology of helminth eggs and larvae, coccidian, and microsporidia are inadequately preserved.
- Unsuitable for acid-fast and safranin stains.
- The reagent is difficult to prepare in the laboratory.

Merthiolate-iodine-formalin (MIF) solution

MIF solution is prepared in two separate stock solutions to be mixed immediately before use:

- **Solution I** is prepared by mixing 250 ml of distilled water, 200 ml of thiomersal, 25 ml of formaldehyde, and 5 ml of glycerol.
- **Solution II** is Lugol's iodine (5% iodine in 10% potassium iodide solution in distilled water).

Before use, 9.4 ml (94 parts) of solution I is mixed with 0.6 ml (6 parts) of solution II. A small amount of the faecal specimen is added to this solution and mixed by stirring and shaking. It stains and fixes all microscopic parasite cysts, eggs, and larvae in the stool without any need for further staining by wet mounts. These are well preserved for 1 year or more.

Advantages

- The reagent components both fix and stain the parasitic forms.
- Preparation is easy and shelf life is long.
- Suitable for concentration procedures.

Disadvantages

- As with formalin preservative, it is not suitable for preparation of permanent trichrome smears.
- The morphology of protozoan trophozoites is poorly preserved.

Schaudinn's solution

It is prepared by mixing 45 gram of mercuric chloride, 310 ml of 95% ethyl alcohol, 50 ml of glacial acetic acid, 15 ml of glycerol and 625 ml of distilled water. In a 20 ml screw-capped vial, 1 ml of stool sample is mixed and stirred in 14 ml of Schaudinn's solution. The vial is then closed and shaken vigorously for 20–30 seconds. It fixes and preserves the specimen for 1 year or more.

Advantages

- Protozoan trophozoites and cysts are well preserved.
- Permanent stained smears are easily prepared.

Disadvantages

- The morphology of helminth eggs and larvae, coccidian oocysts and micrococcidian spores are poorly preserved.
- Less suitable than other preservatives for concentration procedures.
- Mercuric chloride is the main ingredient, making it difficult and expensive to dispose of the fixative.

METHODS OF EXAMINATION

Examination of stool consists of macroscopic and microscopic examination.

Macroscopic examination

Faeces should be examined for its consistency, colour, odour and presence of blood or mucus. Adult intestinal helminths, e.g., *Ascaris lumbricoides* and *Enterobius vermicularis* or segments of tapeworms may be seen in the stool specimen. Blood and mucus may be found in faeces from patients with amoebic dysentery, intestinal schistosomiasis, invasive balantidiasis, and in severe *Trichuris trichiura* infections. Fat-coloured and frothy specimens (containing fat) can be found in giardiasis.

Microscopic examination

Trophozoites of intestinal protozoa are usually found in liquid or soft and occasionally in semi-formed stools. These are not found in formed stools. Cysts are found in formed or semi-formed specimens. Coccidian oocysts and microsporidian spores can be found in any type of faecal specimen; in the case of coccidian oocysts, the more liquid the stool, the more oocysts that are found in the specimen. Helminth eggs may be found in any type of specimen, although the chances of finding of eggs in a liquid stool are reduced by the dilution factor.

Intestinal protozoa, and eggs and larvae of helminths can be detected and identified by microscopic examination of the stool. It includes saline wet mount, iodine wet mount, smear after concentration and permanent stained smear.

Saline wet mount

Saline wet mount is made by mixing a small quantity (about 2 mg) of faeces in a drop of saline placed on a clean glass slide. Remove any gross fibres or particles and cover with a coverslip. Avoid air bubbles by drawing one edge of coverslip slightly into the suspension and lowering it almost to the slide before letting it fall. The mount should be just thick enough that newspaper print can be read through the slide.

The smear is then examined under microscope. Begin at one corner of the smear and systematically examine successive adjacent swaths with the low power of the microscope. When a parasite-like object comes into view, it should be more closely examined and identified under high power. Saline wet mount is used for the detection of trophozoites and cysts of protozoa, and eggs and larvae of helminths. It is particularly useful for detection of live motile trophozoites of *E. histolytica*, *Giardia lamblia* and *Balantidium coli*.

Iodine wet mount

Stool is emulsified in a drop of five times diluted solution of Lugol's iodine on a clean glass slide covered with a clean coverslip and examined under microscope as above. Both saline and iodine wet mounts may be prepared on the same slide. For the preparation of Lugol's iodine, 10 gram of potassium iodide is dissolved in 100 ml distilled water and 5 gram of iodine crystals are then added slowly. *Potassium iodide renders the elemental iodine soluble in water through the formation of triiodide*. The solution is filtered and kept in a stoppered bottle of amber colour. It should be prepared every two weeks.

Iodine wet mount is used for the study of the nuclear character of cysts and trophozoites for the identification of the species. However, iodine immobilizes trophozoites. Iodine stained cysts of *E. histolytica* show pale refractile nuclei, yellowish cytoplasm and brown glycogen mass. The chromidial bars do not stain with iodine. Helminthic eggs and larvae are readily identified without stain, but the iodine stain can be used advantageously in the examination of larvae as it immobilizes and kills them and stains some parts differentially.

Permanent stained smear

Permanent stained smears are essential for cytological details for accurate diagnosis. The detection and identification of *Entamoeba histolytica*, *Giardia lamblia* and other protozoan infections can be greatly enhanced. These can be prepared with both fresh and PVA preserved stool specimens. Iron-haematoxylin, trichrome and modified acid-fast stain are commonly used methods.

1. Iron-haematoxylin stain

A thin smear of faeces is made on a clean glass slide. It is fixed by keeping it in Schaudinn's solution for 15 minutes or longer. The smear is then immersed successively in 70% alcohol, 70% alcohol to which enough iodine has been added to give it a yellow colour, 70% alcohol, and 50% alcohol, 2–5 minutes in each.

It is washed in running tap water for 2–10 minutes and immersed in 2% aqueous ferric ammonium sulphate solution for 5–15 minutes followed by washing in running water for 3–5 minutes. It is then stained in 0.5% aqueous haematoxylin for 5–15 minutes and washed in running water for 2–5 minutes. Then it is differentiated in saturated aqueous solution of picric acid for 10–15 minutes and dehydrated by immersion for 2–5 minutes each in 50%, 70%, 80% and 95% alcohol and 5 minutes each in two changes of absolute alcohol. Stained smear is then cleared in two changes of xylol for 3–5 minutes each, mounted in Canada balsam and covered with coverslip.

2. Trichrome stain

The trichrome stain contains chromotrope 2 R, 0.6 gram; light green SF, 0.3 gram; and phosphotungstic acid, 0.7 gram. These dry components are mixed with 1.0 ml of glacial acetic acid and allowed to stand for 30 minutes, then diluted with 100 ml of distilled water. Faecal smear is prepared and fixed as in case of iron-haematoxylin staining. It is washed in 70% alcohol and in 70% alcohol containing enough iodine, to give it a yellow colour, for 1–5 minutes each. Then it is stained with trichrome solution for 10 minutes and differentiated in acid alcohol (99 parts 90% alcohol: 1 part glacial acetic acid) for 2–3 seconds. It is rinsed in absolute alcohol several times and dehydrated in two changes of absolute alcohol for 2–5 minutes each. Stained smear is then cleared in two changes of xylol for 2–5 minutes each, mounted in Canada balsam and covered with coverslip.

3. Modified acid-fast stain

Modified acid-fast stain is used for detection and identification of *Cryptosporidium parvum*, *Isospora belli* and *Cyclospora cayetanensis*. The staining solution contains:

1. *Carbol fuchsin*: 4 gram basic fuchsin is dissolved in 20 ml 95% ethanol. To this mixture, 100 ml distilled water is added slowly while shaking. Phenol is melted in a water bath at 56°C and 8 ml of this is added to above solution.
2. *Decolouriser*: It is 5% sulphuric acid.
3. *Counter stain*: It is 0.3% methylene blue in distilled water.

A thin smear of faeces is made on a clean glass slide. It is fixed by heat at 70°C for 10 minutes. It is kept on the staining rack and flooded with carbol fuchsin. The slide is heated till carbol fuchsin starts steaming. More carbol fuchsin is added to prevent slide from drying. The slide is allowed to stain for 9 minutes and washed with tap water. It is then decolourised with 5% aqueous sulphuric acid for 30 seconds, followed by washing with tap water and counter staining it with methylene blue for 1 minute. Finally it is washed with tap water, dried, mounted in Canada balsam and covered with coverslip.

Oocysts of *Cryptosporidium parvum*, *Isospora belli* and *Cyclospora cayetanensis* stain red with carbol fuchsin and non-acid-fast background stains blue.

CONCENTRATION METHODS

Eggs, cysts, and trophozoites are often in such low numbers in faecal material that they are difficult to be detected in direct smears or mounts, therefore, concentration procedures should also be performed. Two commonly used methods are:

1. Floatation techniques
2. Sedimentation techniques

Both these methods are designed to separate intestinal protozoa and helminthic eggs from excess faecal debris.

Floatation techniques

Floatation involves suspending the specimen in a medium of greater density than that of the helminthic eggs and protozoan cysts. The eggs and cysts float to the top and are collected by placing a glass slide on the surface of the meniscus at the top of the tube. Following floatation techniques can be used:

Saturated salt floatation technique

- About 1 gram of faeces is placed in a flat-bottomed vial (50 mm tall and 20 mm wide) and a few drops of saturated salt solution (specific gravity 1.200) are added.
- It is then stirred with a glass rod to make an even emulsion.
- More salt solution is added so that the container is nearly full, stirring the solution throughout.
- Any coarse matter, which floats up, is removed. At this stage the container is placed on a level surface.
- The final filling of container is carried out by means of a dropper, until a convex meniscus is formed.
- A glass slide 7.5 cm × 5 cm is carefully laid on the top of the container so that the centre is in contact with the fluid.
- The preparation is allowed to stand for 20–30 minutes, after which the glass slide is quickly lifted, turned over smoothly so as to avoid spilling of the liquid, and examined under the microscope. A coverslip may not be placed over the fluid.

It has been observed that all the helminthic eggs float in the saturated salt solution except unfertilized eggs of *A. lumbricoides*, eggs of *Taenia solium*, *T. saginata* and all intestinal flukes. The *Strongyloides stercoralis* larvae also do not float in salt solution.

Zinc sulphate centrifugal floatation technique

- About 1 gram of faeces is thoroughly mixed in 10 ml of lukewarm distilled water. The coarse particles are removed by straining through gauze.
- The filtrate is poured into a 15 ml conical centrifuge tube and centrifuged at 2,500 revolutions per minute (rpm) for 1 minute.
- The supernatant fluid is poured off and distilled water is added to the sediment. It is shaken well, centrifuged and the process is repeated 2 or 3 times till the supernatant fluid is clear.
- The clear supernatant is poured off and 3–4 ml of 33% zinc sulphate (specific gravity 1.800) is added to the sediment and more zinc sulphate solution is added to fill the tube up to the top and centrifuged again at 2,500 rpm for 1 minute.
- With a platinum wire loop sample is taken from the surface, onto a clean glass slide, a coverslip is put on and examined under microscope.
- For protozoal cysts, one drop of iodine solution is added before the coverslip is put on.

Zinc sulphate centrifugal floatation technique effectively concentrates cysts of protozoa, eggs of nematodes, and small tapeworms. This method is not suitable for unfertilized eggs of *A. lumbricoides* and eggs of most trematodes and large tapeworms. However, the eggs of *Clonorchis sinensis* and *Opisthorchis* spp. are satisfactorily concentrated by this method. High concentration of the zinc sulphate suspension causes the opercula to pop open, fill with fluid, and sink to the bottom of the tube. Therefore, both the surface sample and the bottom sediment should be examined microscopically.

Sedimentation techniques

Concentration of intestinal parasites by sedimentation techniques, using either gravity or centrifugation, leads to a good recovery of cysts of protozoa and eggs of helminths. Cysts and eggs of parasites settle and are concentrated at the bottom because they have greater density than the suspending medium. Following are the commonly used sedimentation techniques:

Simple sedimentation

A sufficient amount of faeces is thoroughly mixed with ten to twenty times its volume of tap water and allowed to settle in a cone-shaped flask for an hour or two. This process is repeated several times till the supernatant fluid is clear. The clear supernatant fluid is discarded and the sediment at the bottom is examined for the eggs. This method is not suitable for protozoal cysts.

Formalin-ether sedimentation

- Half teaspoon of faeces is thoroughly mixed in 10 ml of water and strained through two layers of gauze in a funnel.
- The filtrate is centrifuged at 2,000 rpm for 2 minutes.
- The supernatant is discarded and the sediment is resuspended in 10 ml of physiological saline.
- It is again centrifuged and the supernatant is discarded.
- The sediment is resuspended in 7 ml of formalin saline and allowed to stand for 10 minutes or longer for fixation.
- To this is added 3 ml of ether.
- The tube is stoppered and shaken vigorously to mix.
- Then the stopper is removed and the tube is centrifuged at 2,000 rpm for 2 minutes.
- The tube is allowed to rest in a stand. Four layers become visible, the top layer consists of ether, second is a plug of debris, third is a clear layer of formalin saline and the fourth is sediment.
- The plug of debris is detached from the side of the tube with the aid of a glass rod, and the liquid is poured off leaving a small amount of formalin saline for suspension of the sediment.
- It is poured on a clean glass slide, covered with coverslip and examined under microscope.
- The sediment may also be mixed with a drop of iodine and examined.

Ether dissolves faecal fats and formalin fixes the parasites and removes faecal odour. Risk of laboratory acquired infection from faecal organism is minimized because organisms are killed by formalin solution.

QUANTIFICATION OF WORM BURDEN

For quantitative estimation of worm burden, two methods are commonly used:

- Direct smear egg count
- Stoll's method

Direct smear egg count

- Two mg of faeces is mixed in a small drop of saline on a slide and a coverslip is applied avoiding formation of air bubbles.
- The entire preparation is examined under low power of the microscope and the number of eggs (in 2 mg faeces) is counted and then the number of eggs per gram of faeces is calculated.

Stoll's method

This is commonly used method for determining the number of helminthic eggs in faeces.

- Four gram of faeces is thoroughly mixed with 56 ml of N/10 NaOH in a flask to make a uniform suspension. This is facilitated by adding a few glass beads and closing the mouth with a rubber stopper and then shaking vigorously.
- 0.15 ml of the emulsion is removed with measuring pipette and is placed on a glass slide, a coverslip is put over it and all the eggs in the preparation are counted under low power of the microscope.
- The number of eggs per gram of faeces is calculated by multiplying the count with 100.
- The total egg production per day can then be calculated by multiplying the number of eggs/gram with a 24 hour faecal sample.
- Considering the consistency of faecal specimen, a correction factor (C.F.) is employed to convert the estimate to formed stool. For mushy-formed stool C.F. is 1.5, for mushy stool C.F. is 2, for mushy-diarrhoeic stool C.F. is 3, for frankly diarrhoeic stool C.F. is 4 and for watery stool C.F. is 5.

ANAL SCRAPINGS AND SWABS

- Amoebiasis cutis of the perianal area may be diagnosed by demonstrating motile trophozoites of *E. histolytica* in material scraped from ulcers and examined in saline suspension on a slide under a coverslip.
- *E. vermicularis* infection is usually diagnosed by demonstrating the presence of eggs on the perianal and perineal skin. This can be done by following methods:
  1. Scotch cellulose adhesive tape method
  2. NIH swab

Scotch cellulose adhesive tape method

Hold clear (not frosted) cellophane tape approximately 10 cm long between thumbs and forefingers with sticky surface facing outward. Before the patient has arisen from the bed in the morning (preferably while the child is still asleep), press the sticky side of the tape against the skin across the anal opening with even, thorough pressure. Gently, place the sticky side of the tape down against the surface of a clear glass slide for examination. A drop of toluene may be placed between the tape and slide. The toluene clears essentially everything except eggs and hair. Eggs of other helminths may also be seen in this preparation.

NIH swab

See Chapter 11.

ENTEROTEST

This is a simple and convenient method of sampling duodenal contents that eliminates the need for duodenal intubation. This device consists of a length of nylon string weighted and coiled inside a gelatin capsule.

The string protrudes through one end of capsule. This end of the string is taped to the side of the patient's face. The patient is then asked to swallow the capsule with water. In the stomach, gelatin capsule is dissolved and the weighted string is carried by peristalsis into the duodenum. The string is attached to the weight by a slipping mechanism. It is released and passed out in stool.

The string is recovered after 4 hours. After wearing the gloves bile-stained mucus clinging to the string can be removed by pulling the string between thumb and finger and collected in a small petri dish. The specimen should be examined immediately as a wet mount for motile organisms (trophozoites of *Giardia lamblia* and larvae of *Strongyloides stercoralis*). Iodine may be added later to facilitate the identification of any organism present.

Objects resembling enteric parasites

A large variety of objects that closely resemble various parasite life cycle stages may be seen in faeces. White blood cells, macrophages, and squamous and columnar epithelial cells may resemble amoebae; yeasts and starch granules may resemble protozoal cysts; pollen and fungal conidia may resemble helminth eggs; plant fibres may resemble nematode larvae; and pieces of vegetables or vegetable skin may resemble adult worms or proglottids. Careful differentiation of these objects from real parasites is necessary to prevent inappropriate or unnecessary treatment.

EXAMINATION OF URINE

- *Trichomonas vaginalis* may be recovered in urine sediment from both male and female patients suffering from trichomoniasis.
- Eggs of *Schistosoma haematobium* and *Dioctophyma renale* may also be detected in the sediment of the urine. Samples of large volume should be allowed to settle for 1 or 2 hours. About 50 ml is then taken from the bottom sediment for centrifugation. A drop of sediment is placed on the glass slide covered with coverslip and examined under microscope.
- In case of *Wuchereria bancrofti* and occasionally in case of other filarial worm infections, the microfilariae may be discharged in the urine (chyluria). These may be detected in the centrifuged specimens. Rarely, *S. stercoralis* larvae may also be detected in the urine.

EXAMINATION OF SPUTUM

Sputum is commonly examined for the demonstration of:

- Eggs of *Paragonimus westermani* and *Capillaria aerophila* which reside in the respiratory tract of man.
- In pleuropulmonary amoebiasis, the rupture of the amoebic abscess into a bronchus results in coughing up the contents containing blood, necrotic tissue, and trophozoites of *E. histolytica*.
- Rupture of a pulmonary hydatid cyst is followed by discharge of its contents in which there are fragments of the laminated membrane and usually free scolices of *Echinococcus granulosus*.
- During migratory phase, larvae of *A. lumbricoides*, *Ancylostoma duodenale*, *Necator americanus* and *S. stercoralis* along with eosinophils and Charcot-Leyden crystals may be demonstrated in the sputum.

The sputum is spread in a petri dish and material suspected of bearing eggs (brown streaks) or pus and Charcot-Leyden crystals (opaque white or tan bronchial casts) is placed on a glass slide, covered with a coverslip and examined under microscope. Highly mucoid and gelatinous sputum is examined after the treatment with an equal volume of 3% sodium hydroxide.

EXAMINATION OF ASPIRATES

- The examination of aspirates from the liver is useful in the diagnosis of amoebic liver abscess and hydatid cyst. In amoebic liver abscess, trophozoites of *E. histolytica* are more likely to be found in material aspirated from the wall of the abscess than from the necrotic centre.
- Proctoscopic aspirates and scrapings are useful for the diagnosis of amoebic ulcers in the lower sigmoid colon and rectum.
- Duodenal aspirates may reveal trophozoites of *G. lamblia*, larvae of *S. stercoralis* and parasites in the gall bladder or biliary tract.
- Examination of aspirates (direct and Giemsa stained smears) from lymph nodes, spleen, liver, bone marrow, and spinal fluid is useful for the diagnosis of African trypanosomiasis, visceral leishmaniasis, Chagas' disease, and toxoplasmosis.
- The parasites may also be cultured from the aspirated material.
- The diagnosis of *Leishmania tropica* infection (oriental sore) is made by the microscopic examination of material obtained by puncture of the indurated edge of the sore and stained with Giemsa or Wright stain.

EXAMINATION OF CEREBROSPINAL FLUID

Examination of cerebrospinal fluid by direct microscopic examination of unstained and stained films is useful for the demonstration of:

- *Naegleria fowleri*,
- *Acanthamoeba* spp.,
- *Balamuthia* spp.,
- *Trypanosoma brucei gambiense*, and
- *T. b. rhodesiense*.

EXAMINATION OF BIOPSY MATERIAL

Biopsy is frequently useful, convenient and at times the only method for the diagnosis of a parasitic infection.

Skin biopsy

Skin biopsy can be used to demonstrate *E. histolytica*, *Leishmania* spp., and microfilariae of *Onchocerca volvulus*, *Mansonella streptocerca* and *M. ozzardi*, and encysted procercoid larvae of *Spirometra*.

Lymph node biopsy

Biopsy of an enlarged superficial lymph node may show *T. b. gambiense*, *T. b. rhodesiense*, *T. cruzi*, *Toxoplasma gondii*, *W. bancrofti*, *Brugia malayi* and *B. timori*.

Muscle biopsy

A muscle biopsy may reveal cysticerci of *T. solium*, larvae of *Trichinella spiralis* and *Toxocara*, and sarcocysts of *Sarcocystis lindemanni*.

Gastric biopsy

Gastric biopsy may reveal *Anisakis simplex*.

Small intestinal biopsy

Various life cycle stages of *Cryptosporidium parvum*, *Isospora belli* and *Cyclospora cayetanensis* may be seen in the epithelial cells of the mucosa of small intestine.

Colon and rectum biopsy

Biopsy of colon and rectum may demonstrate the eggs of *S. mansoni* and *S. japonicum*, and the trophozoites of *E. histolytica* and *B. coli*.

Brain biopsy

Brain biopsy may reveal trophozoites of *E. histolytica* and *N. fowleri*, trophozoites and cysts of *Acanthamoeba* spp. and *Balamuthia mandrillaris*, cysticercus cellulosae caused by *T. solium*, hydatid cyst caused by *E. granulosus* and coenurus caused by *Multiceps multiceps*.

Corneal scrapings

Corneal scrapings are helpful in making the diagnosis in cases of suspected *Acanthamoeba* keratitis. Wet mount preparation shows motile trophozoites. Cysts can be seen in stained preparations.

Liver biopsy

Liver biopsy may demonstrate *E. histolytica*, *L. donovani*, *E. granulosus*, *E. multilocularis* and *E. vogeli*.

Lung biopsy

Lung biopsy may demonstrate *E. histolytica*, *E. granulosus*, *P. westermani* and *C. aerophila*.

EXAMINATION OF BLOOD

Next to faeces, the blood provides the most common medium for recovery of various stages of animal parasites, e.g., *Plasmodium* spp., *Babesia* spp., *Leishmania* spp., *T. b. gambiense*, *T. b. rhodesiense*, *T. cruzi*, and microfilariae of *W. bancrofti*, *B. malayi*, *B. timori*, *Loa loa* and *M. ozzardi*. Whenever possible, specimens should be collected before treatment is initiated. When malaria and babesiosis are suspected, blood smears should be obtained and examined without delay. Since the parasitaemia may fluctuate, multiple smears might be needed. These can be taken at 8–12 hours intervals for 2–3 days. Microfilariae exhibit a marked periodicity depending on the species involved, therefore, the time of specimen collection is critical. If a filarial infection is suspected, the optimum collection time for demonstrating microfilariae is:

Loa loa	10 am to 2 pm
Wuchereria bancrofti and *Brugia malayi*	10 pm to 2 am
Mansonella	Any time
Onchocerca	Any time

Following methods can be used for the examination of parasites in the blood:

Wet preparation

A drop of anticoagulated blood can be placed on a clean glass slide, a coverslip put in place and examined microscopically for large, often motile, exoerythrocytic parasites, such as trypanosomes and microfilariae. **Use a suitable anticoagulant, e.g., sodium citrate for microfilariae, and EDTA for malaria parasites and trypanosomes.** Mix the blood well but gently with the anticoagulant. The blood must be examined within 1 hour of collection to avoid morphological changes in the appearance of parasites.

Permanent stained blood smear

Permanent stained blood smear is essential for accurate identification of blood parasites. Two types of blood films are used:

- Thin blood film
- Thick blood film
- Combined thick and thin films on the same slide

Thin blood film

Thin blood film is used primarily for the definitive species identification of plasmodia and other intra-erythrocytic parasites. The pulp of a finger or lobe of an ear is wiped with spirit and allowed to dry. Thereafter, it is pricked with surgical cutting needle under aseptic condition. A drop of blood, about the size of pin head, is taken on a grease-free clean glass slide at about 2 cm from the right end. The drop of blood is touched with the edge of another slide. It is held at an angle of 30 degrees and pushed gently to the left, till the blood is exhausted. As the blood is exhausted, the film begins to form "tails" which end near about the centre of the slide. The film is allowed to dry. The thin film ideally is one cell thick, with erythrocytes lying flat on the glass surface. If the stain to be used is in an aqueous solution, e.g., Giemsa stain, the film must be fixed by covering it with absolute methyl or ethyl alcohol for 2–3 minutes to prevent dehaemoglobinization. For alcohol stains, e.g., Leishman stain, this treatment is not required.

Thick blood film

Thick blood film, many cells thick, contains 6–20 times as much blood per unit area as a thin film. A thick drop of blood is taken on a slide and spread with a needle or with the corner of another slide to form an area of about 12 mm square. It may also be prepared by taking 4 small drops of blood and joining the corners of the drops with a needle. The blood is continuously stirred for about 30 seconds to prevent formation of fibrin clots. If anticoagulated blood is used, stirring is not necessary because fibrin strands do not form. Potassium EDTA is the anticoagulant of choice. The film is allowed to air-dry in a dust-free area. The thickness of the film should be such as to allow a newsprint to be read or the hands of a wrist-watch to be seen through the dry preparation.

Once the film is dry, it should be dehaemoglobinized by placing the film in distilled water in a vertical position in a glass cylinder for 5–10 minutes. When the film becomes white, it is taken out and allowed to dry in an upright position. The disruption of the erythrocytes and the loss of their haemoglobin from the slide permits the remaining structures, including blood parasites, to be seen microscopically even when lying deep in the film. Dehaemoglobinization should be done as promptly as possible to assure total dehaemoglobinization. Thick blood films are especially useful in detecting malaria parasites in light infections.

Combined thick and thin films on the same slide

This method is of special value in survey work. Two drops of blood are taken; one, 1 cm and another, 2.5

cm from the right end of the slide. The former is made into a thick film and the latter into a thin film.

Staining blood film

Both thin and thick smears can be stained by Leishman and Giemsa stains. In addition, thick smear can be stained by Field stain.

Examination of thick smear

Since the erythrocytes (RBCs) have been lysed and the parasites are more concentrated, the thick smear is useful for screening of parasites and for detection of mixed infections.

- First screen the entire smear at low magnification (10× or 20× objective), to detect large parasites such as microfilaria.
- Then examine the smear using the 100× oil-immersion objective lens.
- If you see malaria parasites, make a tentative species determination on the thick smear and then examine thin smear to determine the species.
- NCCLS standards recommend examination of 100 fields using the 100× oil-immersion objective. It takes 5–10 minutes.

Examination of thin smears

Thin smears are useful for species identification of parasites already detected on thick smear, screening of parasites if thick smears are not available, and a rapid screen while thick smear is still drying.

- Screen at low magnification (10× or 20× objective lens) if this has not been done on the thick smears.
- Carefully examine the smear using the 100× oil-immersion objective lens. NCCLS standards recommend examination of at least 300 fields using the 100× oil-immersion objective. It takes 15–20 minutes.

Quantifying parasites

Malaria parasites can be quantified against blood elements such as RBCs or WBCs.

To quantify malaria parasites against RBCs: Count the parasitized RBCs among 500–2,000 RBCs on the thin smear and express the results as % parasitemia.

$$\text{\% Parasitemia} = \frac{\text{Parasitized RBCs}}{\text{Total RBCs}} \times 100$$

If parasitemia is high (e.g., > 10%) examine 500 RBCs; if it is low examine 2,000 or more RBCs. Count asexual blood stage parasites and gametocytes separately. Only the former are clinically important. Gametocytes of *P. falciparum* can persist after elimination of asexual stages by drug treatment.

To quantify malaria parasites against WBCs: On the thick smear, tally the parasites against WBCs until you have counted 500 parasites or 1,000 WBCs, whichever comes first. Express the results as parasites per microlitre of blood using the WBC count, if known, or otherwise assuming 8,000 WBCs per microlitre of blood.

$$\begin{array}{c}\text{Parasites per}\\ \text{microlitre of}\\ \text{blood}\end{array} = \frac{\text{Parasites}}{\text{WBCs}} \times \begin{array}{c}\text{WBC count}\\ \text{per microlitre}\\ \text{(or 8,000)}\end{array}$$

Identification of blood parasites using fluorescent dyes

Fluorescent dyes that stain nucleic acids have been used for the detection of blood parasites. In the Kawamoto technique, blood smears on a slide are stained with acridine orange and examined under fluorescence microscope. This results in a differential staining of nuclear DNA in green and cytoplasmic RNA in red, which allows recognition of parasites. This method has been applied to malaria parasites (and to a lesser extent to African trypanosomes).

Leishman stain

Leishman stain is prepared by dissolving 0.15 gram of Leishman dry powder in 100 ml of absolute methyl alcohol in a bottle. The bottle is shaken until the powder is dissolved and allowed to stand for 48 hours with frequent shaking in between.

The smear is covered with 5–10 drops of stain. After 2 minutes, the stain is diluted by adding twice as many drops of buffered distilled water. The diluted stain is allowed to remain on the slide for 15–20 minutes for staining. The slide is washed with buffered distilled water, dried in air and examined under oil-immersion lens.

Giemsa stain

0.75 gram of Giemsa stain powder is placed in a mortar and 25 ml of glycerol is added to it and is grinded with a pestle until a paste is formed. To this is added 75 ml of methanol and stirred to make a solution. It is then poured in a dark coloured bottle and incubated at 37°C for 24 hours. This is used mainly for staining malaria parasites, trypanosomes, leishmanial parasites, and microfilariae.

The film is fixed by covering it with absolute methyl alcohol for 2–3 minutes. The slide is allowed to dry and immersed in 1:10 dilution of Giemsa stain in buffered distilled water for 30 minutes. It is then washed in buffered distilled water to remove excess stain and allowed to drain by keeping in the upright position and dried in air. The stained film is examined under oil-immersion lens.

Staining of thick and thin films on the same slide

For staining thick and thin films on the same slide, the thick film is first dehaemoglobinized and then stained along with the thin film. A line with a grease pencil is drawn between the films. The undiluted Leishman stain is poured over the thin film and after dilution the stain is flooded over the thick film. If the slide is to be stained with Giemsa stain then the thin part of the film is first fixed with methyl alcohol and after drying, the whole slide is flooded with dilute Giemsa stain and allowed to remain for half to two hours.

Field stain

This is a quick method of staining of malaria parasites in thick films (without fixation). This requires two solutions:

1. Solution A
2. Solution B

Solution A

Methylene blue	0.8 g
Azure I (or azure B)	0.5 g
Disodium hydrogen phosphate (anhydrous)	5.0 g
Potassium hydrogen phosphate (anhydrous)	6.25 g
Distilled water	500 ml

Solution B

Eosin	1.0 g
Disodium hydrogen phosphate (anhydrous)	5.0 g
Potassium hydrogen phosphate (anhydrous)	6.25 g
Distilled water	500 ml

The phosphate salts are first dissolved in water, then the stain is added. Solution of azure I or azure B is facilitated by grinding in a mortar with the phosphate solvent. The solutions are set aside for 24 hours and after filtration are ready for use.

Eosin solution should be renewed as soon as it becomes greenish.

- The thick film is placed in solution A for 1–2 seconds, or till the haemoglobin is removed and no trace of green colour is left.
- It is removed and immediately rinsed by waving gently in clean water for a few seconds until the stain ceases to flow from the film and the glass slide is free from stain.
- It is then placed in solution B for 1 second.
- It is removed and rinsed gently in clean water for 2–3 seconds. It is then allowed to stand upright to drain and dry.

Field stain is useful where large number of blood films have to be examined.

J.S.B. (Jaswant Singh, Bhattacharjee) stain

This is a rapid Romanowsky method of staining malaria parasites by water soluble stain. It consists of two solutions:

1. Solution I
2. Solution II

Solution I

This is prepared by dissolving methylene blue 0.5 gram in 500 ml distilled water in a narrow-mouthed flask. 1% sulphuric acid 3 ml and potassium dichromate 0.5 gram are added one after another, with the formation of a heavy deposit of amorphous purple coloured precipitate of methylene blue chromate. The solution is heated in a water-bath at boiling point for 2–3 hours. At the end of this period the solution turns blue. This indicates almost complete polychroming. The solution is allowed to cool at room temperature and the precipitate appears as steel-blue needle-like branched crystals. At this stage 10 ml of 1% potassium hydroxide is added, drop by drop, with the flask being shaken continuously. The liquid is filtered several times till the dye remaining on the filter paper is completely dissolved. The filtrate is blue having a violet iridescence and is a mixture of the azures with only a trace of methylene blue. It is left to mature at room temperature for 48 hours.

Solution II

This is prepared by dissolving 1 gram eosin in 500 ml distilled water.

Staining of thin film

Thin film is fixed with methyl alcohol for 3–5 minutes and allowed to dry. It is then immersed in solution I for 30 seconds, washed with acidulated tap water (pH 6.2–6.6), stained with solution II for 1 second, washed again with acidulated tap water for 4 seconds, immersed in solution I again for 30 seconds, washed again with acidulated water for 10 seconds, dried and examined under microscope.

Staining of thick film

The procedure for staining thick film is the same as for thin film except that the first step of fixation with methyl alcohol is omitted.

Smears from anticoagulated blood samples should be prepared as soon after collection as possible because the long exposure to the anticoagulant may compromise staining. Morphology of mature schizonts and gametocytes in particular may be altered. Sexual stages continue to develop during storage of blood sample in a warm laboratory environment, or following exposure of the blood sample to air. Gametocytes may exflagellate, releasing gametocytes into plasma. Merozoites, particularly those of *P. vivax*, may be released from mature schizonts and reinvade erythrocytes in which they may appear similar to the small accolé forms of *P. falciparum*.

BLOOD CONCENTRATION METHODS

Several concentration methods can be used for the detection of haemoparasites. These include:

1. Microhaematocrit centrifugation

Blood is collected aseptically by finger prick method in a microhaematocrit tube up to its two-third of the volume. The end of the tube is sealed and centrifuged at 1,500 *g* for 7 minutes. The RBC-plasma interface is then examined under oil-immersion lens for **malaria parasites and trypanosomes**.

2. Triple centrifugation

9 ml of venous blood is mixed with 1 ml of 6% sodium citrate and centrifuged at 100 *g* for 10 minutes. The supernatant is collected and centrifuged at 250 *g* for 10 minutes. The supernatant is centrifuged again at 700 *g* for 10 minutes and the sediment is examined as a wet film or as stained smear. This method is useful for detection of **trypanosomes**.

3. Buffy coat concentration

5 ml of citrated or oxalated blood is centrifuged in a tube. Buffy coat present between the plasma and packed red cells is collected and stained for parasites. Trypanosomes, occasionally *Histoplasma capsulatum* (a fungus which appears as small oval yeast cells resembling those of *Leishmania* amastigote stage), and, in immunocompromised patients, *Leishmania* spp. (*L. infantum*, *L. chagasi* and *L. donovani*) are detected in the peripheral blood. These are found in the large mononuclear cells in the buffy coat. The nuclear material stains dark red-purple, and the cytoplasm stains light blue (*Leishmania* spp.). *H. capsulatum* appears as a large dot of nuclear material (dark red-purple) surrounded by a clear halo area. Trypanosomes in the peripheral blood also concentrate with buffy coat cells.

4. Knott concentration

2 ml of blood is thoroughly mixed with 10 ml of 2% solution of formalin and allowed to stand for 10 minutes or longer. It is then centrifuged at 200 *g* for 2 minutes and the sediment is examined microscopically for microfilariae.

5. Membrane filtration

1 ml of venous blood is drawn into a 10 ml syringe containing 0.1 ml of a 5% solution of sodium citrate. Then in the same syringe, 9 ml of 10% solution of Teepol in physiological saline is drawn and shaken gently for 1 minute. Needle of the syringe is removed and attached to a Swinney filter holder containing a 25 mm membrane filter of 5 μm porosity placed over a supporting filter paper pad of the same size, moistened with saline.

With gentle and steady pressure blood is forced through the filter. Filter is washed three times by passing 10 ml of physiological saline through it. Filter is removed and stained for 5 minutes in hot, but not boiling, Harris' haematoxylin, then it is briefly "blued" in running tap water. It is dried, covered with mounting medium and coverslip, and examined under microscope. This method is used for detection of microfilariae in the peripheral blood.

6. Gradient centrifugation

4 ml of Ficoll-Hypaque solution is mixed with an equal volume of heparinized blood. This is centrifuged at 150 *g* for 40 minutes. This shows three layers – white cell layer in the bottom, Ficoll-Hypaque layer in the middle and plasma layer on the top. Middle layer is examined for **microfilariae**.

CULTURE METHODS

The culture methods are frequently useful for accurate diagnosis of the organism, as a supplement to other methods or to provide positive diagnosis when routine methods have failed. These are also essential for preparation of antigen for immunodiagnosis of parasitic infections and for *in vitro* screening of drugs. Laboratory culture methods are available for many protozoan parasites. These include *E. histolytica*, *B. coli*, *N. fowleri*, *Acanthamoeba* spp., *B. mandrillaris*, *T. vaginalis*, *Leishmania* spp. and *Trypanosoma* spp. Brief methods for cultivation of these parasites are given in corresponding chapters.

SEROLOGIC DIAGNOSIS

The most reliable method for the diagnosis of a parasitic infection is by detection and identification of the infecting organism. However, the serologic approach to the evaluation of parasitic disease is most applicable when invasive techniques other than the routine examination of blood, faeces, or other body fluids are required to establish a diagnosis. For example, infective parasitic forms in toxoplasmosis, extraintestinal amoebiasis, trichinosis, and cysticercosis are often lodged deep within tissues and organs and for the diagnosis either deep-needle or open surgical biopsies are needed. Various serologic tests and their clinical applications are given in Table 13.2.

Table 13.2. Serologic diagnosis of parasitic infections

Test	Disease
Indirect haemagglutination test (IHA)	Amoebiasis, cysticercosis, echinococcosis, filariasis, strongyloidiasis, fascioliasis, Chagas' disease
Fluorescent antibody test (FAT)	African trypanosomiasis
Indirect fluorescent antibody test (IFAT)	Leishmaniasis, malaria, schistosomiasis, toxoplasmosis
Enzyme-linked immunosorbent assay (ELISA)	Toxocariasis, toxoplasmosis, ascariasis
Complement fixation test (CFT)	Chagas' disease, paragonimiasis, leishmaniasis.
Latex agglutination	Echinococcosis
Bentonite flocculation	Trichinellosis, echinococcosis

MOLECULAR BIOLOGY

Molecular assays such as DNA probes and polymerase chain reaction (PCR) are available for the diagnosis of parasitic infections. DNA probe can be used for the diagnosis of malaria and filariasis and PCR can be used for the diagnosis of toxoplasmosis, leishmaniasis, Chagas' disease and onchocerciasis.

CONTROLLING MICROSCOPY

- Clean frequently the lenses of the eyepieces and objectives. The 40× objective can become easily contaminated when examining wet preparation.
- Use appropriate intensity of light for each objective and obtain adequate contrast by adjusting the condenser and iris diaphragm for the type of specimen and objective being used. When contrast is insufficient, parasites will be missed in unstained preparations, particularly trypanosomes in CSF, *T. vaginalis* in discharges, motile *E. histolytica*, *Giardia* trophozoites, and protozoal cysts and oocysts in faecal preparations. When light is insufficient for use with an oil-immersion objective, e.g., use of daylight with a binocular microscope, it will be practically difficult to identify malaria parasites in thick blood films.
- Use both 10× and 40× objectives to examine faecal preparations to avoid missing small parasites.
- Examine specimens for a sufficient length of time to avoid false negative reports and to ensure mixed *Plasmodium* infections, such as *P. falciparum* and *P. malariae*.

Further Reading

1. Beaver, P.C, Jung, R.C. and Cupp, E.W. 1984. Examination of specimens for parasites. *Clinical Parasitology*. Lea & Febiger, Philadelphia: 733–58.
2. Chatterjee, K.D., 1980. Diagnostic Procedures, in: *Parasitology* (*Protozoology and Helminthology*), 11th edn. Chatterjee Medical Publishers, Kolkata, 208–23.
3. Garcia, L.S., 2001. Diagnostic Medical Parasitology, 14th ed., ASM Press, Washington D.C., 581–881.
4. Midha, N., Ichhpujani, R.L., Singh, P., Arora, D.R., Arora, B. and Chugh, T.D. 1981. Evaluation of fluorescent microscopy for the identification of malarial parasites. *J. Com. Dis*., **13**, 241–43.
5. Monica Cheesbrough, 1998. Parasitological tests in District Laboratory Practice in Tropical Countries, Part 1, Cambridge University Press, 178–309.
6. Parija, S.C. 1990. Laboratory diagnosis of parasitic infections at cross roads. *Third Dr. S.C. Dutt memorial lecture*, 1999. Organized by Indian Association for the advancement of Veterinary Parasitology (central chapter) 26-10-1999.

Important Questions

1. Discuss methods of collection and preservation of faecal samples.
2. Describe in detail examination of stool.
3. Discuss various methods of concentration of stool.
4. Discuss biopsy as a method of diagnosis of parasitic infections.
5. Name various parasites which may be present in the blood. Discuss in detail methods of examination of blood.
6. Write short notes on:
   (a) Quantification of worm burden
   (b) Scotch cellulose adhesive tape method
   (c) NIH swab
   (d) Enterotest
   (e) Examination of urine for parasites
   (f) Examination of sputum for parasites
   (g) Examination of CSF for parasites
   (h) Blood concentration methods
   (i) Serologic diagnosis of parasitic infections

Multiple Choice Questions

1. Disadvantage of formalin-fixed stool samples is:
   (a) bacterial overgrowth in the sample.
   (b) further development of helminthic ova.
   (c) unsuitability for the preparation of trichrome-stained smears.
   (d) distortion of cyst morphology.
2. Polyvinyl alcohol is especially suitable for preservation of stool samples for:
   (a) parasitic cysts.
   (b) trophozoite stage.
   (c) helminthic eggs.
   (d) helminthic larvae.
3. Modified acid-fast stain is used for the diagnosis of:
   (a) *Entamoeba histolytica*.
   (b) *Toxoplasma gondii*.
   (c) *Cryptosporidium parvum*.
   (d) *Leishmania donovani*.
4. Which of the following helminthic eggs floats in saturated salt solution?
   (a) Unfertilized eggs of *Ascaris lumbricoides*.
   (b) *Taenia solium*.
   (c) *Taenia saginata*.
   (d) *Ancylostoma duodenale*.
5. Stoll's method is used for:
   (a) determining the number of helminthic eggs in faeces.
   (b) demonstration of *Cryptosporidium* oocysts in faeces.
   (c) concentrating microfilariae in blood.
   (d) staining of lymph node smear for *Leishmania donovani*.
6. Which of the following eggs is found in sputum samples?
   (a) *Paragonimus westermani*.
   (b) *Enterobius vermicularis*.
   (c) *Ascaris lumbricoides*.
   (d) *Ancylostoma duodenale*.
7. Knott concentration method is used for demonstration of:
   (a) malaria parasites in peripheral blood film.
   (b) microfilariae in peripheral blood film.
   (c) *Leishmania donovani* in bone marrow aspirate.
   (d) *Trypanosoma cruzi* in blood.
8. Which of the following is a reason to reject a stool specimen for parasitological examination?
   (a) Specimen was in refrigerator overnight.
   (b) Specimen is diarrhoeic.
   (c) Patient has just been given a barium enema.
   (d) Patient has no symptom of infection.
9. Modified acid-fast staining technique **does not** provide optimum staining for identification of:
   (a) *Cryptosporidium parvum*.
   (b) *Entamoeba histolytica*.
   (c) *Cyclospora cayetanensis*.
   (d) *Isospora belli*.

ANSWERS TO MCQs

1 (c), 2 (b), 3 (c), 4 (d), 5 (a), 6 (a), 7 (b), 8 (c), 9 (b).

14

Medically Important Arthropods

Insects
- *Mosquitoes*
- *Sandflies*
- *Beetles*
- *Reduviid bugs*
- *Fleas*
- *Lice*
- *Other biting flies*
- *Midges*

Arachnids
- *Ticks*
- *Other arthropods*

Arthropods belong to the kingdom Animalia and the phylum Arthropoda. They are animals with jointed legs, segmented bodies and chitinous exoskeletons. There are over one million species in the phylum Arthropoda (insects and their allies). *Arthron* in Greek means jointed and *poda* means feet. Characteristically, arthropods develop from egg to adult by a process known as **metamorphosis**. As they mature, the organisms pass through several distinct morphologic stages, including egg, larva or nymph, pupa (certain insects), and adult. Arthropods are one of the most important sources, other than man himself, of human pathogens. Scientific study of insects is known as *entomology*. *Entom* in Greek means insect and *logas* means scientific study.

Medical entomology is the branch of science that deals with the arthropods, which are involved in the spread of disease in human beings. Medical significance of arthropods is attributed mainly due to their blood sucking habits, and their role as vectors of the agents of bacterial, viral or parasitic infection. The word **vector** means an arthropod or other invertebrate which transmits infection by inoculation into the skin or mucous membrane by biting or by deposit of infective materials on the skin or on food or other objects. They can transmit infection in the following ways:

1. **Mechanical transmission**, in which the arthropod vector merely transports the organisms from one host to another or from the environment to a host and is not a part of the life cycle of the organism.
2. **Biological transmission**, requiring a period of multiplication and/or development in the host. The period of time necessary for the development of the disease agent in the arthropod host is called **extrinsic incubation period**. Biological vector (carrier) is of following types:
   - **Propagative**, where there is multiplication of the parasite with no developmental change, e.g., yellow fever virus in *Aedes aegypti*.

- **Cyclo-propagative**, where the parasite undergoes both multiplication and developmental changes, e.g., *Plasmodium* spp. in female *Anopheles* spp.
- **Cyclo-developmental**, where the parasite undergoes developmental change but no multiplication, e.g., *Wuchereria bancrofti* in *Culex quinquefasciatus*.
- **Transovarian**, where the parasite passes to the progeny arthropods transovarially, e.g., rickettsiae are transmitted transovarially in ticks (spotted fevers) and mites (scrub typhus).

There are five main classes in the phylum Arthropoda (Table 14.1). Insects and arachnids live in close association with man. Other classes include primarily parasites of the animals. Class Insecta includes mosquitoes, flies, fleas, bugs and lice; and class Arachnida includes ticks, mites, spiders and scorpions. The distinctive characters of arthropods of medical importance are given in Table 14.2.

Arthropods of medical interest ingest the pathogenic organisms and convey these to man by following methods:

1. Arthropods may obtain the parasitic organisms in a blood meal from an infected person and deposit them in a vomit-drop in the puncture wound (plague) or in faecal pellets near the puncture wound (epidemic and endemic typhus, trench fever, and Chagas' disease) made in the skin of an uninfected person.
2. Contamination from infected hemolymph may occur when the arthropod is crushed on the skin (epidemic typhus and epidemic relapsing fever).
3. Some arthropods discharge the pathogens (malaria sporozoites and virus particles) through the hypo-

Table 14.1. Classification of medically important arthropods

Class	Order	Common names
1. Insecta	Diptera	Mosquitoes, sandflies, tsetse flies, blackflies, deerflies, botflies, warble flies, house flies, flesh flies, blowflies and kads
	Hemiptera	Bed bugs and assassin bug
	Coleoptera	Beetles
	Siphonaptera	Fleas
	Anoplura	Sucking lice
	Mallophaga	Biting lice
	Hymenoptera	Wasps, honeybees and ants
	Dictyoptera	Cockroaches
2. Arachnida	Acari	Hard ticks, soft ticks, chiggers, itch mites and follicle mites
	Araneae	Spider
	Scorpiones	Scorpions
3. Pentastomida		Tongue worms
4. Myriapoda	Diplopoda	Millipedes
	Chilopoda	Centipedes
5. Crustacea	Copepoda	Water fleas
	Decapoda	Crabs and crayfish

Table 14.2. Distinctive characters of arthropods of medical importance

Characteristic	Insecta	Arachnida	Crustacea
1. Body divisions	Head, thorax and abdomen	Cephalothorax (head and thorax fused) and abdomen	Cephalothorax and abdomen
2. Antennae	One pair	None	Two pairs
3. Legs	Three pairs	Four pairs	Five pairs
4. Wings	One or two pairs; some are wingless	None	None
5. Where present	On land	On land	In water

pharynx in minute droplets of salivary secretion at the time they procure a blood meal. Filarial larvae from the proboscis (labium and mouth area) of the mosquito are deposited on the skin near the site of the puncture. They then enter through puncture wound or penetrate through the skin on their own.

Transmission of parasitic diseases by the bites of arthropod vectors is extraordinarily effective as evidenced by the widespread distribution of diseases such as malaria, trypanosomiasis, and filariasis. In many arthropod-associated diseases, the etiologic agents were undoubtedly parasites of their invertebrate hosts long before man came into the life cycle. In some cases the parasite has been so long and so well adjusted to the arthropod that it produces no obvious injury, namely, *Rickettsia rickettsii* and *Borrelia duttoni* in ticks, and *R. tsutsugamushi* in trombiculid mites.

In the tick and in the mite the respective parasites are even **transmitted vertically (congenitally)** and require no vertebrate host for at least several generations. On the other hand, *R. prowazekii* in the body louse can cause extensive and often fatal damage to this ectoparasite, suggesting that the vector-pathogen relationship is an imperfect one. Vector-borne parasitic human infections are given in Table 14.3 and biting characteristics of medically important arthropods are given in Table 14.4.

INSECTS

Insects comprise more than 90% of all described arthropod species, although few are responsible for transmission of human disease. Members of this class are distinguished from other arthropods by having a

Table 14.3. Vector-borne human parasitic infections

Disease	Causative agents	Vector
PROTOZOAL INFECTIONS		
1. Malaria	*Plasmodium* spp.	*Anopheles* mosquitoes
2. Leishmaniasis	*Leishmania* spp.	*Phlebotomous* spp. (sandflies)
3. Chagas' disease	*Trypanosoma cruzi*	Reduviid bug (*Triatoma* spp., *Panstrongylus* spp., *Rhodinins* spp. and others)
4. East African trypanosomiasis	*Trypanosoma brucei rhodesiense*	Tsetse flies (*Glossina* spp.)
5. West African trypanosomiasis	*T. brucei gambiense*	Tsetse flies (*Glossina* spp.)
6. Babisiosis	*Babessia* spp.	Ticks (*Ixodes damnini* and *I. ricinu*)
HELMINTHIC INFECTIONS		
1. Filariasis	*Wuchereria bancrofti*	*Culex* spp., *Aedes* spp., *Anopheles* spp. and *Mansonia uniformis*
2. Filariasis	*Brugia malayi*	*Anopheles* spp., *Mansonia* spp. and *Aedes* spp.
3. Filariasis	*B. timori*	*Anopheles barbirostris*
4. Filariasis	*Mansonella perstans*	*Culicoides* spp. (biting midges)
	M. streptocerca	*Culicoides* spp.
	M. ozzardi	*Culicoides* spp. and *Simulium* spp. (blackflies)
5. Onchocerciasis	*Onchocerca volvulus*	*Simulium* spp.
6. Loiasis	*Loa loa*	*Chrysops* spp. (mango flies or deerflies)
7. Dog tapeworm infection	*Dipylidium caninum*	Dog flea, cat flea, human flea and dog louse
8. Rat tapeworm infection	*Hymenolepis diminuta*	Rat fleas, beetles and grain beetles
9. Dwarf tapeworm infection	*H. nana*	Grain and flour-eating beetles (*Tribolium* spp., *Tenebrio* spp.), fleas (*Xenopsylla cheopis, Pulex irritans, Ctenocephalides canis*) and moths
10. Dracunculiasis	*Dracunculus medinensis*	*Cyclops* spp.
11. Diphyllobothriasis	*Diphyllobothrium latum*	*Diaptomus* spp. and *Cyclops* spp.
12. Sparganosis	*Spirometra erinacei* and *S. mansonoides*	*Cyclops* spp.
13. Gnathostomiasis	*Gnathostoma spinigerum*	*Cyclops* spp.
14. Paragonimiasis	*Paragonimus westermani*	Freshwater crab and crayfishes

Table 14.4. Biting characteristics of medically important arthropods

Only females bite
- Mosquitoes of genera *Anopheles* and *Culex*
- Sandflies of genera *Phlebotomus* and *Lutzomyia*
- Blackflies (*Simulium* spp.)
- Deerflies or mango flies (*Crysops* spp.)
- Biting midges (*Culicoides* spp.)

Both males and females bite
- Tsetse flies (*Glossina* spp.)

Usually bite at night
- *Anopheles* mosquitoes
- Sandflies of the genera *Phlebotomus* and *Lutzomyia*
- Reduviid bugs

Usually bite during the day time
- *Aedes* mosquitoes
- *Tsetse* flies (*Glossina* spp.)
- Blackflies (*Simulium* spp.)
- Biting midges (*Culicoides* spp.)
- Deerflies or mango flies (*Chryosops* spp.)

Insects those are able to pass through ordinary mosquito net
- Sandflies of the genera *Phlebotomus* and *Lutzomyia*

body divided into three parts (head, thorax, abdomen); one pair of antennae; three pairs of legs; and one, two, or no pairs of wings. This is the only arthropod class in which flight has developed.

MOSQUITOES

Mosquitoes are readily recognised by a long needle-like proboscis. Adult males and females both feed on plant juices, but the female needs blood for the development of her eggs, and is also a voracious predator on a wide variety of vertebrate animals throughout the world. Mosquitoes of importance in human medicine are divided into two broad types:

1. **Anopheline mosquitoes**, numerous species of which transmit malaria.
2. **Culicine mosquitoes**, which are the vectors of many arbovirus infections.

Both anopheline and culicine mosquitoes also act as the intermediate hosts of certain filarial worms. Female mosquitoes lay their eggs on water; larvae and pupae are both aquatic. Most anopheline mosquitoes prefer relatively large expanses of water that do not dry up, but many culicine mosquitoes, particularly *Aedes* spp. will breed in small pockets of water, such as tree holes, water butts, etc. Adults have wide flight range and may be found several kilometres from their breeding ground.

SANDFLIES

Sandflies are tiny flies that are well able to penetrate ordinary mosquito net. They have a restricted flight range, so that the diseases they transmit – notably kala-azar and other forms of leishmaniasis, bartonellosis and sandfly fever – tend to be localized in distribution. Female flies suck blood, usually at night, and breed in dark, moist areas, often in or around human dwellings. Species associated with disease transmission in Africa, the Middle East, Asia and the Mediterranean littoral belong to the genus *Phlebotomus*. In Central and South America, *Lutzomyia* spp. act as vectors of leishmaniasis and Oroya fever.

BEETLES

Some beetles act as intermediate host of the dwarf tapeworm *Hymenolepis diminuta*, an uncommon human parasite of minor importance.

REDUVIID BUGS

Reduviid bugs transmit *Trypanosoma cruzi*, causative agent of Chagas' disease, in South America. They are about 2.5 cm in length – much larger than bed bugs – and unlike them, they have wings. They are usually active at night, settling on the face of an unsuspecting sleeper to take a blood meal and to defecate. The infective trypanosomes are in the hindgut and the bitten person becomes infected by rubbing the bug's faeces into the irritating bite wound.

FLEAS

Fleas are small, wingless insects with laterally compressed bodies and long legs adapted for jumping. Many fleas feed on man if given the opportunity. However, the species that is adapted for life on man is the human flea, *Pulex irritans*. It is common throughout the world. Female fleas of another species, *Tunga penetrans*, attack man once they have been fertilized. The fleas burrow into the skin, or under the toe-nails, of human host and are known as *jiggers*. The abdomen of the gravid female becomes grossly distended *with eggs*, causing pain, irritation and, sometimes secondary infection. Jigger fleas are common in dry, sandy soil, mainly in Africa and parts of Central and South America.

Human fleas are seldom implicated in the transmission of disease, but some other species are important disease vectors. Most notorious is the rat flea, *Xenopsylla cheopis*, which is the most important, but not the sole vector of plague. Some forms of typhus are also transmitted by *X. cheopis* and other fleas.

LICE

Lice are dorsoventrally flattened wingless insects that undergo incomplete metamorphosis during their development. The ones that parasitize man are blood-sucking species with flattened bodies and short legs that are adapted to cling to hair. Body lice and head lice are considered to be variants of the same species, *Pediculus humanus*. Body louse, *P. humanus corporis* is somewhat larger than the head louse, *P. humanus capitis*, and there are other minor differences. A third species *Phthirus pubis* is quite distinct morphologically and is known as 'crab' louse.

Head lice are usually confined to the hair of the scalp, but body lice live in clothing covering the body, rather than on the skin. *Phthirus pubis* is usually found on pubic hair, but may also infest other hairy parts including eyelashes. All types attach their characteristic eggs (*nits*) to body hair and effective treatment involves removal of the *nits* as well as dealing with the adults.

Crab lice are not known to be involved in disease transmission, but body and head lice are classic vectors of epidemic typhus and relapsing fever. Treatment with insecticides such as permethrin, malathion and carbaryl may be effective, but resistance occurs.

OTHER BITING FLIES

The tsetse flies, *Glossina* spp., are found in the so-called 'fly belts' of sub-Saharan Africa, where they are responsible for transmission of trypanosomiasis in man as well as in cattle and other animals. Usually, both male and female feed on blood. Other biting flies responsible for transmission of disease in Africa include species of *Chrysops* (deerflies or mango flies) which act as vectors of *Loa loa* and *Simulium* (blackflies) which act as vectors of onchocerciasis.

MIDGES

Biting midges are tiny flies. The females attack in swarms, usually in the evening , and may give rise to painful reactions. Like mosquitoes, they are mostly aquatic. One genus *Culicoides* spp. transmits filarial worms of *Mansonella* spp.

ARACHNIDS

This group includes spiders, scorpions, ticks and mites. They have four pairs of legs. They do not have wings, nor do they have antennae.

TICKS

Ticks are important vectors of human disease. They are of two types – ***hard (ixodid) ticks***, which have a chitinous shield on the back and ***soft (argasid) ticks***, which lack this feature. Ticks are obligate blood-feeders. They parasitize a wide variety of animals. Ixodid ticks transmit many rickettsiae of the spotted fever group as well as agents of Q fever, Lyme disease, tularaemia, babesiosis and some arboviruses.

OTHER ARTHROPODS

Crustaceans (crabs and crayfish) are of interest in human medicine mainly as intermediate hosts of *Paragonimus westermani*, the lung fluke. Copepods (water fleas) are similarly important only as hosts of guinea worm, *Dracunculus medinensis* and the fish tapeworm, *Diphyllobothrium latum*.

Direct injury due to arthropods

Vectors such as lice, ticks, bugs, fleas, mosquitoes, and blackflies may directly cause injury by their bites, either by hypersensitivity reactions or by toxic effects of their salivary products. Hypersensitivity reactions mainly manifest as itch, with the concomitant potential for secondary infection due to scratching. Bed bug and flea bites may cause immediate type hypersensitivity reactions with itchy erythema greater than 3 cm in diameter. Ticks may induce a chronic local granulomatous lesion, persisting for months, perhaps due to remnants of the mouthparts (denticles) left within the epidermis.

Blackfly bites may produce 'blackfly fever'. Usually, the site of bite becomes oedematous with a golf ball-sized lump and an oozing punctate lesion. Patient develops fever and myalgia lasting for 24 hours. Soft tick bites may immediately cause pain, swelling and irritation at the site of bite, with raised hard wheals. The effects last several days, with irritability of affected part. Certain feeding ticks induce an acute ascending paralysis. Children are usual victims of tick paralysis, with ticks attached at the nape of the neck. Patient develops fatigue, irritability, distal paresthesias, leg weakness with reduced tendon reflexes, ataxia and lethargy. Unless the tick is removed, quadriplegia and respiratory failure may result. Removal of the tick induces a miraculous recovery within 48 hours.

Endoparasitic arthropods

Mites, fleas, fly larvae, and pentastomes invade a host's body and cause scabies, tungiasis, myiasis, and halzoun respectively. The most common of the ectoparasite-caused direct injury is scabies, caused by infestation with the human scabies mite (*Sarcoptes scabiei*). Transmission of scabies is by direct personal contact, and infestations often cluster among groups of people, particularly families. The female scabies mite burrows beneath the stratum corneum, leaving behind eggs and faeces within a track-like trail. A few dozen eggs are deposited, and these hatch within a week. Larvae form new burrows. These may also emerge from the skin and move freely about. Erythematous papules and vesicles first appear on the webs of fingers and spread to the arms, trunk, and buttocks. The burrows contain granular, highly antigenic faeces, which cause both delayed type and immediate type hypersensitivity reactions. In individuals who are immunocompromised, hundreds of female mites may be found, itching is minimal, but a hyperkeratosis is prominent.

Myiasis is the infestation of human or animal tissue by fly larvae, deposited as eggs or first-stage larvae. The larvae develop by feeding on the surrounding tissue, emerge as third-stage larvae, and putate in the environment. Botflies cause follicular lesions or a serpiginous track in the skin. Maggots may invade the nose and accompanying structures, causing nasal or oral myiasis. Maggots may get into ears, producing aural myiasis. Enteric, vaginal, or vesicomyiasis is due to invasion of the gut or genitalia. Treatment is by removal of the maggots using forceps. The lesion may be covered with petrolatum, thereby preventing the maggots from breathing.

Further Reading

Garcia, L.S. 2001. *Diagnostic Medical Parasitology*, 4th edn. Washington DC: American Society for Microbiology Press.

Multiple Choice Questions

1. Which type of vector is *Culex quinquefasciatus* for the transmission of *Wuchereria bancrofti*?
   (a) Propagative.
   (b) Cyclo-propagative.
   (c) Cyclo-developmental.
   (d) Transovarian.
2. Sandflies belong to which of the following classes?
   (a) Insecta.
   (b) Arachnida.
   (c) Pentastomida.
   (d) Crustacea.
3. Both males and females of which of the following genera of arthropods bite?
   (a) *Phlebotomus*.
   (b) *Glossina*.
   (c) *Crysops*.
   (d) *Anopheles*.
4. Which of the following arthropods bites during daytime?
   (a) *Anopheles*.
   (b) Reduviid bugs.
   (c) *Phlebotomus*.
   (d) *Aedes*.
5. Which of the following genera of arthropods can pass through ordinary mosquito net?
   (a) *Phlebotomus*.
   (b) *Culicoides*.
   (c) *Anopheles*.
   (d) *Aedes*.
6. In which of the following arthropods transovarial transmission of pathogens occurs?
   (a) Sandflies.
   (b) Ticks.
   (c) Head lice.
   (d) Reduviid bugs.

ANSWERS TO MCQs

1 (c), 2 (a), 3 (b), 4 (d), 5 (a), 6 (b).

15

Quality Assurance in Parasitology

- *Quality assurance*
  - *Pre-analytical*
  - *Analytical*
  - *Post-analytical*
- *Quality control*
  - *Internal quality control*
  - *External quality assessment*
- *Standard operating procedures*
- *Laboratory accommodation*
- *External services and supplies*
- *Review of contract*
- *Complaints/feedback*
- *Human resource*
- *Safety*

A quality assurance programme for the parasitology section of the laboratory is similar to that for the other laboratory sections and covers all essential aspects of the operations including, among others, a well-written and complete procedure manual that is reviewed annually, guidelines for maintaining all specimen and test result records, complete quality control programme with appropriate technical supervision and participation in an appropriate proficiency testing programme.

The purpose of **quality assurance** (QA) in laboratory practice is to provide test results that are *relevant*, *reliable*, *timely* and *interpreted correctly*. QA includes all those activities both in and outside the laboratory, performance standards, good laboratory practice, and management skills that are required to achieve and maintain a quality service and provide for continuing improvement.

QA has been defined by WHO as the total process whereby the quality of a laboratory report can be guaranteed. It has been summarized as the *right result*, at the *right time*, on the *right specimen*, from the *right patient*, with the result interpretation based on *correct reference data*, and at the *right price*.

The term **quality control** (QC) covers that part of QA which primarily concerns the control of errors in the performance of tests and verification of test results. QC must be *practical, achievable and affordable*.

Effective QA detects errors at an early stage before they lead to incorrect test results. Laboratory personnel need to be aware of the errors that can occur when collecting specimens (pre-examination processes), testing specimens (examination processes), and reporting and interpreting test results (post-examination processes).

Implementing QA requires preparation and use of **standard operating procedures** (SOPs) with details of QC for all laboratory tests and activities. These are required to improve and maintain the quality of laboratory service to patients; to provide laboratory staff with written instructions on how to perform tests;

and to prevent changes in the performance of tests which may occur when new members of staff are appointed. These further facilitate the preparation of a list and inventory of essential reagents, chemicals and equipment.

SOPs must be written and implemented by a qualified and experienced laboratory officer, and followed exactly by all members of staff. For the description of each test mention value of test, principle of test, specimen to be collected, equipment, reagents/stains and controls required. Describe test method in a numbered sequence how to perform the test. Preferred procedures are those that have been published in established/authoritative textbooks, peer reviewed texts or journals. State how the test result is to be reported/interpreted. Summarize important and commonest causes of an incorrect test results.

SOPs should have at least three appendices:

- **First appendix** should have information on stains/reagents – method of preparation and QC; any associated-hazard; labelling; storage and shelf-life; and sources of chemicals and stains.
- **Second appendix** should have information of each item of equipment – name (including model) and supplier; instructions for use; daily QC; maintenance schedule; and troubleshooting and action to be taken if equipment fails.
- **Third appendix** should have information on the safe handling and disposal of specimens; decontamination procedure; personal safety measures; and first-aid measures.

The laboratory accommodation should be dust-free and air-conditioned. The environmental conditions should be monitored daily. For effective quality management system the laboratory should practise **internal quality control** and participate in organized inter-laboratory comparisons such as **external quality assessment schemes**. Before collection of specimen, the contract should be properly reviewed.

External services and supplies should be procured from standard sources. Purchased equipment and consumable supplies should not be used until these have been verified as complying with standard specifications. Contracts to obtain critical supplies should be reviewed regularly to ensure that expectations are met. The laboratory should have a process for receiving and evaluating incoming material and storing consumable material. The laboratory should be furnished with all items of equipment required for provisions of services. These should be properly **calibrated** and major equipment should be on **annual maintenance contract**.

QA of parasitological tests can be divided into pre-examination processes, examination processes and post-examination processes. Pre-examination processes involve selecting parasitology tests appropriately. For specimen collection use specimen containers that are leak-proof, clean, dry and free from traces of antiseptics and disinfectants. If anticoagulated blood specimen is required, **use a suitable anticoagulant, e.g., sodium citrate for microfilariae and EDTA for malaria parasites and trypanosomes**. Mix blood well but gently with anticoagulant. The EDTA blood specimen must be examined within 1 hour of collection to avoid morphological changes in the appearance of parasites.

Specimens must arrive in the laboratory as soon as possible after they are collected. A dysenteric faecal specimen or rectal scrape for detection of motile *Entamoeba histolytica* trophozoites, CSF for detection of motile trypanosomes, and discharge specimen for the detection of motile *Trichomonas vaginalis* require examination within 15–20 minutes after collection. All other specimens should reach the laboratory within 1 hour of collection to avoid loss or distortion of parasites. When needing to transport specimens use suitable preservative.

Label the specimen carefully with the patient's name and identification number, and also the date and time of collection. A correctly completed request form with adequate clinical information and details of any drugs given to or taken by the patient before the specimen was collected must accompany all specimens. In the laboratory check the specimen and request form. It is important to check that the container is not leaking, that the specimen is suitable for the test being requested and has been delivered to the laboratory within the time specified for the particular investigation.

For the QA of examination processes use most suitable method for detecting and identifying a particular parasite and follow exactly the technique as detailed in the SOP. For microscopical examinations, make preparations of the correct thickness, e.g., thick blood films and faecal suspensions. Wipe back of slides clean after staining. Examine slides for a sufficient length of time to avoid false negative reports and to ensure mixed infections are not missed, e.g., mixed *Plasmodium* infections, such as *P. falciparum* and *P. vivax*. Force and length of time of centrifugation are important when sedimenting parasites. Centrifuging at too great a force can destroy trypanosomes or cause the loss of sheath from a pathogenic microfilaria species.

For the QA of post-examination processes write reports clearly and neatly. Communicate immediately any serious result to the medical officer caring for the patient, e.g., finding of trypanosomes in blood or CSF, or a heavy falciparum parasitaemia. Keep written dated records of all the parasitology investigations performed in the laboratory. Actively seek customer feedback. When feedback indicates need for improvement, the laboratory needs to undertake appropriate action for improvement. Complaints/feedback should be addressed and documented.

The performance of individuals responsible for the parasitology section should be monitored periodically with both internal and external unknown specimens, and competency assessment should be up to date, especially for those laboratories that encounter positive specimens infrequently. A variety of reference materials should be readily available for use at the laboratory bench including positive slides.

Unpreserved specimens for parasitologic examination should be considered infectious, and all blood and body fluids should be handled according to universal precautions. In addition to blood-borne viral pathogens, malaria parasites and haemoflagellates may also remain infective. A variety of parasites may remain infective in fresh stool specimens, including cysts of *Entamoeba histolytica* and *Giardia lamblia*, eggs of *Taenia solium*, *Enterobius vermicularis*, and *Hymenolepis nana*, and larvae of *Strongyloides stercoralis*. *Ascaris* eggs can survive and embryonate while in 5% formalin. Faecal specimens may also contain pathogens such as *Salmonella*, *Shigella* and viruses. Strict observance of proper specimen handling techniques and disposal is essential. Personal attention to hand washing is also necessary. Use of ethyl acetate in place of ether in the performance of concentration techniques is recommended to guard against the possibility of explosion.

Acquisition of equipment accounts for only 25% of the solution, training of personnel another 25% and scheduled contracts and preventive maintenance accounts for 50% of equipment functionality. Therefore, it is recommended, a registry of all equipment, schedule of calibration, maintenance and vendor contracts be documented and followed for every piece of equipment. Human resource is the most valuable resource in quality management systems. Policies and processes for obtaining and retaining highly qualified persons should be explicitly indicated by the organization.

Laboratory needs to establish and maintain an environment that provides safety for all. Segregation and disposal of biomedical waste should be strictly according to Bio-Medical Waste Rules. Staff should observe universal precautions and should be offered vaccination against vaccine preventable diseases. Incident/accident reports and action taken should be reviewed and documented.

Further Reading

1. Arora, D.R. 2004. Quality assurance in microbiology, *Indian J. Med. Microbiol*., **47**: 594–95.
2. Cheesbrough, M. 1998. Quality assurance and sources of error in district laboratory practice, in: *District Laboratory Practice in Tropical Countries*, Cambridge University Press, pp. 31–37.
3. ISO 15189: 2012 (E). Medical laboratories – Particular requirements for quality and competence, pp. 1–50.

Multiple Choice Questions

1. Which of the following activities is/are essential to achieve and maintain a quality service?
   (a) Good laboratory service.
   (b) Performance standards.
   (c) Management skills.
   (d) All of the above.
2. For effective quality management system:
   (a) the laboratory should practise internal quality control.
   (b) participate in organized inter-laboratory comparisons.
   (c) monitor environmental conditions daily.
   (d) All of the above.
3. Which of the following test results should be communicated immediately to the medical officer caring for the patient?
   (a) Trypanosomes in blood or CSF.
   (b) Heavy falciparum parasitaemia.
   (c) *Naegleria fowleri* in CSF.
   (d) All of the above.

ANSWERS TO MCQs

1 (d), 2 (d), 3 (d).

16

Ethics in Laboratory Medicine

- *Ethical codes*
- *Informed consent*
- *Privacy*
- *Examination procedures*
- *Results of laboratory examinations*
- *Quality and technical records*

The professional personnel of a medical laboratory are bound by the ethical codes of their respective profession. Personnel responsible for the management of medical laboratories, as with other health professionals, have responsibilities over and above the minimum required by law. Laboratories shall not engage in practices restricted by law and should uphold the reputation of their profession.

The general principle of healthcare ethics is that the patient's welfare is paramount. The laboratory should treat all patients fairly and without discrimination. The laboratory should collect adequate information for the proper identification of the patient, which enables the requested examinations and other laboratory procedures to be carried out, but should not collect unnecessary personal information. The patient should be aware of the purpose for which the information is collected. Safety of staff and other patients are legitimate concerns when communicable diseases are possible and information may be collected for these purposes.

All procedures carried out on a patient require the informed consent of the patient. Forcing some one to undergo medical testing of any kind is an invasion of privacy and a violation of human rights. For most laboratory procedures, consent can be inferred when the patient presents him- or herself at a laboratory with a request form and willingly submits to the usual collecting procedures, e.g., venipuncture. Patient in a hospital bed should normally be given the opportunity to refuse.

Special procedures, including the more invasive procedures, will require a more detailed explanation and, in some cases, written consent. This is desirable when there is likelihood of complications following the procedure. Laboratories performing human immunodeficiency virus (HIV) testing shall follow National AIDS Control Organization (NACO) guidelines, which include pre-test and post-test counselling.

The laboratory shall not perform HIV test unless the individual has been given pre-test counselling and post-test counselling is ensured. Informed consent of the patient will be taken before the blood is collected. The result of HIV test shall be kept strictly confidential.

In emergency situations, consent might not be possible and under these circumstances it is acceptable to carry out necessary procedures provided they are in patient's best interest. The laboratory should endeavour to see that results with serious implications are not communicated directly to the patient without the opportunity for adequate counselling.

Adequate privacy during reception and sampling should be available and appropriate to the type of primary sample being collected and information being requested. If the primary sample arrives in the laboratory in a condition that is unsuitable for the requested examination, it should normally be discarded and referring physician notified.

The laboratory shall use examination procedures, including those for collection of specimens, which meet the needs of the users of laboratory services and are appropriate for the examinations. Preferred procedures are those that have been published in established/authoritative textbooks, peer-reviewed texts or journals or in international, national or regional guidelines. If in-house procedures are used, these shall be appropriately validated for intended use and fully documented. Any fabrication of result is completely unacceptable.

The results of laboratory examinations are confidential unless disclosure is authorized. The results will normally be reported to the requesting physician and may be reported to other parties with the patient's consent or as required by law. The results of laboratory examination that have been separated from all patient identification (unlinked, anonymous) may be used for such purposes as epidemiology, demography or other statistical analyses. In addition to the accurate reporting of laboratory results, the laboratory has an additional responsibility to ensure that, as far as possible, the examinations are correctly interpreted and applied in the patient's best interest.

The laboratory shall establish and implement procedures for identification, collection, indexing, access, storage, maintenance and safe disposal of quality and technical records. All records should be legible and stored such that they are readily retrievable. Records may be stored on any appropriate medium subject to national, regional or local legal requirements. Facilities shall provide a suitable environment to prevent damage, deterioration, loss or unauthorized access. The laboratory shall decide the retention time of records as per the national, regional or local regulations. As per National Accreditation Board for Testing and Calibration Laboratories (NABL) guidelines, the minimum period for retention of test reports issued shall be five years for histopathology and cytopathology, and one year for other disciplines.

Medical laboratories should not enter into financial arrangements with referring practitioners where those arrangements act as an inducement for the referral of patients. Rooms used for primary sample collection should be completely independent and separate from referring practitioners' rooms. Laboratories should try to avoid situations that give rise to a conflict of interest.

Further Reading

1. Arora, D.R. 2007. Ethics in laboratory medicine, *Indian J. Med. Microbiol.*, **25**: 179–80.
2. Arora D.R. and Arora B.B. *Textbook of Microbiology*, 4th edn. CBS Publishers & Distributors, New Delhi; 2012.
3. ISO 15189:2012(E): Medical laboratories – Particular requirements for quality and competence. pp. 1–50.
4. National Accreditation Board for Testing and Calibration Laboratories (NABL) 112. Specific criteria for accreditation of medical laboratories. 2007. pp. 6, 26.

17

Overview of Medical Parasitology

- *Habitat*
- *Morphology*
- *Antigenic variation*
- *Portal of entry*
- *Source of infection*
- *Soil transmitted helminths*
- *Life cycle*
- *Obligate intracellular parasites*
- *Symptomatology*
- *Parasites causing autoinfection*
- *Parasites causing opportunistic infections in AIDS*
- *Parasites causing common tropical parasitic diseases*
- *Parasitic infection considered to be life-threatening*
- *Most lethal helminth infection of man*
- *Clinical samples*
- *Parasites which can be cultured in the laboratory*
- *Skin tests*
- *Classification of nematodes*
- *Nematode occurring both in adult and larval form in man*
- *Nematodes which do not show systemic migration in man*
- *Types of microfilariae*
- *Parasitic causes of traveller's diarrhoea*
- *Concomitant immunity*
- *Life-long immunity*
- *Universal precautions*
- *Most lethal of all helminthic infections of man*
- *Both male and female worms remain coiled together*

Parasites affect over half the world's population and are a major cause of mortality in the developing world. In the developed world, they represent a threat to those undergoing immunosuppressive therapy or suffering from HIV infection. A large number of parasites can invade human body and these may localize in different organs and tissues. Presence of the parasites in these locations leads to the host response including inflammatory reaction. The infective forms of the parasites may be present in stool, urine, sputum, blood, etc. from where they are acquired by healthy individuals. This saves their race from extinction.

The parasites causing human disease have been described in the preceding chapters. The purpose of this chapter is to (1) quickly revise medical parasitology, and (2) detect areas of weakness in your understanding of the subject matter. The following pages will provide an interesting challenge as well as an opportunity to determine your ability to read, digest, and comprehend the vast accumulation of knowledge.

HABITAT

PARASITES RESIDING IN SMALL INTESTINE

Protozoa

- *Giardia lamblia*
- *Isospora belli*
- *Sarcocystis hominis*
- *Cryptosporidium parvum*
- *Cyclospora cayetanensis*
- *S. suihominis*

Cestodes

- *Diphyllobothrium latum*
- *T. saginata*
- *Hymenolepis nana*
- *Taenia solium*
- *T. asiatica*

Trematodes

- *Fasciolopsis buski*
- *Metagonimus yokogawai*
- *Heterophyes heterophyes*

Nematodes

- *Ascaris lumbricoides*
- *Necator americanus*
- *Trichinella spiralis*
- *Trichostrongylus* spp.
- *Ancylostoma duodenale*
- *Strongyloides stercoralis*
- *Capillaria philippinensis*

PARASITES RESIDING IN LARGE INTESTINE

Protozoa

- *Entamoeba histolytica*
- *Balantidium coli*

Nematodes

- *Enterobius vermicularis*
- *Trichuris trichiura*
- *Ternidens deminutus*
- *Oesophagostomum* spp.

PARASITES RESIDING IN BODY CAVITIES

- *Mansonella perstans*
- *M. ozzardi*

PARASITES RESIDING IN LIVER

Protozoa

- *Entamoeba histolytica*
- *Plasmodium* spp.

Trematodes

- *Fasciola hepatica*
- *Clonorchis sinensis*

Cestodes

- *Echinococcus granulosus*
- *E. multilocularis*

Nematodes

- *Capillaria hepatica*

PARASITES RESIDING IN LUNGS

Trematodes

- *Paragonimus westermani*

Nematodes

- *Capillaria aerophila*
- *Dirofilaria immitis*

Cestodes

- *Echinococcus granulosus*

PARASITES RESIDING IN KIDNEYS

- *Dioctophyma renale*

PARASITES RESIDING IN SUBCUTANEOUS TISSUE

- *Loa loa*
- *Onchocerca volvulus*
- *Dracunculus medinensis*
- *Dirofilaria* spp.

PARASITES RESIDING IN THE DERMIS

- *Mansonella streptocerca*

PARASITES RESIDING IN LYMPHATIC SYSTEM

- *Wuchereria bancrofti*
- *Brugia malayi*
- *B. timori*

PARASITES RESIDING IN PORTAL VENOUS SYSTEM VENULES

- *Schistosoma* spp.

MORPHOLOGY

LARGEST PROTOZOAL PARASITE INHABITING LARGE INTESTINE OF MAN

- *Balantidium coli*

LONGEST TAPEWORM INFECTING HUMANS

- *Diphyllobothrium latum*

SMALLEST TAPEWORM INFECTING HUMANS

- *Hymenolepis nana*

LARGEST NEMATODE PARASITIZING HUMAN INTESTINE

- *Ascaris lumbricoides*

SMALLEST NEMATODE KNOWN TO CAUSE INFECTION IN MAN

- *Strongyloides stercoralis*

LARGEST TREMATODE KNOWN TO CAUSE INFECTION IN MAN

- *Fasciolopsis buski*

OPERCULATE EGGS

- *Diphyllobothrium latum*
- *Fasciola hepatica*
- *F. gigantica*
- *Fasciolopsis buski*
- *Clonorchis sinensis*
- *Paragonimus westermani*
- *Gastrodiscoides hominis*
- *Watsonius watsoni*
- *Opisthorchis felineus*
- *O. viverrini*
- *Heterophyes heterophyes*
- *Metagonimus yokogawai*

AMOEBAE FORMING CYSTS IN TISSUES

- *Acanthamoeba* spp.
- *Balamuthia mandrillaris*

PARASITES SHOWING ANTIGENIC VARIATION

- *Trypanosoma brucei gambiense*
- *T. b. rhodesiense*
- *Plasmodium* spp.
- *Giardia lamblia*

ACID-FAST OOCYSTS AND EGGS

Oocysts:

- *Cryptosporidium parvum*
- *Isospora belli*
- *Cyclospora cayetanensis*

Eggs:

- *Schistosoma intercalatum*

PORTAL OF ENTRY

PARASITES ENTERING THROUGH MOUTH

Protozoa

- *Entamoeba histolytica*
- *Giardia lamblia*
- *Balantidium coli*
- *Sarcocystis hominis*
- *S. suihominis*
- *Isospora belli*
- *Cyclospora cayetanensis*
- *Cryptosporidium parvum*
- Microsporidia

Trematodes

- *Fasciola hepatica*
- *Fasciolopsis buski*
- *Clonorchis sinensis*
- *Opisthorchis felineus*
- *Paragonimus westermani*
- *Gastrodiscoides hominis*

- *Watsonius watsoni*
- *Heterophyes heterophyes*
- *Metagonimus yokogawai*

Cestodes

- *Taenia solium*
- *T. saginata*
- *T. asiatica*
- *T. multiceps*
- *Diphyllobothrium latum*
- *Spirometra* spp.
- *Echinococcus granulosus*
- *E. multilocularis*
- *E. vogeli*
- *Hymenolepis nana*
- *H. diminuta*
- *Dipylidium caninum*

Nematodes

- *Ascaris lumbricoides*
- *Trichuris trichiura*
- *Enterobius vermicularis*
- *Trichinella spiralis*
- *Dracunculus medinensis*
- *Capillaria* spp.
- *Angiostrongylus* spp.
- *Trichostrongylus* spp.
- *Ternidens deminutus*
- *Oesophagostomum* spp.
- *Anisakis simplex*
- *Gnathostoma* spp.

PARASITES TRANSMITTED BY SEXUAL CONTACT

- *Trichomonas vaginalis*
- *Entamoeba histolytica*
- *Giardia lamblia*

PARASITES TRANSMITTED CONGENITALLY

- *Toxoplasma gondii*
- *Plasmodium* spp.
- Microsporidia
- *Trypanosoma cruzi*

PARASITES TRANSMITTED BY BLOOD TRANSFUSION

- *Plasmodium* spp.
- *Babesia* spp.
- *Trypanosoma cruzi*

PARASITES ENTERING THROUGH SKIN

Direct

- *Ancylostoma duodenale*
- *A. braziliense*
- *A. caninum*
- *Necator americanus*
- *Strongyloides stercoralis*
- *Schistosoma haematobium*
- *S. japonicum*
- *S. mansoni*

Through blood-sucking insects

Protozoa

- *Leishmania* spp.
- *Trypanosoma* spp.
- *Plasmodium* spp.
- *Babesia* spp.

Nematodes

- *Wuchereria bancrofti*
- *Brugia malayi*
- *B. timori*
- *Loa loa*
- *Mansonella streptocerca*
- *M. ozzardi*
- *M. perstans*
- *Onchocerca volvulus*
- *Dirofilaria* spp.

SOURCE OF INFECTION

RAW/UNDERCOOKED PORK IS THE SOURCE OF:

- *Taenia solium*
- *T. asiatica*
- *Trichinella spiralis*
- *Sarcocystis suihominis*

RAW/UNDERCOOKED BEEF IS THE SOURCE OF:

- *Taenia saginata*
- *Sarcocystis hominis*
- *Toxoplasma gondii*

AQUATIC VEGETATIONS ARE THE SOURCE OF:

- *Fasciola hepatica*
- *Gastrodiscoides hominis*
- *Fasciolopsis buski*
- *Watsonius watsoni*

FRESHWATER FISHES ARE THE SOURCE OF:

- *Diphyllobothrium latum*
- *Metagonimus yokogawai*
- *Clonorchis sinensis*
- *Heterophyes heterophyes*
- *Capillaria philippinensis*
- *Gnathostoma spinigerum*
- *Dioctophyma renale*

MARINE FISH IS THE SOURCE OF:

- *Anisakis simplex*

CRAB AND CRAYFISHES ARE THE SOURCE OF:

- *Paragonimus westermani*
- *Angiostrongylus cantonensis*

CYCLOPS ARE THE SOURCE OF:

- *Spirometra*
- *Dracunculus medinensis*

RAW AND POORLY COOKED AMPHIBIANS AND REPTILES ARE THE SOURCE OF:

- *Spirometra* spp.
- *Gnathostoma spinigerum*
- *Angiostrongylus cantonensis*
- *Dioctophyma renale*

DOG IS THE SOURCE OF:

- *Echinococcus granulosus*
- *E. multilocularis*
- *Toxocara canis*
- *Taenia multiceps*

CAT IS THE SOURCE OF:

- *Toxoplasma gondii*
- *Toxocara cati*
- *Cryptosporidium parvum*

SOIL TRANSMITTED HELMINTHS

- *Ascaris lumbricoides*
- *Necator americanus*
- *Trichuris trichiura*
- *Strongyloides stercoralis*
- *Ancylostoma duodenale*

LIFE CYCLE

PARASITES REQUIRING ONE INTERMEDIATE HOST

Pig

- *Taenia solium*
- *T. asiatica*
- *Trichinella spiralis*
- *Sarcocystis suihominis*

Cow

- *Taenia saginata*
- *Sarcocystis hominis*

Man

- *Plasmodium* spp.
- *Echinococcus granulosus*
- *E. multilocularis*
- *Taenia multiceps*
- *Spirometra* spp.

Flea

- *Dipylidium caninum*
- *Hymenolepis diminuta*

Reduviid bug

- *Trypanosoma cruzi*

Mosquito

- *Plasmodium* spp.
- *Brugia malayi*
- *Mansonella streptocerca*
- *M. perstans*
- *Wuchereria bancrofti*
- *B. timori*
- *M. ozzardi*
- *Dirofilaria* spp.

Snail

- *Schistosoma* spp.

Copepod

- *Dracunculus medinensis*

Sandfly

- *Leishmania* spp.

Tsetse fly

- *Trypanosoma* spp.

Chrysops

- *Loa loa*

Simulium

- *Onchocerca volvulus*

PARASITES REQUIRING TWO INTERMEDIATE HOSTS

Freshwater snail and freshwater crayfish or crab

- *Paragonimus westermani*

Copepods and fresh-water fish

- *Diphyllobothrium latum*

Snail and freshwater fish

- *Clonorchis sinensis*

Snail and aquatic vegetation

- *Fasciola hepatica*
- *Fasciolopsis buski*

PARASITES REQUIRING NO INTERMEDIATE HOST

Protozoan

- *Entamoeba histolytica*
- *Chilomastix mesnili*
- *Balantidium coli*
- *Isospora belli*
- Microsporidia
- *Giardia lamblia*
- *Trichomonas vaginalis*
- *Cryptosporidium parvum*
- *Cyclospora cayetanensis*

Helminths

- *Enterobius vermicularis*
- *Ascaris lumbricoides**
- *Necator americanus**
- *Trichuris trichiura*
- *Ancylostoma duodenale**
- *Hymenolepis nana*

MAN IS INTERMEDIATE HOST IN

- *Plasmodium* spp.
- *Sarcocystis lindemanni*
- *Echinococcus granulosus*

BOTH ADULTS AND LARVAE OCCURRING IN THE SAME HOST

- *Trichinella spiralis*
- *Taenia solium*

CESTODE WHICH COMPLETES ITS LIFE CYCLE IN ONLY ONE HOST

- *Hymenolepis nana*

NEMATODES WHICH COMPLETE THEIR LIFE CYCLE IN TWO HOSTS

- Filarial nematodes
- *Dracunculus medinensis*

OBLIGATE INTRACELLULAR PARASITES

- *Plasmodium* spp.
- *Babesia* spp.
- *Leishmania* spp.
- *Trypanosoma cruzi* (amastigote form)
- *Toxoplasma gondii*
- Microsporidia

SYMPTOMATOLOGY

PARASITES CAUSING DIARRHOEA

Protozoa

- *Entamoeba histolytica*
- *Cryptosporidium parvum*
- *Isospora belli*
- *Giardia lamblia*
- *Cyclospora cayetanensis*

Cestodes

- *Taenia solium*
- *T. asiatica*
- *T. saginata*

Trematodes

- *Fasciolopsis buski*
- *Paragonimus westermani*
- *Metagonimus yokogawai*
- *Clonorchis sinensis*
- *Heterophyes heterophyes*
- *Gastrodiscoides hominis*

Nematodes

- *Trichinella spiralis*
- *Strongyloides stercoralis*
- *Necator americanus*
- *Trichostrongylus* spp.
- *Trichuris trichiura*
- *Ancylostoma duodenale*
- *Capillaria philippinensis*

PARASITES CAUSING BLOOD AND MUCUS IN STOOL

- *Entamoeba histolytica*
- *Schistosoma japonicum*
- *Trichuris trichiura*
- *Balantidium coli*
- *S. mansoni*

PARASITE CAUSING FAT-COLOURED AND FROTHY STOOL

- *Giardia lamblia*

PARASITE IN URETHRAL AND VAGINAL DISCHARGE, AND PROSTATIC SECRETIONS

- *Trichomonas vaginalis*

* Require a period of maturation in the soil after passage before they are infective.

PARASITES CAUSING ANAEMIA

- *Plasmodium* spp.
- *Leishmania donovani*
- *Schistosoma haematobium*
- *Necator americanus*
- *Ternidens deminutus*
- *Babesia microti*
- *Diphyllobothrium latum*
- *Ancylostoma duodenale*
- *Trichuris trichiura*

PARASITES CAUSING INFECTION OF EYE

- *Acanthamoeba* spp.
- *Onchocerca volvulus*
- *Toxoplasma gondii*
- *Encephalitozoon* spp.
- *Toxocara* spp.
- *Loa loa*
- *Echinococcus granulosus*
- *Trypanosoma cruzi*
- *Thelazia callipaeda*
- *Nosema* spp.
- *Angiostrongylus cantonensis*
- *Dirofilaria conjunctivae*
- *Taenia solium*

PARASITES CAUSING SKIN ULCERS

- *Leishmania tropica*
- *L. braziliensis*
- *L. major*
- *L. mexicana complex*
- *L. peruviana*
- *Dracunculus medinensis*

PARASITES CAUSING CNS INFECTION

Protozoa

- *Entamoeba histolytica*
- *Acanthamoeba* spp.
- *Plasmodium falciparum*
- *Trypanosoma brucei gambiense*
- *T. cruzi*
- *Naegleria fowleri*
- *Balamuthia mandrillaris*
- *Toxoplasma gondii*
- *T. b. rhodesiense*
- Microsporidia

Cestodes

- *Taenia solium*
- *T. multiceps*
- *E. multilocularis*
- *Spirometra* spp.
- *Echinococcus granulosus*
- *E. vogeli*

Trematodes

- *Schistosoma japonicum*
- *Paragonimus westermani*

Nematodes

- *Trichinella spiralis*
- *Gnathostoma spinigerum*
- *Toxocara canis*
- *Angiostrongylus cantonensis*
- *Strongyloides stercoralis*
- *Toxocara cati*

PARASITES ASSOCIATED WITH MALIGNANCY

- *Schistosoma haematobium*
- *Opisthorchis viverrini*
- *Clonorchis sinensis*

PARASITES CAUSING TROPICAL EOSINOPHILIA

- *Wuchereria bancrofti*
- *Brugia malayi*

PARASITES CAUSING LARVA MIGRANS

Cutaneous larva migrans

- *Ancylostoma braziliense*
- *Bunostomum phlebotomum*
- *Gnathostoma spinigerum*
- *G. doloresi*
- *A. caninum*
- *Uncinaria stenocephala*
- *G. hispidum*
- *G. nipponicum*

Visceral larva migrans

- *Toxocara canis*
- *T. cati*
- *Angiostrongylus cantonensis*
- *Gnathostoma spinigerum*
- *Anisakis simplex*
- *Baylisascaris procyonis*

PARASITES CAUSING PNEUMONIA, PNEUMONITIS, OR LOEFFLER'S SYNDROME

- Migrating larval stages of:
  - *Ascaris lumbricoides*
  - *Ancylostoma duodenale*
  - *Necator americanus*
  - *Strongyloides stercoralis*
- Eggs of *Paragonimus westermani*
- *Echinococcus granulosus* hooklets
- *Entamoeba histolytica*
- *Cryptosporidium parvum*

PARASITES CAUSING AUTOINFECTION

- *Strongyloides stercoralis*
- *Capillaria philippinensis*
- *Enterobius vermicularis*
- *Taenia solium*
- *Hymenolepis nana*
- *Cryptosporidium parvum*

PARASITES CAUSING OPPORTUNISTIC INFECTION IN AIDS CASES

- *Toxoplasma gondii*
- *Isospora belli*
- *Entamoeba histolytica*
- Free-living protozoa
- *Leishmania* spp.
- *Cryptosporidium parvum*
- Microsporidia
- *Giardia lamblia*
- *Cyclospora cayetanensis*
- *Strongyloides stercoralis*

PARASITES CAUSING COMMON TROPICAL PARASITIC DISEASES

Food- and water-borne

- *Entamoeba histolytica*
- *Cryptosporidium parvum*
- *Cyclospora cayetanensis*
- *Giardia lamblia*
- *Isospora belli*

Vector-borne

- *Plasmodium* spp.
- *Wuchereria bancrofti*
- *Onchocerca volvulus*
- *T. cruzi*
- *Leishmania donovani*
- *Brugia malayi*
- *Trypanosoma brucei*

Soil transmitted

- *Ascaris lumbricoides*
- *A. braziliense*
- *Trichuris trichiura*
- *Ancylostoma duodenale*
- *A. caninum*
- *Strongyloides stercoralis*

PARASITIC INFECTION CONSIDERED TO BE LIFE-THREATENING

- *Plasmodium falciparum* malaria

CLINICAL SAMPLES

PARASITES FOUND IN THE STOOL

Cysts/Trophozoites/Oocysts/Sarcocysts/Sporocysts/Spore

Protozoa

- *Entamoeba histolytica*
- *Balantidium coli*
- *S. suihominis*
- *Cyclospora cayetanensis*
- Microsporidia
- *Giardia lamblia*
- *Sarcocystis hominis*
- *Isospora belli*
- *Cryptosporidium parvum*

Eggs

Cestodes

- *Diphyllobothrium latum*
- *T. saginata*
- *Hymenolepis nana*
- *Dipylidium caninum*
- *Taenia solium*
- *T. asiatica*
- *H. diminuta*

Trematodes

- *Schistosoma mansoni*
- *Fasciolopsis buski*
- *F. gigantica*
- *Opisthorchis* spp.
- *Watsonius watsoni*
- *Metagonimus yokogawai*
- *S. japonicum*
- *Fasciola hepatica*
- *Clonorchis sinensis*
- *Gastrodiscoides hominis*
- *Heterophyes heterophyes*

Nematodes

- *Ascaris lumbricoides*
- *Ancylostoma duodenale*
- *Enterobius vermicularis*
- *Trichostrongylus orientalis*
- *Trichuris trichiura*
- *Necator americanus*
- *Capillaria philippinensis*

Larvae

- *Strongyloides stercoralis*
- *Trichinella spiralis* (rarely)

Adult worms

Cestodes

- *Taenia solium*
- *T. asiatica*
- *T. saginata*
- *Diphyllobothrium latum*

Nematodes

- *Ascaris lumbricoides*
- *Necator americanus*
- *Trichinella spiralis*
- *Ancylostoma duodenale*
- *Enterobius vermicularis*

PARASITES FOUND IN URINE

- *Trichomonas vaginalis*
- *Wuchereria bancrofti*
- *Schistosoma haematobium*
- *Dioctophyma renale*

PARASITES FOUND IN CSF

- *Trypanosoma brucei gambiense*
- *T. b. rhodesiense*
- *Acanthamoeba* spp.
- *Angiostrongylus* spp.
- *Naegleria fowleri*
- *Balamuthia* spp.

REFRIGERATION OF CSF IS NOT RECOMMENDED BECAUSE THIS MAY KILL:

- *Naegleria fowleri*

PARASITES FOUND IN SPUTUM

- *Paragonimus westermani*
- *Capillaria aerophila*
- *Entamoeba histolytica*
- Fragments of laminated membrane and free scolices of *Echinococcus granulosus*

Rarely, migrating larvae of

- *Ascaris lumbricoides*
- *Ancylostoma duodenale*
- *Strongyloides stercoralis*
- *Necator americanus*

PARASITES WHICH CAN BE SEEN IN BIOPSY

Protozoa

- *Leishmania* spp.
- *Balantidium coli*
- *Acanthamoeba* spp.
- *Toxoplasma gondii*
- *Isospora belli*
- *Giardia lamblia*
- *Entamoeba histolytica*
- *Naegleria fowleri*
- *Balamuthia* spp.
- *Sarcocystis lindemanni*
- *Cryptosporidium parvum*

Cestodes

- *Taenia solium*
- *E. multilocularis*
- *Taenia multiceps*
- *Echinococcus granulosus*
- *E. vogeli*
- *Spirometra* spp.

Trematodes

- *Schistosoma haematobium*
- *S. japonicum*
- *S. mansoni*

Nematodes

- *Wuchereria bancrofti*
- *B. timori*
- *Anisakis simplex*
- *Mansonella streptocerca*
- *Trichinella spiralis*
- *Brugia malayi*
- *Capillaria aerophila*
- *Onchocerca volvulus*
- *M. ozzardi*

PARASITES FOUND IN PERIPHERAL BLOOD FILM

Protozoa

- *Plasmodium* spp.
- *Babesia* spp.
- *Leishmania* spp.
- *Trypanosoma brucei gambiense*
- *T. b. rhodesiense*
- *T. cruzi*

Nematodes

Microfilariae of:

- *Wuchereria bancrofti*
- *Brugia malayi*
- *B. timori*
- *Loa loa*
- *Mansonella ozzardi*

INFECTIOUS PARASITES WHICH MAY BE PRESENT IN THE FAECAL SPECIMEN RECEIVED IN THE LABORATORY

- *Entamoeba histolytica*
- *Cryptosporidium parvum*
- *Enterobius vermicularis*
- *Hymenolepis nana*
- *Giardia lamblia*
- *Strongyloides stercoralis*
- *Taenia solium*

PARASITES WHICH CAN BE CULTURED IN THE LABORATORY

- *Entamoeba histolytica*
- *Acanthamoeba* spp.
- *Leishmania* spp.
- *Trichomonas vaginalis*
- *Balantidium coli*
- *Naegleria fowleri*
- *Balamuthia mandrillaris*
- *Trypanosoma* spp.
- *Giardia lamblia*

SKIN TESTS

Showing immediate hypersensitivity in

- Hydatid disease
- Schistosomiasis
- Strongyloidiasis
- Filariasis
- Ascariasis

Showing delayed hypersensitivity in

- Leishmaniasis
- Toxoplasmosis
- Trypanosomiasis
- Amoebiasis

CLASSIFICATION OF NEMATODES

OVIPAROUS NEMATODES

Laying unsegmented eggs

- *Ascaris lumbricoides*
- *Trichuris trichiura*

Laying eggs with segmented ova

- *Ancylostoma duodenale*
- *Trichostrongylus* spp.
- *Oesophagostomum* spp.
- *Necator americanus*
- *Ternidens deminutus*

Laying eggs containing larva

- *Enterobius vermicularis*

VIVIPAROUS NEMATODES

- *Dracunculus medinensis*
- *Brugia malayi*
- *Trichinella spiralis*
- *Wuchereria bancrofti*
- *B. timori*

OVO-VIVIPAROUS NEMATODES

- *Strongyloides stercoralis*

NEMATODES WHICH DO NOT SHOW SYSTEMIC MIGRATION IN MAN

- *Trichuris trichiura*
- *Enterobius vermicularis*

TYPES OF MICROFILARIAE

SHEATHED MICROFILARIAE FOUND IN BLOOD

- *Wuchereria bancrofti*
- *B. timori*
- *Brugia malayi*
- *Loa loa*

UNSHEATHED MICROFILARIAE

Found in blood

- *Mansonella ozzardi*
- *Dirofilaria* spp.
- *M. perstans*

Found in skin

- *M. streptocerca*
- *Onchocerca volvulus*

PARASITIC CAUSES OF TRAVELLER'S DIARRHOEA

- *Entamoeba histolytica*
- *Cryptosporidium parvum*
- *Giardia lamblia*
- *Cyclospora cayetanensis*

CONCOMITANT IMMUNITY

- *Plasmodium* spp.

LIFE-LONG IMMUNITY

- Cutaneous leishmaniasis

LABORATORY WORKERS MUST ADHERE TO UNIVERSAL PRECAUTIONS WHEN HANDLING SPECIMENS FROM PATIENTS WITH SUSPECTED:

- African trypanosomiasis
- Chagas' disease

MOST LETHAL OF ALL HELMINTHIC INFECTIONS OF MAN

- Alveolar or multilocular hydatid cyst

BOTH MALE AND FEMALE WORMS REMAIN COILED TOGETHER AND IT IS DIFFICULT TO SEPARATE THEM.

- *Wuchereria bancrofti*

RELATIVE SIZES of morphological forms of various PROTOZOA

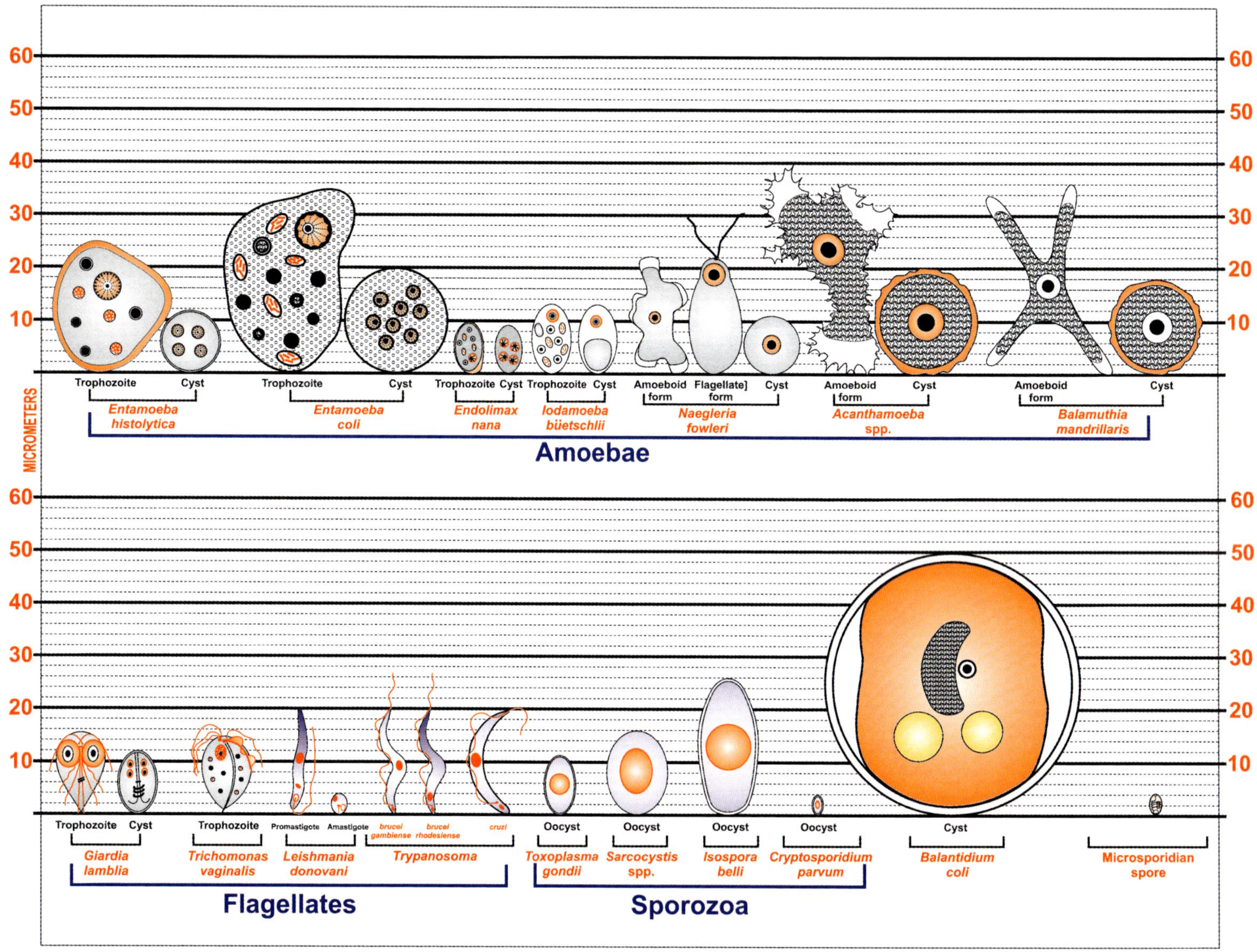

RELATIVE SIZES of HELMINTH EGGS

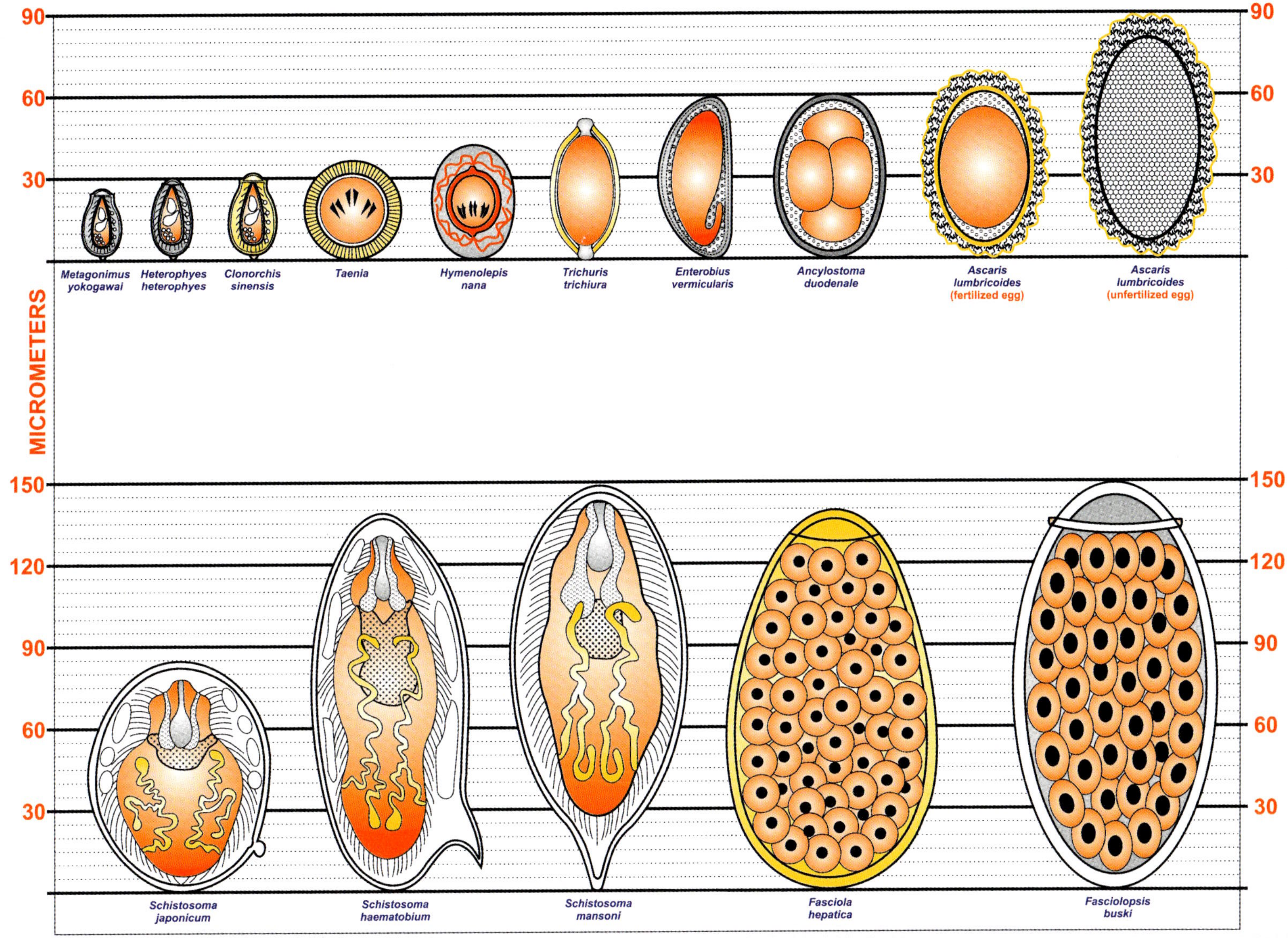

Index

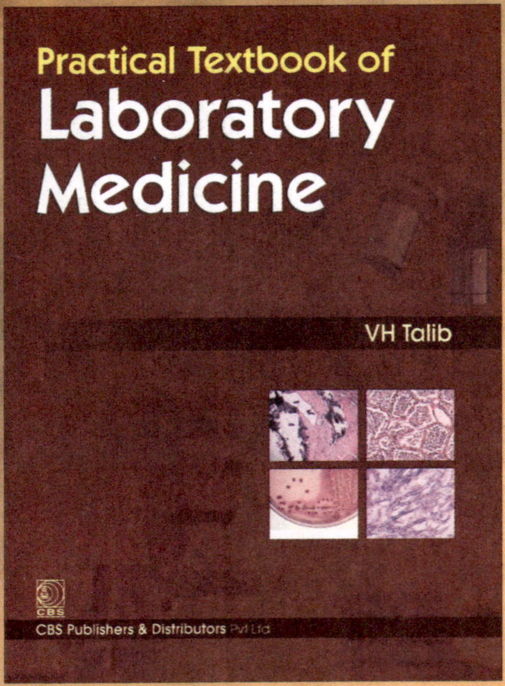
Practical Textbook of
Laboratory Medicine
VH Talib
CBS Publishers & Distributors Pvt Ltd

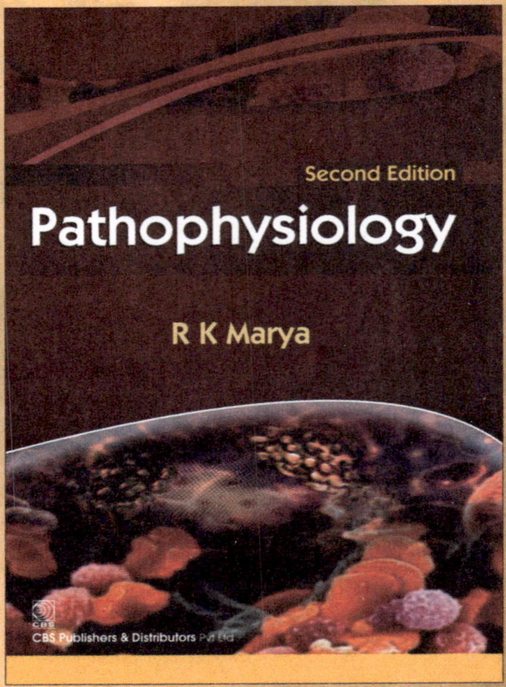
Second Edition
Pathophysiology
R K Marya
CBS Publishers & Distributors Pvt Ltd

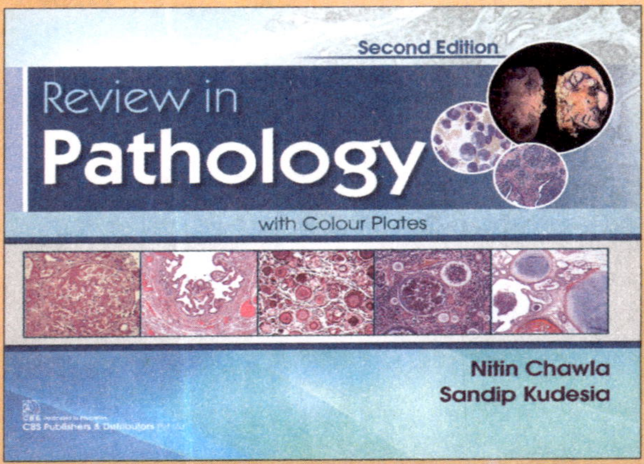
Second Edition
Review in
Pathology
with Colour Plates
Nitin Chawla
Sandip Kudesia
CBS Publishers & Distributors

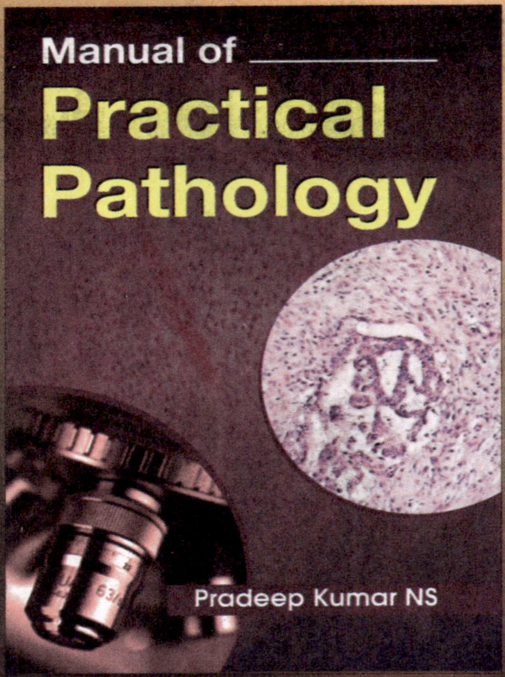
Manual of
Practical
Pathology
Pradeep Kumar NS

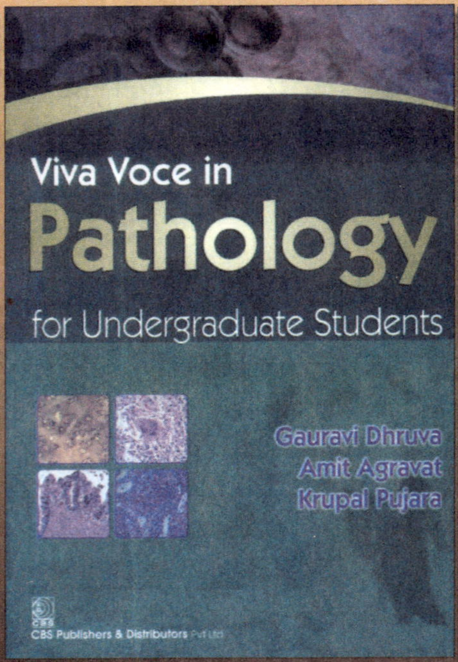
Viva Voce in
Pathology
for Undergraduate Students
Gauravi Dhruva
Amit Agravat
Krupal Pujara
CBS Publishers & Distributors Pvt Ltd

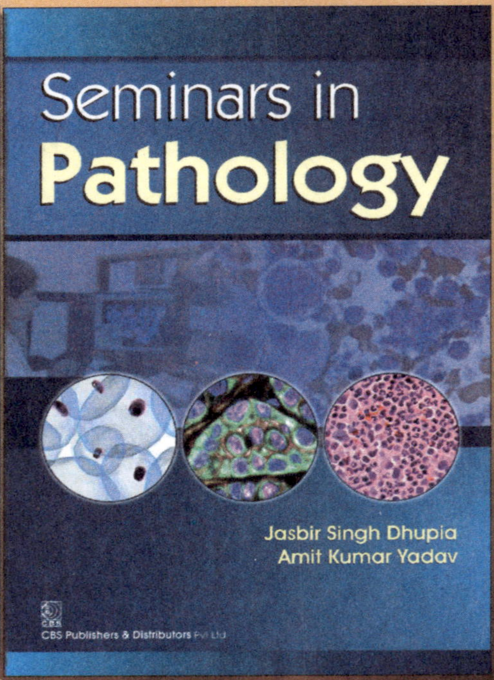
Seminars in
Pathology
Jasbir Singh Dhupia
Amit Kumar Yadav
CBS Publishers & Distributors Pvt Ltd